To Kimberly,

Thanks for all
of your hard work
& dedication to
the transplant
program

7/3/03

Clinical Management of the Transplant Patient

Edited by

Paul C. Kuo MD, MBA

*Department of Surgery, Duke University Medical Center,
Durham, North Carolina, USA*

Rebecca A. Schroeder MD

and

Lynt B. Johnson MD

*Departments of Anesthesia and Surgery, Georgetown University Medical Center,
Washington, DC*

A member of the Hodder Headline Group
LONDON • NEW YORK • NEW DELHI

First published in Great Britain in 2001 by
Arnold, a member of the Hodder Headline Group,
338 Euston Road, London NW1 3BH

http: //www.arnoldpublishers.com

Distributed in the USA by
Oxford University Press Inc.,
198 Madison Avenue, New York, NY10016
Oxford is a registered trademark of Oxford University Press

Whilst the advice and information in this book are believed to be true and
accurate at the date of going to press, neither the authors nor the publisher
can accept any legal responsibility or liability for any errors or omissions
that may be made. In particular (but without limiting the generality of the
preceding disclaimer) every effort has been made to check drug dosages;
however, it is still possible that errors have been missed. Furthermore,
dosage schedules are constantly being revised and new side-effects
recognized. For these reasons the reader is strongly urged to consult the
drug companies' printed instructions before administering any of the drugs
recommended in this book.

British Library Cataloguing in Publication Data
A catalogue record for this book is available from the British Library

Library of Congress Cataloging-in-Publication Data
A catalog record for this book is available from the Library of Congress

ISBN 0 340 76127 X

1 2 3 4 5 6 7 8 9 10

Commissioning Editor: Nick Dunton
Development Editor: Michael Lax
Production Editor: Wendy Rooke
Production Controller: Martin Kerans
Typeset in 10/11.5 pt Palatino by Cambrian Typesetters, Frimley, Surrey
Printed and bound in Great Britain by MPG Books, Bodmin, Cornwall

What do you think about this book? Or any other Arnold title?
Please send your comments to feedback.arnold@hodder.co.uk

Contents

Contributors

Elsie Allen MD
Department of Medicine, University of Maryland Medical Center, Baltimore, MD

John V. Conte Jr MD
Department of Surgery, Johns Hopkins Hospital, Baltimore, MD

E. Darrin Cox MD
Naval Medical Research Center, Bethesda, MD

Eric A. Elster MD
Naval Medical Research Center, Bethesda, MD

Alan Farney MD
Department of Surgery, University of Maryland Medical Center, Baltimore, MD

Ronald Freudenberger MD
Department of Medicine, University of Maryland Medical Center, Baltimore, MD

Lynt B. Johnson MD
Department of Surgery, Georgetown University Medical Center, Washington, DC

Allan D. Kirk MD, PhD
Naval Medical Research Center, Bethesda, MD

David K. Klassen MD
Department of Medicine, University of Maryland Medical Center, Baltimore, MD

Paul C. Kuo MD
Department of Surgery, Duke University Medical Center, Durham, NC

Jacqueline C. Lauren MD
Department of Medicine, University of Maryland Medical Center, Baltimore, MD

Peter N. Madras MD
Department of Surgery, Rhode Island Hospital, Providence, RI

Anthony P. Monaco MD
Department of Surgery, Beth Israel-Deaconess Medical Center, Boston, MA

Paul E. Morrissey MD
Department of Surgery, Rhode Island Hospital, Providence, RI

Jonathan Orens MD
Department of Medicine, Johns Hopkins Hospital, Baltimore, MD

Jeffrey S. Plotkin MD
Department of Anesthesia, Georgetown University Medical Center, Washington, DC

Sandra Rosen-Bronson PhD
Department of Pediatrics, Georgetown University Medical Center, Washington, DC

Vinod K. Rustgi MD
Departments of Medicine and Surgery, Georgetown University Medical Center, Washington, DC

Rebecca A. Schroeder MD
Department of Anesthesia, Georgetown University Medical Center, Washington, DC

Eugene Schweitzer MD
Department of Surgery, University of Maryland Medical Center, Baltimore, MD

Matthew R. Weir MD
Department of Medicine, University of Maryland Medical Center, Baltimore, MD

James B. Whiting MD
Department of Surgery, Maine Medical Center, Portland, ME

Preface

Significant advances in the perioperative management of transplant patients have transformed solid organ transplantation from an experimental procedure to accepted therapies for end-stage organ disease. The current outcomes associated with organ transplantation are the result of multidisciplinary contributions by surgeons, physicians, anesthesiologists, pharmacists, nutritionists, psychiatrists, social workers, administrators and nurses. The need to train students and residents in these various specialties as well served as the motivation for writing this book.

This volume introduces the broad science and art of transplantation to this wide audience. Although it is by no means a complete treatise, this work will serve as a fundamental guide or manual. Additional specifics can be garnered from any number of definitive texts.

We dedicate this book to our students, residents and trainees who continually inspire our admiration and dedication.

Paul C Kuo MD

History of solid organ transplantation

Paul E. Morrissey, Peter N. Madras and
Anthony P. Monaco

Early history

The story of transplantation dates back to the early recordings of
mankind. The fact that despite tremendous biologic diversity there
are common anatomical and functional structures between man
and beast led to tales of half-man, half-animal creatures imbued
with various mystical or superhuman powers. These so-called
'chimeras' were the primitive conceptualization of modern allotransplantation and hopefully of tomorrow's successes in xenotransplantation. Allotransplantation in humans was first conceived
in the Middle Ages. In this account, the leg of the sacristan Deacon
Justinian was amputated to treat a cancerous lesion. According to
legend, the leg of a recently slain Ethiopian Moor gladiator was
retrieved from the battlefield and transplanted to the amputation
site. Cosmas and Damian, twin Arab brothers who were converts
to Christianity, performed the operations. In addition to the famed
transplant, these saintly brothers performed miraculous cures and
feats of medicine and surgery for which they are aptly considered
to be the patron saints of medicine and transplantation. Their
achievements have been chronicled in countless paintings, litho-
graphs and artists' depictions throughout the centuries. The saints,
martyred in the third century, were honored by the construction of
the Basilica of SS Cosmas and Damian in sixth-century Italy.

The modern history of transplantation is even more fascinating.
The first phase occurred at the turn of the century. The surgical
clinics of Europe were ripe with development and experimentation. The potential of surgery had been recognized decades before,
and it erupted with the successful implementation of general anesthesia. Many conditions formerly considered to be uniformly fatal

were being treated and cured. Like today, surgery was primarily directed at patching or removing what had been disrupted in the organism. However, during this era, several investigators hypothesized that organ replacement could be applied as a therapy for organ failure. The earliest recordings of solid organ transplantation date to the turn of the century, when crude experiments in renal transplantation were undertaken in large animal models and in humans. These procedures took the form of autotransplantation in animals and of allo- and xenotransplantation in humans. A wide array of procedures was undertaken with the aim of achieving technical success with a viable organ, evaluating organ function and eventually attaining clinical success by prolonging survival in individuals with end-stage renal failure. Ultimately, an inadequate scientific foundation to pursue the postulates of early graft loss resulted in years of clinical failures.

Transplantation is the story of surgical pioneers with a single goal of organ replacement to treat end-stage irreversible organ failure. The early history largely involves technical aspects of organ recovery and replacement. Success in cadaver organ transplantation was achieved in the 1960s. However, disappointing results in large populations of patients tempered early enthusiasm. The field proliferated, spurred on by the dismal outlook for patients with end-stage disease and by continued progress in the areas of surgical technique, organ preservation and, most importantly, transplant immunology. The co-operation of basic scientists and surgeons led to the remarkable success story of modern solid organ transplantation. Since the modest and largely unsuccessful beginnings of solid organ transplantation in the 1950s (kidney only) and 1960s (liver, lung, pancreas and heart), there has been a continuous rise in the annual number of transplants and the success of the procedures. As of 1996, over 400 000 kidney transplants, 52 000 liver transplants, 40 000 heart transplants, 9000 pancreas transplants, 2000 lung transplants and 300 islet-cell transplant procedures had been performed. All of the solid organ transplants have met with remarkable success, but consistent good results for cellular transplantation and xenografts remain elusive.

Kidney

Kidney transplantation without immunosuppression

Emerich Ullmann (1861–1937) performed the first well-recorded studies of organ transplantation in Vienna at the turn of the century. In several large animal models he was able to carry out successful autotransplants as well as allografts. Perhaps his most remarkable achievement was the transplantation of a dog kidney to the carotid vessels of a goat with function. At this time, function was defined as urine output, and Dr Ullmann's success in xeno-transplantation was openly demonstrated at a meeting of the local surgical society. Not long afterward, Alexis Carrel began his early experiments on transplantation and the suturing of blood vessels. He transplanted a variety of organs, including kidney, bowel, spleen, ovary, segments of blood vessels, limbs, and reportedly a complete head on to the neck of another dog. His initial studies were conducted in France, but he continued his research in the USA, first in Chicago and shortly thereafter at the Rockefeller Institute (c. 1905) in New York. There he established what remains as an invaluable model for studying allografts, namely the bilateral nephrectomized, unilateral transplanted animal which he published as a single case in *Science* under the title 'Successful transplantation of both kidneys from a dog into a bitch with removal of both normal kidneys from the latter'. Although the initial procedure was considered a success by Carrel, a later publication revealed that the animal only survived for 8 days after surgery. Carrel enjoyed better success with renal allografts in cats, where one subject was a healthy survivor at 21 days. Based on these 'technical' successes, he correctly hypothesized that differences in autograft vs. allograft survival were due to 'biological factors'. For his historic efforts and vision he was awarded the Nobel Prize for Medicine in 1912. The suturing of vessels and transplantation of organs was described at the Nobel ceremony as 'the boldest and most difficult of operations' (Table 1.1). As evidence of the developing surgical confidence of the era, and in a desperate attempt to offer some therapy to patients with renal failure, several xenotransplants (termed heterografts) were performed from animal donors to man. Pig, goat, lamb and monkey donors were used. The transplants were carried out heterotopically, usually in the groin. The list of those who attempted these procedures reads like an international *Who's Who* of surgical history, including Ullmann, Jaboulay, Unger and others. Success was non-existent, and this dampened the enthusiasm for transplantation, except for a brief rekindling by Dr Williamson of the Mayo Clinic in 1923. While working in the laboratories of Frank C. Mann, he performed a series of successful auto- and allotransplants in dogs and he followed renal clearance as a marker of function, dispelling the notion that urine output alone equated with renal function.

The claim to the first renal allograft in humans and the first successful solid organ allograft spans 43 years of medical history, beginning with a case reported in the lay press and culminating

Table 1.1 Nobel Prize awards in physiology or medicine relevant to transplantation

Date	Recipient(s) of award	Research development
1908	Paul Ehrlich Elie Metchnikoff	Antibody secretion and phagocytosis as cellular defenses
1912	Alexis Carrel	Suturing of vessels and transplantation of organs termed 'the boldest and most difficult of operations'
1960	Sir Peter Medawar Sir Frank Macfarlane Burnet	Immunologic basis of failed transplants Concept of self and non-self, clonal deletion
1980	Baruj Benacerraf Jean Dausset George D. Snell	HLA and histocompatibility Genetic control of immune responses (HLA) Resistance to transplanted tumors genetically determined
1988	George H. Hitchings Gertrude Elion	Important principles in drug therapy (azathioprine)
1990	Joseph E. Murray E. Donnall Thomas	Successful kidney transplantation in humans Bone-marrow transplantation
1996	Rolf M. Zinkernagel Peter C. Doherty	Discovery of how the immune system recognizes virus-infected cells (T-cell receptor)

with the identical twin transplant at the Peter Bent Brigham Hospital. The first attempted renal transplantation in humans took place at the Methodist Episcopal Hospital in Philadelphia on 14 November 1911. According to a report in the *New York Times* (there is no account in the medical literature), a pedestrian was struck dead by a carriage outside the hospital. Inside resided a patient who was dying as a result of renal failure. The cadaver donor organ was quickly procured and transplanted by Dr L.J. Hammond. Although the organ did not function, the brief newspaper article addressed many of the key issues in solid organ transplantation, including the need for improved methods of organ preservation, the shortage of organs and the ethics of cadaver organ donation. Yu Yu Voronoy, in Kiev, described the next human renal allograft in 1933. A cadaver renal transplant was performed across the ABO barrier in a man with mercury poisoning. The kidney never functioned and the patient died within less than 48 hours. In 1947, the Peter Bent Brigham Hospital was the premier center in the world for the study of renal diseases. Hemodialysis, initially conceived and developed by Dr Willem Kolff in the Nazi-occupied Netherlands, was under intense development and the earliest phases of application. The surgical laboratory was pursuing studies in renal and adrenal transplantation. During that year, a pregnant woman with uterine sepsis and shock developed renal tubulopathy. After a prolonged period of anuria it was decided to attempt a renal transplant, and the surgical team undertook the task of locating a cadaver donor. Fortunately, one was found and David Hume procured the kidney. The recipient had lapsed into coma from sepsis and renal failure. The kidney was 'transplanted' extracorporeally to the brachial artery and median cubital vein by Drs Huffnagel (vascular surgery), Landsteiner (urology) and Hume (general surgery/transplantation). The kidney functioned for a period sufficient for the patient to clear the renal waste products, awaken from the coma and recuperate her native renal function. Although the functional success of the transplant was limited to a few days, this transplant probably represents the first life-saving allograft. R.H. Lawler, in Chicago, reported the first intra-abdominal transplant and long-term success in 1950. A young patient with polycystic kidney disease underwent an orthotopic renal transplant. The patient was not anuric prior to transplantation. However, early function was proved by dye excretion. The allograft functioned for several months, presumably until shortly prior to its removal seven months after transplantation. Shortly after this reported 'success' a number of groups attempted renal homografts. Most prominent among these efforts were those of three individual groups in Paris and the group at the Peter Bent Brigham Hospital, which consisted of both medical and surgical specialists dedicated to the application of renal replacement therapies. In 1951, eight renal allografts were performed in France by Marceau Servelle, Charles Dubost and Rene Kuss. Some of these donor kidneys were retrieved from criminals executed by guillotine. Kuss described the first transplant from a live donor that involved transplanting a healthy kidney removed for therapeutic purposes. On Christmas morning in 1952, a team at the Hospital Necker under the direction of Jean Hamburger performed a living related renal transplant (mother to son) in Paris. The recipient was a 16-year-old boy who underwent a nephrectomy for trauma. Postoperatively it was discovered that he had a congenital solitary kidney. Six days after the nephrectomy, his mother donated a kidney, which enjoyed early function. After 22 days of function the graft was lost, probably to acute rejection. Hamburger and Kuss in France and the group at the Peter Bent Brigham Hospital reported similar experiences. Of 10 initial transplants performed by Rene Kuss, there were seven early deaths and three prolonged survivals, none longer than 18 months. In 1955, David Hume reported nine cadaver renal transplants performed without immunosuppression. Four of the nine allografts functioned briefly. One particularly successful cadaver renal transplant was performed at the Peter Bent Brigham Hospital on 11 February 1953. The kidney was revascularized in the right thigh after 180 minutes of warm ischemia. Following a prolonged period of acute tubular necrosis, the allograft functioned and the patient was discharged home after 81 days as the first patient ever to be discharged with a functioning allograft. Unfortunately, success was limited and the patient died three months later of acute renal failure and hypertensive crisis.

The combined experiences of the Peter Bent Brigham Hospital and several groups in France confirmed the laboratory experience – that transplantation without immunosuppression was doomed to failure. The immunologic barrier surpassed the technical ability of the surgeons. At the time, without hemodialysis, physicians persevered in their efforts to salvage patients with renal failure. Morale must have been low in the early 1950s until two events, one scientific (acquired tolerance) and the other surgical (identical-twin renal transplantation) rejuvenated those in the field. Eventually, both primary investigators – Sir Peter Medawar of England and Joseph Murray at the Peter Bent Brigham Hospital – were awarded the Nobel Prize for Medicine and Physiology for these contributions.

The early history of transplantation science

The term immunity ('freedom from burden') derives from the Latin *immunis* and is defined in modern terms as an inherited, acquired or induced condition to a specific pathogen (antigen). The concepts of self and non-self grew from the skin-grafting experiments of Dr Emil Holman which were performed at the Johns Hopkins Hospital in the 1920s. These clinical studies demonstrated the uniqueness of the individual. The concept was refined by Sir Frank Macfarlane Burnet, who originated the theory of clonal deletion as an immunologic explanation for differentiating between self and non-self. This concept established the hallmarks of immunology, namely recognition, tolerance and memory. The modern era of transplantation science was ushered in by the classical studies of Peter Medawar, who began studying the fate of skin homografts in the late 1930s while completing his graduate studies in zoology at Oxford. During World War Two, his efforts were accelerated in an attempt to solve 'the homograft problem' and establish a successful therapy for grafting burn victims from the war. Working with Thomas Gibson, a plastic surgeon, at the Clarks

Surgical Unit in the Glasgow Royal Infirmary, Medawar established the special role of lymphocytes in rejection. The 'second set phenomenon' alluded to in the studies of Holman was refined in the descriptions of accelerated rejection occurring in soldiers in whom a second skin graft was placed. These results were confirmed in carefully controlled experiments in rabbits. Grafts from third-party donors confirmed the individual-specific nature of the effect.

Medawar's most significant contribution, namely acquired immunologic tolerance, for which he shared the Nobel Prize in 1960, arose from his reputation in the study of skin grafts and serendipity. While at a dinner party, Medawar was confronted with the problem of differentiating betweem dizygotic and monozygotic cattle twins. This was of some concern to small dairy farmers, because female dizygotic cattle were sterile and this had serious economic consequences for the individual farmer. Medawar reasoned that simple skin grafting could differentiate between the cattle twins. To his surprise, skin grafts placed on male–female twin pairs (dizygotic twins) were permanently accepted. Grafts from parents or siblings of separate birth were rejected as expected. The explanation of this finding lay in the earlier work of Ray Owen, who established that the shared placental blood supply of bovine twins resulted in blood group chimerism. Medawar and his colleagues Rupert Billingham and Leslie Brent embarked on a lengthy series of studies that involved manipulating the fetal immune system. Six years later they published their classic article in *Nature*, in which they described acquired tolerance by the infusion of donor splenocytes into fetal mice. When the mice matured, they accepted skin grafts from the original donor strain, but they rejected third-party grafts. The simplicity of the project belies the importance of the finding, but it deserves mention. In prior experiments the group had shown that skin grafts from A-line mice to CBA mice survived for 11 days. Second grafts survived for less than 6 days, confirming earlier observations of accelerated rejection. In this study, six CBA fetal mice were injected with 0.01 mL of A-line tissue cells. Five mice were born alive 4 days later and skin grafted 8 weeks later. Two of the skin grafts failed. Skin grafts were accepted for more than 50 days in three mice, and one mouse received a second skin graft on day 50, which was also accepted. It was concluded that antigen presented to an immunologically immature host produced tolerance, while the same antigen presented to an immunocompetent host (adult) resulted in immunity.

Medawar was cautious about the significance of these findings,

Table 1.2 'Firsts' in human organ transplantation

Date	Organ	Principal investigator
23 December 1954	Kidney*	Joseph Murray
22 March 1961	Cadaver kidney*	Joseph Murray
15 April 1963	Lung	James Hardy
1 March 1963	Liver	Thomas Starzl
17 December 1966	Pancreas	William Kelly and Richard Lillehei
5 April 1967	Intestine	Richard Lillehei
3 December 1967	Heart	Christian Barnard
1981	Heart–lung*	Norman Shumway

*First successful cases – other attempts made previously.

commenting sometime later that the fetal studies of acquired tolerance would have little impact on the practicality of clinical transplantation. In the spring of 1954, the New York Academy of Sciences sponsored the First International Conference on Transplantation, entitled 'The Relation of Immunology to Tissue Homotransplantation'. The link between laboratory investigations in immunology and clinical transplantation was established, and it stimulated continued interest in kidney transplantation, which resulted in the first largely successful kidney transplant 10 months later at the Peter Bent Brigham Hospital (see Table 1.2).

Modern renal transplantation

Frequent failures and occasional short-term function characterized renal transplantation from 1950 to 1954. Long-term allograft function was never achieved. Several lessons were learned from the laboratory and the unsuccessful clinical attempts at transplantation. Hemodialysis, newly introduced during this period as a life-saving therapy for acute renal failure, was available at only a few centers, and the lack of options for the patient with failed kidneys allowed the surgical groups to pursue their studies. Several principles were established in animal experiments, including an assurance that a functioning kidney transplant could restore biochemical values to normal, and the preferred intra-abdominal location of the transplant with ureterocystostomy. The role of uremia in abrogating acute rejection was appreciated, and the failed transplants provided valuable specimens for the pathologists to study the immunologic nature of graft failure. Around the time that enthusiasm for renal transplantation may have been declining, fate brought forth the circumstance of the historic renal transplant between identical twin brothers at the Peter Bent Brigham Hospital. On 23 December 1954, Richard Herrick underwent living related renal transplant from his twin brother Ronald, followed a few days later by bilateral nephrectomy for persistent hypertension. He survived for 8.5 years and represents the first 'successful' renal transplant. By 1958, the Peter Bent Brigham Hospital had reported seven living related renal transplant procedures from twin donors. In addition, identical twin transplants were performed in Paris, Montreal and Oregon, igniting enthusiasm for the field. Interestingly, 30 years previously, the German surgeon, K.H. Bauer, had exchanged skin grafts between twins during the surgical repair of webbed fingers. These allografts and a control set of autografts were sustained perfectly, providing strong evidence that the failure of allografts was dependent on individuality. Unfortunately, twins result from only 1 in 270 pregnancies, making such recipient–donor combinations a rarity. Realizing this, investigators in the field took the next major step, namely transplantation under immunosuppression.

Equipped with the knowledge that rejection was an immunologic phenomenon, efforts were made to weaken the immune system. Prior to the publication of acquired tolerance, Medawar and others reported on the immunosuppressive effects of total body irradiation and of the newly synthesized hormone cortisone. One year later, Frank Dixon reported in the *Journal of Immunology* that X-rays could depress immune responsiveness. The first use of clinical immunosuppression was at the Peter Bent Brigham Hospital (1958–1960) using total body irradiation with subsequent reconstitution by a bone-marrow allograft. Protocols were derived from experimental studies conducted by Murray and others in skin-grafted rabbits. The initial cases were associated with short-term success and a high rate of complications related to the transplant operation, renal failure or bone-marrow suppression. One patient with profound thrombocytopenia succumbed to bleeding complications one month after renal transplantation. Post-mortem examination failed to demonstrate any evidence of rejection. In the group's sixth case, the protocol was modified for a living related renal transplant from a fraternal twin. A lack of identity was clinically apparent, and immunologic disparity was proved by applying preoperative and postoperative skin grafts, which were rapidly rejected. Given the closeness of the relation, 450 Gray of total body irradiation (a reduction compared to earlier transplants), was administered 8 days preoperatively. The allograft was accepted, representing the first successful living related renal transplant under immunosuppression. The success was soon repeated, first by Hamburger in the identical setting of living related renal fraternal twins, and a year later by Kuss in a sister-to-brother combination. Several other long-term successes resulted from protocols with total body irradiation by these two investigators, and Hamburger showed that further radiation could be given to reverse acute rejection in the allograft. This strategy was soon widely applied at Denver, UCLA, the University of Minnesota, Edinburgh, Hammersmith, the Massachusetts General Hospital and the Medical College of Virginia. The following year, a second strategy in clinical immunosuppression arose from the development of 6-mercaptopurine in the laboratory. Subsequently, azathioprine was developed in collaboration with clinicians who were interested in transplantation, and was applied to the clinical arena after careful experiments in animal models.

In 1959, Schwartz and Darneshek showed that the compound 6-mercaptopurine was capable of blocking antibody production in rabbits that had been injected with human albumin. These findings were applied to transplantation in the animal laboratory the following year by Roy Calne, who was visiting the laboratories at the Peter Bent Brigham Hospital, and by Charles Zukoski at the Medical College of Virginia, where David Hume had recently established the program in renal transplantation. The group at the Peter Bent Brigham Hospital used 6-mercaptopurine clinically on 14 April 1960 and its imidazole derivative, azathioprine, on 22 March 1961. In 1962, under drug (azathioprine) immunosuppression, the team at the Peter Bent Brigham Hospital succeeded in another first, namely cadaver renal transplantation. The allograft survived for one year, and the success quickly produced a flurry of international transplant activity, ushering in the present era of transplantation under drug immunosuppression.

In short course, steroids were introduced to clinical immunosuppression. The subsequent combination of azathioprine and steroids brought kidney transplantation into the mainstream. During the next year, 25 renal transplant programs began in the USA. Renal transplantation still remained a formidable undertaking, and this outburst of enthusiasm was tempered by the difficult hospital course of the majority of patients in this era. Many of the new programs in transplantation were short-lived. The clinical introduction of antilymphocyte globulin (ALG) combined with drug therapy resulted in an encouraging 45% one-year graft survival. Refinements in patient selection, postoperative care and antibiotics eventually resulted in close to 80% one-year graft survival following living related renal transplantation, although one-year graft survival for cadaver renal transplantation remained closer to 50%. Given these continued unsatisfactory results and the limited number of cadaver donors several groups made attempts at heterotransplantation (xenotransplantation) under immunosuppression. Starz1 in Denver, Reenitsma in New Orleans and Hardy in Mississippi reported a limited series of baboon or chimpanzee to human heterografts. Amazingly, both the New Orleans group and James Hardy reported a patient with more than six months of function from a chimpanzee donor. Overall, the results were discouraging even with optimal immunosuppression, which consisted of azathioprine, actinomycin C, steroids and graft irradiation.

The transplant community owes a great debt to the early experience at the Peter Bent Brigham Hospital. When receiving the Nobel Prize in 1990, Murray stated that

> If gold medals and prizes were awarded to institutions instead of individuals, the Peter Bent Brigham Hospital of 30 years ago would have qualified. The ruling board . . . did not falter in their support of the quixotic objective of treating end-stage renal disease despite a long list of tragic failures that resulted from these early efforts − leavened only by occasional encouraging notations such as those in the identical twin case.

The rich academic environment at the Peter Bent Brigham Hospital enabled so many transplant firsts to take place, including the first successful renal transplant, the first successful non-identical-twin transplant, the first successful transplant under drug immunosuppression and the first successful cadaver renal transplant. The tenures of George Thorn, Chief of Medicine, and Francis Moore, Chief of Surgery, at that hospital represent a three-decade commitment to renal replacement therapies. In addition to the successes in renal transplantation, hemodialysis was refined and clinically developed at the Peter Bent Brigham Hospital. Laboratory investigations of immunosuppression by radiation and drugs with immediate clinical application led to the series of notable 'firsts'. This commitment to end-stage renal disease, which had been uniformly fatal in the early 1950s, represents one of the greatest institutional achievements in medical history. Joseph Murray established the first transplant registry in 1964. The compilation of 342 non-twin renal transplants summarizes the early world experience − the birth of clinical transplantation. Twenty-five years later, Starzl revisited this registry to produce a list of 24 patients who had survived longer than 25 years after renal transplantation. Although desperation and bold initiatives characterized this era, these long-term survivors and today's burgeoning field of transplantation are the fruits of these labors.

Recent progress in renal transplantation

By the end of the 1970s, living related renal transplantation was an accepted and effective therapy for end-stage renal dialysis. However, some of the earlier enthusiasm for cadaver renal transplantation had diminished. Surgical expertise in hemodialysis access and medical improvements in the delivery of dialysis increased the attractiveness of this modality. The 5-year cadaver renal allograft survival rate was only 35%. Azathioprine and prednisone were routinely used, but antilymphocyte globulin was not readily available. The morbidity of massive infusions of methylprednisolone was prohibitive. Some centers performed thoracic duct drainage to deplete the recipient lymphocyte pool, although the effectiveness was unproved and the technique was cumbersome. It was widely perceived that efforts in histocompatibility matching and the 'transfusion' effect contributed only slightly towards improved cadaver renal transplantation. Some physicians in the field expressed a measure of pessimism about that level of success.

A Symposium on Organ Transplantation was compiled in the *Surgical Clinics of North America* published in 1978. Felix Rapaport summarized this sentiment in the section on immunobiology:

> Transplantation immunobiology appears to be alive and well ... Progress in clinical kidney transplantation appears, however, to suffer from a hopefully temporary frost. The continued absolute dependence of the transplant surgeon upon azathioprine and prednisone, and the plateau at which human kidney transplantation results have flattened, provide a clear illustration of the problem. Indeed, a significant prolongation of the present impasse may hold the very considerable hazard of depriving the transplant surgeon of his therapeutic credibility.

Fortunately, Rapaport's prediction was soon followed by the next quantum leap in transplantation science and medicine, namely the clinical introduction of cyclosporine.

Cyclosporine, a fungal peptide, was discovered in a soil sample retrieved during a holiday expedition to the Arctic Circle by researchers from the Sandoz Laboratories. Jean Borel demonstrated its immunosuppressive properties *in vitro* and in a mouse skin graft model. Oral administration of cyclosporine in mice abrogated antibody formation, prolonged skin allograft survival, delayed the onset of graft-vs.-host disease and prevented paralysis in rats with allergic encephalomyelitis. Sir Roy Calne proved its utility in experimental solid organ transplantation in the rat heterotopic cardiac allograft model and in canine renal allografts, and correctly predicted that this single agent was far more potent than previous combinations of immunosuppressive drugs. Only two years later, Calne reported the first use in human renal transplantation. Unfortunately, the animal studies had not predicted the nephrotoxicity of cyclosporine in humans. Cyclosporine was first used as monotherapy at a dose of 25 mg/kg. No assay was available to monitor blood levels. Many of the recipients of cadaver renal transplants in this era suffered significant allograft dysfunction or loss due to cyclosporine toxicity. Protocols were quickly devised to overcome this toxicity, and soon lower doses of cyclosporine were employed in combination with azathioprine and steroids. The results were astounding. Lower doses of all of the immunosuppressive agents resulted in a marked decrease in drug-related side-effects. Furthermore, the regimens were effective. First-year survival rates after cadaver renal transplantation exceeded 80% in many centers. The success in kidneys spread to other organs, enabling the routine transplantation of lung and pancreas.

Liver

The early history of liver transplantation dates back to animal experiments in the 1950s. At that time, C. Stuart Welch in Albany described auxiliary liver transplantation and Jack Cannon at UCLA briefly reported the technique of liver transplantation in dogs. Shortly thereafter, two groups emerged, one in Boston under the direction of Francis Moore, and Tom Starzl's group in Chicago, to study liver transplantation in a dog model in the hope of developing liver transplantation in humans. The focus of the Boston group was on the immunologic feasibility of liver replacement, having already achieved institutional success in kidney transplantation. Starzl and his colleagues focused on the technical aspects of liver replacement (core cooling for preservation and veno-venous bypass for hemodynamic support) and hepatic physiology. In addition to establishing the technical possibility of orthotopic liver engraftment, these studies contributed significantly to our understanding of the liver in relation to gut hormones, and established the concept of hepatotrophic factors in the portal circulation. Starzl's laboratory moved to the Denver Veteran's Administration Hospital and functioned at an inexhaustible pace. Persistence with the dog model and the introduction of azathioprine resulted in the first long-term survival in an animal model of liver transplantation. These experiments provided the technical and immunologic groundwork that would in 1968 result in the first descriptions of long-term survival after liver transplantation in humans. Human liver transplantation began in Denver, at the University of Colorado, on 1 March 1963. The recipient was a ventilator-dependent 3-year-old boy with biliary atresia. The donor was a child who died during an open heart operation. The complexity of the procedure was recounted by Starzl:

> Although we had performed nearly 200 liver transplantations in dogs, nothing could have prepared us for the difficulties in the recipient which were caused by portal hypertension, scarring from previous operations, and a complete lack of clotting. The patient bled to death.

Other attempts in Boston and Paris were similarly disappointing, and all clinical trials were halted until October 1966. However, the lack of options for patients with end-stage liver disease and the perseverance of early investigators provided the framework for continued attempts at liver replacement in the face of failure. More than a dozen liver transplants were performed over a 5-year period until a single long-term success was achieved. Of the first nine, the longest survivor was 23 days, while for the next seven liver transplants survival was for 2, 3.5, 4.5, 6 days and greater than 1, 2.5 and 9 months. In the discussion of that paper, Dr Moore, reflecting on the development of liver transplantation, stated that 'This is a magnificent achievement, and liver surgery as of this day has an entirely new look from hither forward'. Ultimately, the three surviving children described in that paper died 13, 15 and 30 months after transplantation, two succumbing to recurrent hepatoma and the other to chronic rejection. The series demonstrated the feasibility of liver transplantation in humans. Tom Starzl in the USA and Sir Roy Calne in Cambridge, England, pioneered human liver transplantation in the late 1960s. Progress in clinical liver transplantation was slow due to the poor initial results. Significant controversy arose in the medical and political arenas with regard to the practicality of the procedure and the enormous economic cost of these clinical experiments. Between 1963 and 1979, 170 patients were transplanted by Starzl's group. These early years of animal experimentation and clinical liver transplantation are chronicled in Starzl's autobiography, *The Puzzle People*. Over the next decade, case reports and small series were reported from several centers worldwide, the largest series coming from Starzl's team in the USA, Sir Roy Calne and Williams at King's College, London, in England and R. Pichlmayr and C. Broelsch in West Germany.

Of necessity, the surgical teams involved in the transplantation of extrarenal organs developed core cooling and refined organ procurement. In the early years of transplantation, organs were recovered from non-heart-beating donors or, in the case of kidney transplantation, from live donors. Live donor kidneys were often removed for medical reasons (a small parenchymal lesion or a ureteropelvic obstruction that could be corrected *ex vivo*). No live donor source existed at the time for extrarenal organs. As mentioned earlier, the first allografted kidney was obtained from a man who was killed in a carriage accident directly in front of the Philadelphia hospital with a waiting recipient. At the old Peter Bent Brigham Hospital, surgeons waited in-house for a patient to expire so that their kidneys could be quickly procured for lifesaving renal transplants. Some of the early transplants in Paris were performed with kidneys retrieved from prisoners who had consented to post-mortem donation prior to execution by the guillotine for heinous crimes. Clinical liver transplantation pre-dated brain death legislation. The recipient operation was commenced prior to withdrawing life support from the donor, who suffered irreversible brain injury. Following cessation of the donor heartbeat, the liver was rapidly procured in order to limit the warm ischemic time and was then transported to the nearby operating-theater to the waiting recipient. The limitations of warm ischemia and organ availability imposed by this system contributed to the high failure rate of early liver transplantation. Two developments in the late 1960s, namely established criteria for brain death, and organ preservation by cooling, provided the solution to this problem.

Lillehei and his associates developed core cooling and first applied it to intestinal transplantation. Shortly thereafter, Starzl's group embraced this concept. Starzl and his colleagues were the principal advocates of organ cooling and the efficient procurement of organs for transplantation. When brain death was established, organs could be recovered and preserved for periods sufficient to allow transport to a waiting recipient at distant centers. Multiple organ harvesting, which was rare in the early days of transplanta-tion, developed out of necessity to meet the growing demand. Although now commonplace, it did not start until 1978 – when two kidneys, the heart and the liver, were procured from a single donor – that being a collaborative effort of teams from the University of Colorado and the University of Minnesota.

Although the technical aspects of liver transplant surgery were of paramount importance to the Starzl team, their innovative applications of drug immunosuppression to clinical renal and liver transplantation remain important contributions to the field. Because of the tremendous technical limitations imposed by liver transplantation, the pharmacology of liver replacement was adapted from the experience obtained in renal transplantation. Starzl can be credited with the combined use of azathioprine and steroids, the first large-scale application of antilymphocyte globulin (ALG), and more recently, the development of tacrolimus for clinical use. An early observation from the first canine liver transplants was that engraftment of the liver, although technically more challenging, was immunologically more easily achieved than a kidney transplant. This raised the issue that the liver may be less immunogenic than the kidney, and that rejection may therefore be easier to control. Sir Roy Calne confirmed this observation and further demonstrated that the transplanted liver might be tolerogenic. Starzl in the USA and Calne in Cambridge, England, persevered with orthotopic liver transplantation throughout the 1970s. Their efforts were rewarded with the introduction of cyclosporine-based immunosuppressive regimens. Clinical application to liver transplantation by Calne and Starzl, now in Pittsburgh, demonstrated the clinical efficacy of this agent, thereby ushering in the modern era of liver transplantation. Before cyclosporine A, the best results for liver transplantation under ALG, azathioprine and steroid immunosuppression were in the range 24–33% one-year survival. In the 2 years following the introduction of cyclosporine A, survival rates approached 70%.

Liver transplantation has continued to progress along two lines – one technical and the other immunologic. To meet the needs of patients with end-stage liver disease, technical innovations have been driven by the shortage of suitable organs and the resulting attrition due to death while on the liver transplant waiting-list. Among the recent technical innovations has been the use of reduced-size liver transplants in pediatric liver transplantation. Back-table liver reduction soon led to living related segmental liver transplantation. These innovations have reduced the waiting time for pediatric livers, and in so doing have decreased the mortality of pediatric liver disease. A further development has been the application of 'split-liver' transplantation to children and small adults. Immunologic advances came largely from the Pittsburgh Transplant Institute. The clinical introduction of tacrolimus (FK506) was largely limited to this single institution. While the contributions of this agent over cyclosporine-based immunosuppression are still being elucidated for most solid organs, there appeared to be an immediate benefit in the difficult area of small bowel transplantation. A second seminal observation from this group, having accumulated a large number of long-term survivors of kidney and liver allografts, was that of donor chimerism and its relationship to host adaptation.

The demonstration of donor microchimerism deserves special mention. The role of chimerism in allograft acceptance dates back to the freemartin cattle studies of R.D. Owen and later studies by Medawar. Medawar showed that allografts survived in blood group chimeras. Eighteen years later, Starzl's group demonstrated the development of chimerism in humans following successful liver transplantation, and 23 years later, Starzl revisited the phenomenon with new zeal. Using *in-situ* hybridization and karyo-typing to identify the Y-chromosome from male donors to female liver transplant recipients, the Pittsburgh group showed that nine of nine long-term liver allograft survivors had cells of donor origin (microchimerism). Furthermore, the cells were identified not only in the allograft, but also in peripheral blood, skin and lymph node tissue. Similar findings were made in long-term recipients of renal allografts. Finally, the recognition that clinical graft-vs.-host disease occasionally accompanies liver transplantation established the basis for the 'two-way paradigm', by which bidirectional cellular trafficking between donor and host tissues enables the development of the chimeric state. The clinical importance of these findings has yet to be elucidated, but the results of early studies promoting chimerism through donor bone-marrow or stem-cell infusion (the 'Monaco model') offer further hope for improvement in organ transplantation.

Pancreas

Transplantation of the pancreas, like that of other solid organs, began in surgical laboratories and was introduced with limited success in the clinical arena shortly thereafter. For two decades pancreas transplantation remained an experimental therapy for insulin replacement, rather than a cure for diabetes. With the advent of stronger immunosuppression, the refinement of surgical techniques, the development of interventional radiology techniques to diagnose and treat early complications, and an improved understanding of pancreatic allograft physiology, the procedure is currently performed with success rates that compare favorably with cadaver renal transplantation. Efforts are in progress to demonstrate the effectiveness of the procedure in preventing and potentially reversing the secondary complications of insulin-dependent diabetes mellitus.

The origin of many of the practices of modern-day transplantation can be found in canine experiments performed over five decades. Five years after the discovery of insulin by Banting and Best, pancreas transplantation was performed in pancreatectomized dogs. Endocrine function of the allograft was documented hours after surgery. In 1936, Bottin reported a canine pancreatic allograft perfused by the cervical circulation for 6 days. However, he did not describe the functional success of this experiment. Following the limited functional survival of whole-organ allografts, the majority of efforts focused on the function of auto- and allografts of pancreatic tissue and isolated islets. Pockets of pancreatic tissue were transplanted subcutaneously or intramuscularly in animals with chemically induced diabetes and, after a period of neovascularization, function was evaluated. Transplantation of pancreatic islets into the immunologically privileged sites of the testis or the anterior chamber of the eye lowered blood glucose levels, and endocrine function could be demonstrated at 30 days. However, none of these techniques resulted in a durable result that could be applied in large animal models or humans. Canine studies were resumed with segmental and whole-organ pancreas allografts being placed heterotopically in the groin or abdomen of pancreatectomized dogs. Studies of pancreatic duct ligation, portal venous drainage and enteric drainage of exocrine secretions were undertaken. For a period orthotopic grafts, which required pancreatic exocrine and biliary drainage, were placed with some success by the group at the University of Minnesota. Ultimately, intra-abdominal heterotopic placement of the allograft became the experimental and early clinical standard. DeJode and Howard initially described the technique of external catheter drainage of the exocrine secretions. The procedure was modified by Idezuki and colleagues at Minnesota to include internal enteric drainage, and it became the early standard for clinical transplantation. Prior to undertaking transplantation in humans, investigators had demonstrated endocrine function by documenting serum glucose and circulating insulin levels, and had worked out some of the basic principles of the effect of acute rejection on exocrine function of the gland. Graft histology in non-immunosuppressed recipients showed the typical lymphocytic infiltrates characteristic of acute rejection beginning on the fourth postoperative day. The Minnesota group, which was already active in the area of organ preservation, had defined the time course of *in-vivo* and *in-vitro* pancreatic allograft function following cold perfusion. Successful canine allotransplantation under azathioprine and steroid immunosuppression established the feasibility of the procedure in humans.

Human pancreas transplantation was pioneered by William Kelly and Richard Lillehei on 17 December 1966. This also represented the first combined solid organ transplant in humans. The graft was placed intra-abdominally and vascularized via the iliac blood supply. A long segment of duodenum accompanied the pancreas and was brought out as a cutaneous duodenostomy. The initial allograft – a partial pancreatic allograft – was lost to a pancreatic leak, a complication which did not arise in the next nine kidney–whole organ pancreas transplants performed over 2 years. Eight of the original 10 recipients (age range 26–44 years) died within seven months of transplantation, the majority of sepsis. In only one patient did both allografts function for longer than a year. However, solid organ transplantation surgery in diabetic patients, which was previously thought to be too risky for routine application, was gaining acceptance as a viable alternative to insulin therapy and/or hemodialysis. At the time, the authors incorrectly concluded that the majority of the complications arose from the heightened antigenicity and subsequent rejection of the kidney allograft, and postulated that pancreas transplantation alone might offer a safer alternative to combined kidney–pancreas grafting. After these early clinical experiments, whole-organ pancreas transplantation was temporarily abandoned in favor of clinical studies of isolated islet transplantation. Although islet cells functioned well in the laboratory, none of the first 24 patients became euglycemic, although the requirement for insulin in a few patients was reduced. In fact, islet-cell transplantation remains a dismal procedure, with less than 2% of grafted islets resulting in long-term survival and insulin independence. Enthusiasm for pancreas transplantation at the University of Minnesota returned in 1978 with the development of partial pancreatic transplantation with pancreatic duct obliteration. At the same time, David Sutherland founded the International Transplant Registry. New life was breathed into these failed projects with the advent of cyclosporine A.

Quantum improvements were noted in pancreas transplantation with the use of better immunosuppression. However, a high rate of morbidity was still associated with the procedure. In an effort to decrease the perioperative morbidity, a number of technical innovations were developed to improve the procedure. Surgical innovations were aimed at treating the metabolic, mucosal and duodenal complications associated with pancreatic exocrine secretion. Urinary drainage of the pancreatic exocrine secretions via the recipient ureter was introduced by Gleidman and modified by Sollinger, who anastomosed a button of duodenal tissue directly to the bladder. Corry and Nghiem developed the current practice of duodenocystostomy several years later. Further modifications included the injection of synthetic polymers into the pancreatic duct to obliterate the exocrine secretions, and at many centers an enthusiastic return to enteric exocrine drainage combined with portal venous drainage, a technique first attributed to Roy Calne.

With these modifications, the success rate of pancreas transplantation approximates to that of cadaver renal transplantation. Despite the early predictions of Lillehei and colleagues, 85% of cases are performed as combined kidney–pancreas transplants, while pancreas transplant alone presents a greater immunologic challenge. At present the surgical techniques are well established, although no consensus is available on the preferred approach. Many clinical studies are in progress to evaluate the end-organ benefits of euglycemia achieved by pancreas transplantation and the vascular effects of hyperinsulinemia.

Heart

Like the history of renal transplantation, the advent of cardiac transplantation had its origin with the early experiments of Alexis Carrel conducted at the University of Chicago. The concept of heart and heart–lung transplantation began with the heterotopic (cervical) transplantation of allografts in large animal models. These experiments established the feasibility of vascular anastomosis and demonstrated that the ventricle could function as a pump in a denervated heart. Frank Mann at the Mayo Clinic and V.P. Demikhov in the Soviet Union furthered these studies during the 1930s and 1940s. Orthotopic cardiac transplantation was not achieved in animal models until the 1950s, and was not performed with any degree of success until the development of cardiopulmonary bypass in 1953. In 1964, James Hardy performed a cardiac xenotransplant (chimpanzee to human) in an individual who could not be weaned from bypass. The xenograft functioned, but the pump function was inadequate to support the individual, who succumbed after several hours. Two years later a human-to-primate xenograft was performed in the laboratory by Lower, demonstrating that the transplanted heart could support hemodynamic function. These seminal discoveries are described in Reitz's detailed account of cardiac and heart–lung transplantation. Eventually the technique of orthotopic cardiac transplantation that would usher in clinical transplantation was reported by Cass and Brock in 1959, and was adopted by Lower and Shumway at Stanford University. The Stanford group reported on eight dogs that underwent successful orthotopic cardiac transplantation by suture of atrial cuffs, aorta and pulmonary artery. Five of the eight dogs survived for 6 to 21 days, until their transplanted hearts failed due to biopsy-proven acute rejection. Later the same group achieved one-year allograft function in this model with azathioprine and prednisone immunosuppression.

In the public's view the greatest achievement in solid organ transplantation must be the advent of successful cardiac transplantation. Despite years of experimentation in the Stanford Medical School laboratories, Christian Barnard shocked the world by performing the first human heart transplantation in Capetown, South Africa. The surgery, which was performed without public fanfare on 3 December 1967, was a technical success. The donor was a 24-year-old woman who had been injured in a car accident. The donor and recipient operations proceeded simultaneously, with both patients on cardiopulmonary bypass. In the absence of accepted brain-death criteria, the donor was removed from the ventilator and progressed to asystole prior to cardiac cooling and recovery. The cardiac transplant was performed as described by Lower and Shumway. Then, with the world watching, Louis Washansky, a diabetic who suffered from ischemic cardiomyopathy, recovered and ultimately survived for 18 days before he succumbed to infectious complications. During the next 3 years, the South African group transplanted six more patients. Four of these individuals survived for longer than 18 months, including two patients who survived for more than 12 and 21 years, respectively. A truism in life that is often validated in the scientific world, a cardiac transplant performed days later at Maimonades Hospital in New York City went almost unrecognized. Three days after the historic first, Adrian Kantrowitz transplanted the heart of a 2-day-old anencephalic donor to a 17-day-old infant with Ebstein's anomaly. Despite years of experience and experimental success with large animals, the child died within hours of the procedure. On 2 January 1968, Barnard performed a second transplant with a 20-month survival. Four days later, Shumway transferred his efforts from the canine model to the clinical arena. Denton Cooley followed suit four months later with what is widely regarded as the first successful cardiac transplant in the USA. Public awareness of transplantation medicine soared, and cardiac surgeons caught up in this infectious enthusiasm performed 167 cardiac transplant procedures at 58 centers during the next two years. Unrecognized or under-appreciated in these efforts was the fact that in those centers where cardiac transplantation would flourish there was a strong interest and understanding of transplant immunology and the management of immunosuppression to maintain the cardiac allograft. For although the technical aspects of cardiac transplantation were within the capabilities of many surgeons, the clinical and immunologic aspects of patient care necessary for successful cardiac transplantation were only appreciated by a few select centers during this nascent period. Indeed, Barnard had made a year-long journey through the transplant centers of the USA prior to the initial cardiac transplant. He visited the clinics and laboratories of the Medical College of Virginia, the University of Colorado and Stanford. There he learned the nuances of allograft rejection, the use of antilymphocyte antibodies and the technical aspects of cardiac transplantation. Equipped with this knowledge, he undertook the historic first transplant surgery. Pre-dating this event was a decade of interest and careful research by the group at Stanford.

The initial enthusiasm of the cardiac surgery community was tempered by the nemeses of transplantation, namely rejection and infection. Under azathioprine and prednisone immunosuppression the initial results were poor and the majority of clinical outcomes were disappointing, despite the 'technical success' of the surgery. During the ensuing decade, approximately 20–30 heart transplant operations were performed annually, around one-third of them at Stanford University. Among the better early results, Cooley and colleagues at the Texas Heart Institute performed 23 cardiac transplants, with the longest survivor maintaining cardiac allograft function for 18 months. Long-term survivors (more than 10 years), as reported by Barnard and Shumway, were rare. Overall, 35% of cardiac transplant recipients survived for 3 months and only 10% had a durable result. Shumway and his colleagues persevered. In 1982, their group reported 227 cardiac transplant operations in 206 patients. Not surprisingly, their results were among the best, with one-year survival rates approaching 50%. Among the significant contributions made by the Stanford team was the development of transvenous endomyocardial biopsy. The Stanford team established the criteria and grading system for acute cardiac allograft rejection, and advanced the concept of protocol cardiac biopsies. With the use of endomyocardial biopsy to monitor the graft and the clinical introduction of cyclosporine, cardiac transplantation entered a second phase of growth in the 1980s. In 1981, for the first time since 1968, over 100 transplants were performed.

Since the early 1980s successful cardiac transplantation has been performed at numerous centers worldwide. The results improved dramatically, with one-year graft survival rates exceeding 80% under current immunosuppression. The clinical problem of graft atherosclerosis (chronic rejection) is now the primary cause of long-term failure. Several advances in surgical and medical therapy for those afflicted with end-stage cardiac disease have been developed in parallel with cardiac transplantation. The shortage of donor organs and the death of potential recipients on the waiting-list provided much of the impetus for these efforts. Despite creative procedures such as ventricular aneurysmectomy and skeletal cardiomyoplasty, transplantation remains the preferred therapy for the failing heart in most patients.

Lung

Although the first pulmonary allografts were probably performed in dogs by the Russian physiologist Demikhov, the technique was first published by Metras in France and was revised by Hardin and Kittle in the USA. Amazingly, the concepts of bronchial vascularization and preferential use of a left atrial anastomosis rather than the left pulmonary vein were elucidated in these early studies. However, the complex nature of lung transplantation could not have been appreciated in Jackson, Mississippi when James Hardy performed the first lung allograft in a human. Despite the fact that literally hundreds of canine lung auto- and allotransplants had been performed by the group prior to attempting the procedure in humans, the surgical, postoperative infectious and immunologic challenges that lay ahead were immense. Even today, despite three decades of clinical experience, numerous surgical innovations, improved immunosuppression and better patient selection, the long-term results for lung transplantation (approximately 55% three-year survival rate) are poor compared to those for other organ transplants. The lack of success in the few lung transplantation procedures performed in the 1960s is not surprising given the evolution of lung transplantation surgery and intensive care.

Based on the clinical success of cadaver renal transplantation, Hardy and his colleagues began studies of canine lung replacement. Lung replantation and transplantation had been described in 1950. In fact, the techniques developed by these investigators, including the preference for left lung transplantation and the use of an atrial cuff to incorporate the pulmonary veins, underwent little change during the next 30 years. Hardy's initial experiments consisted of autograft specimens removed for varying lengths of time, evaluated after a variety of preservation techniques and then reimplanted. Elaborate physiologic studies of the denervated lungs were undertaken in an attempt to elucidate the fate of the divided bronchiolar blood supply and the pulmonary lymphatics. Allografts were then performed under various immunosuppressive regimens. Initial studies were conducted with azathioprine, hydrocortisone, methotrexate or azathioprine plus actinomycin C. Azathioprine provided the best results, extending survival to 30.4 days, compared to 7.4 days for untreated control animals. Encouraged by these results, screening began for a suitable candidate for lung 'homotransplantation'.

After several months an appropriate candidate was identified in an unfortunate man with a near-obstructing squamous-cell carcinoma of the left mainstem bronchus, whose lung tissue had been destroyed by a series of necrotizing pneumonias. The patient was admitted on 15 April 1963. The left lung was removed from a cadaver donor who had succumbed to a massive myocardial infarction and pulmonary edema. The procured lung was venti-lated extracorporeally in a cold bath until transplantation. Immediately after transplantation the oxygen saturation improved (from 87% to 98%), indicating that the allograft was participating in gas exchange. The patient survived for 3 weeks before succumb-ing to renal failure. At autopsy, no evidence of acute rejection was found. MaGovern and Yates performed the second lung transplant in humans that same year. Over the next two decades approxi-mately 40 lung transplantation procedures were undertaken worldwide. No patient survived long term, and only one patient survived to discharge from the hospital. That patient was a 23-year-old man who underwent lung transplantation for silicosis. He died 2 months later as a result of chronic rejection and pulmonary sepsis. In other patients who survived the initial surgery, death was usually attributable to bronchial disruption and infection. In 1981, the Stanford group extended their experience with heart transplantation, announcing the first series of patients to undergo successful heart–lung transplantation. This report demonstrated the potential of long-term survival with allografted lung tissue.

Lung transplantation alone remained a discouraging venture until two critical observations were made by Joel Cooper and his colleagues in Toronto. First, the limitation of the bronchial anasto-mosis could be overcome by the introduction of cyclosporine A. Second, with the use of cyclosporine, the dose of steroids could be dramatically reduced. This reduction of the steroid dose and devel-opment of the technique of bronchial omentopexy improved heal-ing at the bronchial anastomosis site. The benefits of these modifications were realized immediately. In total, 16 of Cooper's next 20 lung transplant recipients were discharged home without supplemental oxygen. Within a short time, the majority of patients with lung disease (most of whom had normal biventricular func-tion) underwent successful single-lung transplantation. Further modifications included the use of bilateral bronchial anastomoses for double-lung transplantation. This trend, together with the domino heart transplant procedure (utilizing the healthy heart of a heart–lung transplant recipient for isolated heart transplantation) highlighted the critical nature of the organ shortage.

As a result of technical advances in lung transplantation, the greatest challenges in the field are now increasing organ availabil-ity and preventing early chronic rejection. The indications for single-lung transplantation have been extended beyond emphy-sema and pulmonary fibrosis to include primary pulmonary hypertension and some congenital lung diseases. In 1982, two lung allografts were performed. In 1987, there were 17 lung transplantation procedures. By contrast, in 1995 a total of 871 procedures were performed, representing a 4700% increase. Unfortunately, cadaver lung donors are limited by the susceptibility of the lung to infection and edema coincident with head injury and brain death. Death on the recipient waiting-list remains a harsh reality, especially given the technical feasibility of the operation. As with liver transplantation, surgical innovation has provided an alternative in some cases in the form of live donor (segmental) lung allografts. The expansion of this area of solid organ transplantation has been remarkable.

Further reading

Billingham R, Brent L and **Medawar PB**. 1953: Actively acquired tolerance of foreign cells. *Nature* **172**, 603–6.

Broelsch CE, Emond JC, Whitington PF, Thistlethwaite JR, Baker AL and **Lichtor JL**. 1990: Application of reduced-size liver transplants as split grafts, auxillary orthotopic grafts, and living related segmental transplants. *Annals of Surgery* **212**, 368.

Carrel A. 1906: Successful transplantation of both kidneys from a dog into a bitch with removal of both normal kidneys from the latter. *Science* **23**, 394–5. This paper established the model, implicit in the title, for evaluating the functional success of renal transplants.

Hamburger J. 1991: Memories of old times. In Terasaki PI (ed.), *History of transplantation: thirty-five recollections*. Los Angeles, CA: UCLA Tissue Typing Laboratory, 63–72. Compiled by Terasaki, this work represents 35 personal recollections from outstanding contributors to the field of organ transplantation.

Medawar PB. 1944: The behaviour and fate of skin autografts and homografts in rabbits. *Journal of Anatomy* **78**, 176–99. Medawar carefully repeated in outbred rabbits the observations made with Gibson in homografted soldiers following extensive burn injury. He identified the lymphocyte as the effector of rejection, documented the accelerated rejection accompanying presensitization and, in grafting the skin from third-party donors, clarified the role of specificity.

Merrill JP, Murray JE and **Takacs F**. 1963: Successful transplantation of a kidney from a human cadaver. *Journal of the American Medical Association* **185**, 347–9. Although the twin transplant remains the best known, these first successful renal transplantations with immunosuppressive drugs form the basis of modern organ transplantation – the real 'landmark' case.

Moore FD. 1972: *Transplant: the give and take of organ transplantation*. New York: Simon and Schuster. This book is fascinating reading. The inner workings of the Peter Bent Brigham Hospital are disclosed as the problem of renal replacement is tackled from all angles. Included are the clinical development of hemodialysis and 30 years of laboratory and clinical work in renal transplantation. Success ultimately derived from the collaborative efforts of physicians in medicine and surgery and their colleagues in the laboratory.

Murray JE, Merrill JP and **Harrison JH**. 1955: Renal homotransplantation in identical twins. *Surgical Forum* **6**, 432.

New York Times. 1911: **14 November**, **2** and **15 November**, 10 (editorial). This is the first account of human-to-human renal transplantation. The editorial in the next day's issue discussed many salient issues, including organ preservation by cooling, cadaver organ donation and overcoming the shortage of cadaver organs by xenotransplantation.

Owen R. 1945: Immunogenetic consequences of vascular anastomoses between bovine twins. *Science* **102**, 400.

Reitz BA. 1990: The history of heart and heart–lung transplantation. In Baumgartner WA, Reitz BA and Achuff SC (eds), *Heart and heart–lung transplantation*. Philadelphia, PA: W.B. Saunders. Cardiac transplantation is chronicled by one of the pioneers of Shumway's team, from the laboratory to the clinics. A detailed account of the first years of clinical cardiac transplantation is followed by some of the innovations that led to the widespread acceptance of and general good results obtained in current practice.

Starzl TE, Todo S, Fung J, Demetris AJ, Venkataramanan F and **Jain A**. 1989: FK506 for human liver, kidney and pancreas transplantation. *Lancet* **2**, 1000.

Ullmann E. 1902: Experimentielle Nierentransplantation. *Wiener Klinische Wochenschrift* **15**, 281. An account of kidney allografts and xenografts in dogs and goats.

Williamson CS. 1926: Further studies on the transplantation of the kidney. *Journal of Urology* **16**, 231. These studies at the Mayo Foundation furthered the experimental model of renal transplantation by quantifying renal allograft function.

Immunosuppression 2

Matthew R. Weir

Introduction

The principal strategies of clinical immunosuppression are to provide adequate suppression of immunologic activity yet to avoid immunodeficiency and non-immune toxicity of the drugs. Clinical immunosuppression remains an empiric and imprecise science as there is no adequate *in-vitro* mechanism for determining the adequacy of the immunosuppressive agents being employed. Inadequate immunosuppression results in rejection of the transplanted organ, whereas over-immunosuppression results in immunodeficiency and adverse clinical consequences such as infection, lymphoproliferative disease or even malignancy. In addition, non-immune toxicity related to the individual drugs either alone or in concert with one another requires close patient follow-up and individual adjustments of medications as necessary. Thus a delicate balance needs to be achieved, which can vary substantially from one patient to another. Although protocols exist to guide direction with regard to immunosuppression, these are only templates which may require substantial adjustment. No two patients are alike. Substantial differences exist with regard to patient tolerability of medications. Likewise, the capacity of medications to suppress differences in immunologic responsiveness between donor and recipient alloantigens ultimately requires individualization of immunosuppressive strategy.

The practice of immunosuppression is based on the belief that tolerance will occur in time because the host immune system will adjust or adapt to the presence of the antigens on the transplanted allograft. Our ability to provide initial protection against the immediate response during the first few weeks post-transplantation requires much higher levels of induction immunosuppression. Most post-transplantation protocols steadily reduce the doses of immunosuppressive drugs during the first year post-transplant in an effort to minimize the likelihood of toxicity while at the same time providing the necessary immunosuppression. The ability to taper medication may vary substantially from one patient to another. As previously mentioned, an objective *in-vitro* method of determining the adequacy of immunosuppression is lacking. Consequently, we tend to over-immunosuppress patients during their first few months post-transplantation, necessitating close follow-up and often the use of prophylactic antibiotics and antiviral medications to limit infections in the recipient.

The development of immunosuppressive agents has undergone substantial evolution in the last several decades. Many new therapies are now available that specifically target immune activation events. However, despite the sophistication of newer interventions, we are still unable to induce antigen-specific immune quiescence, as opposed to global immunosuppression. In this regard, current immunosuppressive strategies do not differ from those used in the late 1950s and early 1960s, when thoracic duct drainage and total lymphoid radiation were used. As mentioned previously, one of the key axioms of immunosuppression is to balance the immunosuppressive effect against the immunodeficient complications and non-immune toxicities. The ratio between the immunosuppressive benefit and the complications and toxicity is the therapeutic index. This should be the goal of our therapeutic approach. For this reason, strategies have been developed using lower doses of more drugs to knock out immune activation pathways individually in order to provide better immunosuppression and yet avoid the toxicity associated with higher doses of the individual therapies. Drug combination therapy may thus provide equal levels of immunosuppression, but with substantially less non-immune toxicity.

In the next section we shall review the course of events following T-cell activation. Each step in this process provides an opportunity to intervene pharmacologically.

Pharmacological inhibition of the immune response

The immune response can be conceptualized as a series of interrelated events which occur over a period of minutes to days. The first event to initiate rejection is the presentation of alloantigen to the T-cell by the antigen-presenting cell. Engagement of the T-cell receptor/CD_3 complex with presented alloantigen leads to a complex series of immunologic events. Activation of tyrosine kinases subsequently occurs, which is followed by the synthesis of a variety of transcription factors for cytokine production. Once the cytokines are produced there are subsequent waves of cell division ending in clonal expansion of specific alloantigen-directed lymphocytes. During the ensuing days immune cytotoxic effector cells are produced together with a series of effector molecules, including granzymes, perforins, serine esterases and tumor necrosis factor.

Corticosteroids

Corticosteroids have been the mainstay of clinical immunosuppression for more than 30 years. There is still no general consensus with regard to their optimal therapeutic use, and protocols continue to change with regard to the amount and duration of their dosing, largely due to non-immune toxicities associated with high-dose or long-term use of these drugs. Corticosteroids provide broad non-specific immunosuppressant anti-inflammatory series effects. They exert their most important immunosuppressive effect by blocking the expression of several cytokine genes, the most important of which are interleukin-1 and 2, but also interleukin-3, interleukin-6, tumor necrosis factor α, and γ interferon. The blockade of interleukin-1 and interleukin-6 gene expression by the antigen-presenting cell is particularly important because these cytokines provide critical costimulation for interleukin-2 production by activated T-cells. Consequently, corticosteroids can block interleukin-2 production both directly and indirectly. The inhibition of interleukin-1 production is probably responsible for the abrogation of fever that is observed with these drugs.

Corticosteroids also cause lymphopenia due to redistribution of lymphocytes from the vascular compartment back to lymphoid tissue, and in addition they interfere with the migration of monocytes. The synthesis, release and action of a variety of chemotactants and permeability-increasing agents may also be inhibited by corticosteroids. In clinical immunosuppression, corticosteroids can be used in a variety of different ways. High-dose intravenous steroids can be used to initiate induction immunosuppression or to treat rejection. Oral steroids can be given in high doses as part of induction immunosuppression or as part of a steroid pulse for rejection followed by a slow taper to a chronic maintenance dose (either daily or every other day).

Complications associated with long-term corticosteroid use include cataracts, diabetes, hypertension, hyperlipidemia, obesity, striae, avascular necrosis of bone and poor wound healing (see Box 2.1). Short-term abnormalities are predominantly related to abnormalities of glycemic control or possibly even the development of depression or psychosis and dysregulation of the normal sleep–wake pattern. Abrupt discontinuation of corticosteroids may also result in adrenal insufficiency.

Prednisolone or its 11-ketone metabolite prednisone are the commonest oral preparations, whereas methylprednisolone is the most commonly used intravenous preparation. There are both branded and generic preparations available for clinical use. Comparative clinical trials have not been conducted to evaluate

Box 2.1 Corticosteroid toxicity

Acne (face, abdomen, back)
Avascular necrosis of bone (usually weight-bearing joints)
Cataracts
Glucose intolerance
Skin fragility and striae
Impaired wound healing
Gastritis, peptic ulcer disease
Hyperlipidemia
Central obesity, cushingoid facies, buffalo hump
Hypertension
Emotional lability, insomnia, psychosis
Colonic perforation
Growth retardation in children

comparative potency in branded and generic formulations. Corticosteroids are metabolized by hepatic microsomal enzyme systems. As such, drugs such as phenytoin, rifampin or barbiturates may lower plasma prednisolone levels, whereas oral contraceptives or ketoconazole may increase prednisolone levels. There is no available method of measuring plasma prednisolone levels for clinical use. Empirical adjustments are frequently made.

Azathioprine

Azathioprine is an imidazole derivative of 6-mercaptopurine. It has been used for more than 30 years in clinical transplantation. As will be discussed later, newer-generation antimetabolites will decrease the use of this drug in clinical practice. Azathioprine is a purine analog that is incorporated into cellular DNA, where it inhibits purine nucleotide synthesis. It also interferes with the synthesis and metabolism of RNA. This drug does not prevent gene activation but inhibits at a more distal step by inhibiting gene replication and consequent T-cell activation and clonal expansion. Azathioprine inhibits myelocyte maturation and decreases the numbers of circulating leukocytes and monocytes. There is a consequent reduction in the number of functional macrophages, which may help to interfere with antigen processing and presentation to T-cells. Thus these drugs are helpful in preventing the onset of acute rejection, as opposed to treating rejection once the immune response has occurred.

In clinical immunosuppression, azathioprine is used for maintenance immunosuppression to prevent rejection. The side-effects of

---

Box 2.2 Azathioprine toxicity

Leukopenia
Macrocytic anemia
Thrombocytopenia
Neoplasia (particularly cutaneous malignancy)
Hepatitis (non-cholestatic)
Pancreatitis
Nausea
Alopecia

---

azathioprine are most often hematologic (see Box 2.2). Bone-marrow suppression, including leukopenia, thrombocytopenia and anemia, can occur, and it responds quickly when the drug is reduced or stopped. Hepatitis, pancreatitis and cholestasis may occur with chronic azathioprine use.

The azathioprine dosage needs to be adjusted when allopurinol is given concomitantly, as allopurinol interferes with the metabolism of azathioprine. Azathioprine can be given either intravenously or orally. The IV dose is usually equivalent to half the oral dose. Blood levels are not valuable clinically, as the effectiveness of the drug is not dependent on blood level.

Cyclosporine

Cyclosporine is a cyclic polypeptide of fungal origin (*Tolypocladium inflatum Gams*). It is lipophilic. The immunosuppressive effect of this drug depends on its ability to bind to a cytoplasmic receptor protein called cyclophylin, which in turn binds to an intracellular protein known as calcineurin. Inhibition of calcineurin impairs the activation of several genes that are critical for interleukin expression, most importantly interleukin-2. Cyclosporine also upregulates the expression of transforming growth factor β, which also inhibits the production of interleukin-2 and the generation of cytotoxic T-lymphocytes. In addition, cyclosporine has other inhibitory properties. However, none of them are as important as its effects on dampening the production of interleukin-2.

Cyclosporine is commercially available in three forms, namely Sandimmune oral solution, Sandimmune gel capsules, and a newer micro-emulsion formulation in a capsule called Neoral. The latter formulation provides a much more bioavailable preparation than the absorption of the original Sandimmune liquid or gel capsule formulations (10–30%). Both branded and generic formulations of cyclosporine will be available for commercial use shortly. The gastrointestinal absorption of cyclosporine is incomplete and variable. The time to peak concentration is also variable. The improved gastrointestinal absorption of the micro-emulsion formulation and the reduced dependence on a functional enterohepatic circulation and bile for absorption makes this the preparation of choice for clinical immunosuppression. This newer micro-emulsion formulation also has substantial advantages over the older formulations in patients with impaired gastrointestinal absorption, such as those with uremia, diabetic gastroparesis, cholestasis, malabsorption or diarrhea. The dose required to achieve an equivalent trough level with the micro-emulsion formulation is approximately 10% less than with the older Sandimmune preparations. The soft gel capsule forms are available in 25 mg and 100 mg strengths. This drug is most commonly taken twice daily, preferably on an empty stomach.

Cyclosporine is also available in an intravenous formulation. Conversion between the oral and intravenous forms is an approximately 3:1 dose relationship. The intravenous preparation is most commonly used immediately post-transplant or during periods when the gastrointestinal tract is non-functional. This is optimally given as a constant IV infusion over 24 h. Cyclosporine dosing is best monitored by using trough levels. The relationship between levels, drug toxicity and episodes of rejection is inconsistent. However, more often than not drug levels are beneficial when monitoring clinical immunosuppression with this drug. More sophisticated monitoring techniques have been developed using a pharmacokinetic profile in order to calculate the area under the curve of the drug. However, these techniques are not popular due to their complexity and cost. The concentration of cyclosporine can be measured in the serum, plasma or whole blood. Whole-blood levels are used in most centers as there is no temperature dependence. Several different assays are used to measure cyclosporine, including the high-performance liquid chromatography (HPLC) assay, which specifically measures the unmetabolized parent compound. The INCSTAR technique employs a radioimmunoassay method to determine cyclosporine parent compound levels. The Abbott TDX fluorescence polarization assay is the most popular technique, as it is consistent and rapidly performed. The TDX assay can measure either the parent compound and metabolites, or the parent compound alone. Cyclosporine is primarily used as a maintenance immunosuppressant in order to prevent rejection. Occasionally it may be used as part of rescue immunosuppression therapy if a patient has not previously received the drug.

The major side-effects of cyclosporine are related to the kidney.

Box 2.3 Cyclosporine toxicity

Non-renal
Cholestatic hepatitis
Hypertrichosis
Gingival hyperplasia
Hyperlipidemia
Glucose intolerance
Hypertension
Tremor
Headache
Thrombo-embolic events
Lymphoma

Renal
Intrarenal vasoconstriction
Salt sensitivity of blood pressure
Reversible renal dysfunction from vasoconstriction of afferent
   glomerular arteriole
Irreversible renal dysfunction from fibrosis (chronic, more common) or
   arteriolopathy (acute, relatively uncommon)
Hemolytic uremic syndrome (relatively uncommon)
Hyperkalemia
Hypomagnesemia
Hyperuricemia

The drug can provoke acute and chronic nephrotoxicity
syndromes, as outlined in Box 2.3. The acute syndrome is related to
a functional decrease in renal blood flow and glomerular filtration
rate due to intrarenal vasoconstriction. This may be either related
to the drug itself or due to second mediators such as endothelin or
vasoconstrictor prostaglandins. The drug may also cause chronic
renal damage by provoking the development of interstitial fibrosis.
This may be related to chronic hypertension, chronic intrarenal
vasoconstriction or stimulation of transforming growth factor β,
which enhances the soluble mediators of fibrosis and overproduc-
tion of extracellular matrix within the kidney. Cyclosporine may
also induce a thrombotic microangiopathy which, although rare,
when it occurs is very damaging to the kidney.

Non-renal toxicity of cyclosporine can manifest itself as
cholestatic hepatitis, hypertrichosis, gingival hyperplasia, hyperlipidemia, glucose intolerance and mild neurotoxicity, manifested
primarily as tremor. Hyperuricemia, hypomagnesemia and hyperkalemia may also occur.

Cyclosporine concentrations may also be altered substantially
by different types of drug. Drugs that reduce cyclosporine concentrations by augmenting hepatic P450 activity include rifampin,

isoniazid, phenytoin, carbamazepine and barbiturates. Drugs that may increase cyclosporine levels by inhibition of P450 include verapamil, diltiazem, nicardipine, amlodipine, ketoconazole, fluconazole, itraconazole, erythromycin, clarithromycin and azithromycin.

Tacrolimus

Tacrolimus (Prograf) is a macrolide antibiotic compound, derived from a fungus (*Streptomyces tsukubaenis*), which shares many of the immunosuppressive and toxic properties of cyclosporine. It is highly lipophilic and has a large volume of distribution. Although structurally unrelated to cyclosporine, it primarily inhibits T-cell function by interfering with the release of interleukin-2. Like cyclosporine it also binds to a specific intracytoplasmic binding protein (the FK binding protein), which in turn binds to calcineurin and impairs its ability to stimulate gene activation for cytokine production.

Tacrolimus is commercially available in intravenous and oral formulations. The oral formulation has consistent gastrointestinal absorption and can be administered via a nasogastric tube. Consequently, the intravenous preparation is seldom needed. It is also much more nephrotoxic and needs to be started at a lower dose (0.05–0.1 mg/kg/day as a continuous infusion over 24 h). The recommended oral starting dose is 0.15–0.3 mg/kg/day administered in a divided dose every 12 h. It is metabolized primarily by the liver and excreted via the biliary system. Tacrolimus is mainly used to prevent rejection as part of a maintenance immunosuppressive regimen. It has also been used successfully to help to rescue patients with recurrent rejection who have not previously received the drug.

Primary toxicity of tacrolimus is related to the kidney (see Box 2.4). Like cyclosporine, it produces an acute functional deterioration in renal function that is largely due to intrarenal vasoconstriction. In addition, it can cause a chronic interstitial fibrosis which is irreversible. Despite the similarities to cyclosporine, tacrolimus causes substantially less systemic hypertension and hypercholesterolemia. It causes more glucose intolerance and neurotoxicity, primarily manifested by headaches and tremor, compared to cyclosporine. A hemolytic uremic syndrome manifested by microangiopathy is seen rarely, as with cyclosporine. Hyperkalemia and hypomagnesemia are not uncommon.

Drug interactions with tacrolimus are very similar to those described previously for cyclosporine.

Box 2.4 Tacrolimus toxicity

Non-renal
Headache
Tremor
Parasthesias
Glucose intolerance
Gastrointestinal (nausea, vomiting, diarrhea)
Major neurotoxicity (rare) (encephalopathy, coma, seizures, psychosis,
  autism)

Renal
Intrarenal vasoconstriction
Reversible renal dysfunction from vasoconstriction of afferent
  glomerular arteriole
Irreversible renal dysfunction from fibrosis (chronic, more common) or
  arteriolopathy (acute, relatively uncommon)
Hemolytic uremic syndrome
Hyperkalemia
Hypomagnesemia

Mycophenolate mofetil

Mycophenolate mofetil (Cellcept) is a reversible inhibitor of the enzyme inosine monophosphate dehydrogenase. This is a critical and rate-limiting enzyme in the *de-novo* synthesis of purines which is necessary for the formation of guanosine nucleotides from inosine. As lymphocytes rely on the *de-novo* purine synthesis pathway, rather than using salvage pathways like other cells, they are selectively sensitive to the effects of *de-novo* purine synthesis inhibition. The active component of mycophenolate mofetil is mycophenolic acid. It functions as an antimetabolite like azathioprine, and will probably replace this drug in clinical immunosuppression because it is more powerful and more selective for white cells, particularly lymphocytes. Mycophenolate blocks the proliferation of both T- and B-cells and cytotoxic T-cells. It also downregulates the expression of adhesion molecules on lymphocytes. In addition, it may inhibit the recruitment of mononuclear cells into rejection sites.

The primary purpose of mycophenolate, like that of azathioprine, is to prevent acute rejection. Two large studies, one conducted in the USA and the other in Europe, demonstrated that mycophenolate, whether dosed at 1 g or 1.5 g twice a day, reduced the incidence of acute rejection by about 50% compared to placebo or azathioprine in cyclosporine- and prednisone-treated recipients of cadaveric renal transplants. The drug has also been used with success to help rescue patients with recurrent rejection who have not previously received the drug.

After ingestion, the drug is rapidly absorbed and converted to mycophenolic acid. It has 90% bioavailability and a half-life of about 12 h. Its major limiting side-effects are diarrhea and abdominal cramps. Leukopenia and anemia are unusual but can occur. In contrast to cyclosporine and tacrolimus, nephrotoxicity, neurotoxicity and hepatotoxicity do not occur.

There do not appear to be any known drug interactions, although recent reports suggest that tacrolimus may increase drug levels. With more significant degrees of renal insufficiency the drug (mycophenolic acid) will accumulate and dosing may need to be adjusted, although there are no consistent data on how best to adjust for progressive renal dysfunction. Drug levels are not yet commercially available.

Sirolimus

Sirolimus (Rapamune) is a macrolide antibiotic whose structure is very similar to that of tacrolimus. The immunosuppressive activity is unique compared to the previously discussed drugs, although it does bind at the same cytoplasmic binding protein as tacrolimus (FK binding protein). It does not bind to calcineurin but targets a protein called RAFT and impairs the capacity of previously synthesized cytokines to activate T-cells to enter the cell division cycle.

Early clinical trials with sirolimus plus cyclosporine in renal transplant patients are under way. Preliminary results suggest that sirolimus and cyclosporine can reduce acute rejection in renal transplant recipients from 10% to 25%. However, there was an outbreak of *Pneumocystis carinii* pneumonia in some of the phase two studies, suggesting that this potent combination may produce excessive immunodeficiency.

The principal drug-related toxicity of sirolimus is hypertriglyceridemia and mild thrombocytopenia. There is no evidence of nephrotoxicity. The place of sirolimus in clinical immunosuppression will be further clarified when more clinical trials have been completed. This drug is now commercially available.

Polyclonal and monoclonal antibodies

Polyclonal antibodies have been used in clinical immunosuppression for more than two decades. The only commercially available agents at present are antithymocyte globulin (ATGAM) and thymoglobulin. However, many others have been used as part of research protocols, including Minnesota antilymphocyte globulin, which is no longer commercially available. They are primarily used for induction immunosuppression where greater immuno-suppression is needed, or to spare the use of cyclosporine or tacrolimus in kidneys with impaired function, or for the treatment of acute rejection.

The mode of action of polyclonal antibodies is related to the clearance of lymphocytes in the reticulo-endothelial system, or through lysis after the antibodies have bound to the T-cells. It is also possible that due to lymphocyte binding by the antibody the surface antigens are masked and may no longer be able to bind to donor antigens. In addition, there are theories that suppressor-cell production may be responsible for the prolonged immunosup-pressive effect of these drugs after administration. Polyclonal anti-bodies are usually given daily in an approximate dose of 10–20 mg/kg/day for 7 to 14 days when being used for induction or rejection. They are generally given in normal saline in a large volume, usually 500–1000 mL through a central vein.

Allergic reactions are the commonest problem. Patients frequently need to be premedicated with intravenous methylpred-nisolone, 50 mg of diphenhydramine hydrochloride and oral aceta-minophen (see Box 2.5). Side-effects include thrombocytopenia, chills, fever, arthralgias and myalgias (see Box 2.6). Rarely there can be anaphylaxis or a serum sickness syndrome.

The potency of each batch of polyclonal antibodies may vary. Side-effects may occur more commonly with some batches than with others. Similarly, under- or over-immunosuppression may also occur. Monitoring of total lymphocyte counts is necessary in order to identify the optimal therapeutic dose in patients. Adjusting the dose to keep the total CD_3+ lymphocyte count below 50 cells/mm^3 has been shown to be effective in our hands for ensuring adequate immunosuppression. The most common infectious complication related to polyclonal antibody administration is cytomegalovirus infection. Concomitant intravenous ganciclovir should be given during administration of polyclonal antibody preparations.

Monoclonal antibody preparations produced by the hybridiza-tion of murine antibody-secreting B-lymphocytes with myeloma cells permit the secretion of specific unique antibody in perpetuity. The OKT3 antibody is specifically directed against the CD_3–anti-gen complex found on all mature human T-cells. This is the only commercially available monoclonal antibody for therapeutic use. Like polyclonal antibodies, this agent can be used for induction immunosuppression or for the treatment of rejection.

OKT3 specifically reacts with the CD_3 complex on human T-cells. Once bound, the T-cell receptor undergoes endocytosis and disappears from the cell surface. Thus the T-cells become ineffec-

---

Box 2.5 ATGAM administration: patient preparation

Before administering first dose of ATGAM:
1. ensure that the patient is continuously monitored with a *pulse oximeter* for the first two doses;
2. ensure that the patient has no allergy to horse serum, or a history of anaphylaxis after administration of ATGAM;
3. if the test dose results in a significant wheal and flare reaction, discuss it with a staff physician before proceeding with the regular dose of ATGAM;
4. if there is no wheal and flare reaction, give the regular dose of ATGAM (usually 15 mg/kg);
5. the ATGAM dose is usually given over 4–6 h by a central line, but it can also be given by a peripheral line;
6. administer premedications 30 min prior to ATGAM:

Dose of ATGAM	Hydrocortisone	Benadryl	Tylenol
First	100 mg IV	50 mg IV/PO	650 mg PO/PR
Second/third	0	50 mg IV/PO	650 mg PO/PR
Subsequent	0	As required	As required

7. the dose of azathioprine and cyclosporine should be reduced by half during ATGAM administration. Normal doses should be resumed about 3 days prior to discontinuing ATGAM;
8. draw baseline T-cell counts: (a) CBC with differential blood count for calculating absolute lymphocyte count; (b) T-cell subsets, especially absolute CD3 count;
9. peripheral line – add 1000 U of heparin to each bottle of ATGAM. Use a central line with no heparin.

---

tual and unable to bind antigens. In addition, they may be opsonized and removed from the circulation into the reticuloendothelial system. This results in a significant depletion of CD_3-positive cells. Daily monitoring of CD_3 counts demonstrates the efficacy of the infused monoclonal antibody. The dose is adjusted from 2.5 to 10 mg/day in order to keep the CD_3+ lymphocyte count below 5% of the total lymphocyte count. The usual course of therapy is in the range 7–14 days. The standard dose for induction immunosuppression is 2.5–5 mg/day given as an IV bolus through a millipore filter after a test dose of 1 mg. Anti-rejection therapy requires doses of 5–10 mg/day. OKT3 administration can be performed through a peripheral IV line and does not require extra intravenous fluid.

The major toxicity associated with OKT3 administration is a potentially life-threatening adverse reaction, usually within the first 24–48 h, which is related to a cytokine release syndrome (see

Box 2.6 Antilymphocyte antibody toxicity

Polyclonal antibodies (ATGAM)
Chills, fever
Arthralgia
Serum sickness (rare)
Thrombocytopenia
Leukopenia
Hemolytic anemia
CMV infection, herpes simplex infection
Volume overload (associated with large fluid administration)
Pruritis

Monoclonal antibodies (OKT3)
Cytokine release syndrome
Chills, fever
Pulmonary edema, capillary leak syndrome
Hypotension
Acute renal dysfunction
Aseptic meningitis
Episcleritis
Diarrhea
Headache
Recurrent rejection
CMV infection, herpes simplex infection
EBV infection (post-transplant lymphoproliferative disorders)

Box 2.6). Fever, chills and a pulmonary capillary leak syndrome may occur. Patients may wheeze, become dyspneic, and even develop pulmonary edema and require intubation. Volume-overloaded patients should not be given OKT3. Acutely, renal function may deteriorate and a variety of neurologic complications may occur, including headache and even aseptic meningitis. It is mandatory to pre-treat patients receiving OKT3 with intravenous hydrocortisone (100 mg) and diphenhydramine hydrochloride (50 mg) and oral/per rectum indomethacin (50 mg) or tylenol (650 mg) for the first three doses. In addition, in renal transplant patients their weight should be reduced to within 3% of dry weight either by dialysis or by diuresis prior to starting treatment in order to avoid respiratory embarrassment (see Box 2.7). OKT3 administration reduces the threshold for developing a cytomegalovirus infection, and prophylaxis with intravenous ganciclovir is strongly recommended.

OKT3 monitoring is designed to assess the percentage of CD_3-positive cells in the circulation during the course of therapy. Initially there is a rapid fall within the first 24–48 h to less than 5%.

Box 2.7 OKT3 administration: patient preparation

Before administering first dose of OKT3:
1. ensure that current weight is less than 3% over the dry weight;
2. ensure that chest X-ray shows no evidence of fluid overload;
3. ensure that there is minimal or no peripheral edema;
4. ensure that the patient is continuously monitored with a *pulse oximeter* for the first three doses;
5. if the patient has a history of OKT3 administration, they may have antimurine antibodies, which could interfere with the action of OKT3. Patients with a history of OKT3 administration should be tested for these antibodies before being given OKT3;
6. Solu-Medrol 500 mg IV is given 2–6 h prior to the first dose of OKT3;
7. administer premedications 30 min prior to OKT3:

Dose of OKT3	Hydrocortisone	Benadryl	Tylenol	Indocin
First hour		50 mg IV	650 mg PO/PR	50 mg PO/PR every 8 h
Second hour	100 mg IV	50 mg IV	650 mg PO/PR	50 mg PO/PR every 8 h
Third hour	100 mg IV	50 mg IV	650 mg PO/PR	0
Fourth hour +	0	As required	As required	0

8. usual dose of OKT3 is 5 mg IV pushed over 1 min (do not drip in) via syringe filter;
9. the dose of azathioprine and cyclosporine should be reduced by half during OKT3 administration. Normal doses should be resumed about 3 days prior to discontinuing OKT3;
10. draw baseline T-cell counts: (a) CBC with differential blood count for calculating absolute lymphocyte count; (b) T-cell subsets, especially absolute CD3 count.

This reduction should be maintained throughout the course of the therapy. The failure of the CD_3-positive cells to disappear from the circulation may indicate the appearance of blocking antibodies. This is particularly important during retreatment when antimurine postantibodies have developed. If blocking antibodies are present, the dose of the OKT3 can be doubled to 10 mg four times a day. A low titer of antibody may be overcome by this treatment. However, it is critical to monitor the CD_3 percentage in order to determine the effectiveness of the drug.

Patients can receive repeat treatment with ATGAM or OKT3. Additional courses of therapy may lead to immunodeficient complications or even malignancy. Adverse events can be as serious as during initial treatment.

An explosion in monoclonal antibody technology has led to the development of newer biological agents which are currently being tested in controlled clinical trials.

Humanized monoclonal antibodies exploit the benefit of a rodent-derived antibody-binding site with a human antibody framework. Genetic engineering techniques have facilitated this technology such that rodent antigen-binding sites can be grafted on to human antibody structures. Two humanized anti-interleukin-2 receptor antibodies (antiCD25) have recently been approved and show great promise as induction agents. Another interesting strategy is the development of monoclonal antibodies which will block costimulatory pathways in lymphocyte activation, which will result in the development of tolerance. An example of this is the CTLA4Ig fusion protein.

A CD45 monoclonal antibody has been developed to bind against leukocyte common class 1 and class 2 antigens on dendritic cells or passenger leukocytes. Thus cadaveric kidneys can be treated with these monoclonals prior to transplantation to deplete them of their dendritic cells or leukocytes and remove their immunogenicity. Other monoclonals developed against adhesion molecules in order to diminish their immunogenicity, such as antiLFA 1 and antiICAM 1, may be helpful in preventing rejection. Monoclonal antibodies are also being developed and targeted against the a chain of the interleukin-2 receptor and other parts of the T-cell antigen–receptor complex. Immunotoxins are being attached to monoclonal antibodies to deliver poisons such as the diphtheria toxin to activated T-cells, specifically those which have expressed high-affinity interleukin-2 receptors. Hopefully, much of this technology will have the potential to induce tolerance as opposed to broad immunodepression.

Induction immunosuppression

Induction immunosuppressive strategies can be used in immunological high responders or as a means of minimizing the early nephrotoxicity caused by calcineurin inhibitors. The risk of acute rejection is maximal during the first few weeks to months post-transplant, and immunosuppression is usually at its highest level during this period, which may predispose to infection or non-immune toxicity. Delayed kidney graft function may complicate early transplant management, since there may be a need for dialysis, kidney biopsies, and lack of an adequate means to monitor graft function closely due to the lack of urine output or the measurement of serum creatinine levels.

Induction immunosuppression strategies have been designed to minimize the likelihood of delayed graft function by sparing the use of nephrotoxic drugs such as cyclosporine or tacrolimus until the graft is functioning adequately. Antilymphocyte therapies with either polyclonal or monoclonal antibodies or antiCD25 monoclonal antibody in conjunction with corticosteroids and mycophenolate mofetil are preferred until adequate graft function is evident. The antilymphocyte therapy should be monitored for effectiveness, as previously discussed, and it should not be discontinued until fully therapeutic levels of either cyclosporine or tacrolimus are achieved. The maximal duration of antilymphocyte induction therapy is 14 days, so cyclosporine or tacrolimus are usually started on day 12 or sooner in order to ensure that therapeutic levels of drug are evident by day 14.

Cyclosporine or tacrolimus are started immediately post-transplant in patients with adequate urine output and falling serum creatinine levels. Cyclosporine is administered at a dose of approximately 10 mL/kg/day orally as a twice daily dose aiming for 12-h trough levels of approximately 350–400 ng/mL using the TDX assay.

Azathioprine has been the traditional third drug added to cyclosporine- and prednisone-based immunosuppression. However, there is no clinical evidence that azathioprine provides additional immunosuppressive benefit when these two drugs are employed. The usual dose is 1–2 mg/kg/day, and it needs to be adjusted on the basis of the white blood cell count. The introduction of mycophenolate mofetil essentially replaced the use of azathioprine.

Maintenance immunosuppression

The basis of maintenance immunosuppression is to provide long-term immunoquiescence of the host vs. the transplanted allograft, yet not to interfere with normal host responses to infections or immunosurveillance against the malignant transformation of cells. In kidney and/or pancreas transplantation, a decision is made at the outset to use either cyclosporine- or tacrolimus-based immunosuppression in conjunction with long-term use of corticosteroids and mycophenolate mofetil. The decision as to which drug to use must be based on personal experience, patient tolerability of side-effects, and propensity for rejection. High immune responders, such as regrafts, usually receive tacrolimus, particularly if they rejected an earlier graft while receiving cyclosporine. The doses of all medications need to be adjusted carefully in order to avoid acute and chronic toxicity. For example, corticosteroids need to be carefully adjusted and decreased as necessary in order to avoid complications related to impaired glycemic control, obesity or complications related to wound healing or bone disease. Mycophenolate mofetil may need to be adjusted in order to avoid complications related to crampy abdominal pain, diarrhea or recurrent infectious disease syndromes, such as cytomegalovirus.

If the gastrointestinal tract is not functioning properly, cyclosporine may be administered intravenously at approximately one-third of the oral dose given as a constant infusion over 24 h. A reduction in the dose may be required in order to avoid progressive nephrotoxicity or other non-immune toxicity.

Tacrolimus, since it has much better oral bioavailability, can be used orally or via a nasogastric tube, even if there is some gastrointestinal tract dysfunction. The recommended starting dose is 0.15–0.3 mg/kg/day administered in a split dose every 12 h. Initial target levels post-transplantation should be in the range 15–20 ng/mL, as outlined in Table 2.1. The approximate therapeutic range for tacrolimus dosing also decreases over time, and tacrolimus levels also may need to be adjusted if there is progressive deterioration of renal function which cannot be ascribed to either technical problems or rejection.

On the first day of transplantation corticosteroids are started intravenously with methylprednisolone, usually 500 mg IV, followed by a tapering schedule as outlined in Table 2.2. The majority of patients are reduced to 0.3 mg/kg/day by day 15. At approximately 1 year post-transplant most patients are on 0.1 mg/kg/day or 0.2 mg/kg every other day. The rapidity of the taper partly depends on the stability of graft function and on non-immune toxicity of the steroids. For example, patients with steroid-induced diabetes may benefit from a more rapid reduction in corticosteroids, particularly if there is no evidence of rejection.

Adjustments in cyclosporine and tacrolimus are usually necessary in order to avoid acute and chronic nephrotoxicity. The therapeutic index of cyclosporine and tacrolimus declines substantially once the serum creatinine level is higher than 2.0–2.5 mg/dL, when

Table 2.1 Sample cyclosporine and tacrolimus levels for kidney transplantation

Time (months)	Cyclosporine (ng/mL)	Tacrolimus (ng/mL)
0–3	350 ± 25	18 ± 2
4–6	300 ± 25	16 ± 2
7–9	275 ± 25	14 ± 2
10–12	250 ± 25	12 ± 2
>12	200 ± 25	10 ± 2

Table 2.2 Sample corticosteroid dosing
for kidney transplantation

Day	Dose (mg/kg/day)
1, 2	2.0
3–5	1.5
6–8	1.0
9–11	0.75
12–14	0.5
≥15	0.3

the likelihood of non-immunologic processes such as intrarenal vasoconstriction, and stimulation of soluble mediators of fibrosis by these drugs, leads to progressive graft injury. This is a process that was once termed chronic rejection and is now more properly referred to as chronic allograft nephropathy, since it has both an immunologic and a non-immunologic basis. As outlined in Boxes 2.5 and 2.7, a progressive reduction in the doses of all of the drugs with the exception of mycophenolate mofetil occurs during the first year post-transplant. An additional reduction in drug dosing may occur after the first year. However, as yet there are no data on the optimal two-drug regimen to employ in the long term without increasing the risk of development of acute rejection or chronic rejection related to enhanced immunologic responsiveness. Steroid withdrawal may be appropriate in some patients, particularly if they develop insulin-dependent diabetes mellitus or avascular necrosis of bone. Similarly, either mycophenolate mofetil, cyclosporine or tacrolimus may be removed after 1 or 2 years of a stable post-transplant course due to problems with non-immune toxicity or recurrent infection. However, these adjustments should only be made on an as-needed basis, since no long-term safety has been demonstrated with these maneuvers.

Acute rejection

Most first rejections are treated with pulse methylprednisolone therapy, usually 500–1000 mg/day for 3 days, followed by an oral steroid taper (see Box 2.7). This treatment is sufficient to reverse in excess of 75% of first acute rejection episodes. Pulse steroid therapy is usually well tolerated. However, some patients may experience significant fluid retention or lose glycemic control, which may require more aggressive medical intervention. The taper schedule is based on weight, and is usually completed within 2 weeks after the rejection episode.

If a very severe rejection process occurs or there is recurrent rejection, then OKT3 is the preferred agent. Patients are always hospitalized and placed in a monitored setting in order to evaluate closely their response to the first-dose effect of OKT3. A dose of 5 mg every day is then administered for 10–14 days, with daily monitoring of the total CD_3 percentage to ensure that it remains below 5%. After the first three doses, patients can usually complete their course as outpatients unless there are problems related to fever or recurrent symptoms due to the medication, such as headache, myalgias, arthralgias, or chills. On completion of the OKT3 course, 250 mg of IV methylprednisolone are given in order to prophylax against the likelihood of spontaneous recurrent rejection, which can occur in a substantial proportion of OKT3-treated patients. OKT3 is an extremely effective anti-rejection therapy, and over 90% of rejections are reversed. However, there is also a much greater likelihood of immunodepression. Consequently, all patients should be prophylaxed with IV ganciclovir therapy during treatment.

Recurrent or refractory rejections may require repeat administration of OKT3. Prior to embarking on treatment it is imperative to ensure that OKT3 blocking antibodies have not developed due to the prior treatment (Transtat OKT3 assay). If so, OKT3 may still be effective if it is given at a higher dose (10 mg/day or higher). Polyclonal antilymphocyte therapy with ATGAM can also be substituted, or a repeat pulse with intravenous corticosteroids may be helpful. Switching patients either from cyclosporine to tacrolimus, or from tacrolimus to cyclosporine, may also help to prophylax against the development of recurrent rejection. In addition, if the patient is not already receiving mycophenolate mofetil, this should be substituted instead of azathioprine.

During antilymphocyte therapy treatment for acute rejection, it is wise to reduce the dose of cyclosporine or tacrolimus by approximately 50%. One might also decrease the dose of the mycophenolate mofetil or azathioprine in order to avoid over-immunosuppression.

Living related transplantation

The only major adjustments for living related transplants compared to cadaveric transplants are that cyclosporine or tacrolimus can be started 5–7 days before the transplant in order to provide fully therapeutic levels at the time of transplantation. A progressive reduction in the dosing of the steroids and cyclosporine or tacrolimus occurs during the first year in an identical manner to that with the cadaveric transplants. However, individualization for steeper reductions in immunosuppression may occur, particularly with HLA identical matched transplants, where smaller amounts of immunosuppression may be required in order to maintain immune quiescence.

Chronic allograft nephropathy

Chronic allograft nephropathy is another important clinical situation where revisions in the immunosuppressive regimen may be critical for protecting long-term allograft function. A slow, progressive increase in serum creatinine levels of 0.5 mg/dL or more over 6 months to 1 year could indicate smoldering acute rejection which would require anti-rejection treatment, structural abnormalities leading to hydronephrosis, or chronic fibrosis and vascular sclerosis. The latter problem may respond to an alteration in immunosuppression. Recent therapeutic efforts have focused on reducing cyclosporine and tacrolimus levels by 50% in patients with biopsy-proven chronic allograft nephropathy and deteriorating renal function. Patients can be successfully maintained on low-dose prednisone together with full-dose mycophenolate mofetil, without increasing the risk of acute rejection. The stabilization of renal function is related to a reduction in renal exposure to cyclosporine or tacrolimus. A high index of suspicion for this type of insidious deterioration of graft function is important in order to identify it early on and so prevent a progressive loss of allograft function.

Immunosuppressive strategies in kidney–pancreas or pancreas transplantation

Due to the greater frequency and intensity of rejection in patients receiving pancreas transplants alone or with a kidney, immunosuppressive strategies are designed to be more intensive with a greater overall immunosuppressive effect. The principles of induction and maintenance immunosuppression are similar to those for kidney transplantation alone. Post-transplant, all patients receive induction immunosuppression with OKT3 monoclonal antibody. This is continued for 10 days, prior to starting either cyclosporine or tacrolimus. Pancreas transplants alone receive tacrolimus, whereas simultaneous pancreas–kidney transplant patients receive either cyclosporine or tacrolimus as the foundation for their chronic immunosuppression. Mycophenolate mofetil, 1000 mg twice a day IV, followed by oral prednisone is administered in a similar manner to that described earlier for renal transplants.

During the first year post-transplant, cyclosporine and tacrolimus levels are identical to those used for kidney transplantation (see Boxes 2.6 and 2.7). Corticosteroids are tapered but rarely discontinued. Mycophenolate mofetil is routinely used as the third immunosuppressive agent.

Long-term immunosuppression beyond the first year post-transplant almost always involves the use of three drugs. Clinical trials are currently in progress to determine whether steroids can be safely removed, particularly in patients with a quiescent first year post-transplant.

Acute rejection almost always requires antilymphocyte therapy for resolution, unlike the majority of rejections in kidney transplant recipients. Recurrent rejection is also more common, frequently necessitating the use of ATGAM or recurrent use of OKT3.

Future considerations

The prospects for the future role of immunosuppression are bright, as newer technology and understanding of the immune system will enable the development of more sophisticated forms of immunosuppression specific to transplanted alloantigens or possibly xenoantigens. The goal is to reduce non-immune toxicity and global immunodepression in favor of selective immunosuppression or tolerance.

The development of in-vivo monitoring techniques for assessing the adequacy of immunosuppression is also a critical factor with regard to improving our existing techniques. This will allow transplant physicians a more objective means of determining the adequacy of medications that are currently being employed. Chronic immunosuppression, which is now customarily employing three agents, will need to be studied with two or fewer agents in order to determine whether satisfactory long-term immunoquiescence can be maintained with less risk. On the other hand, lower doses of two or more drugs may provide a better therapeutic index than higher doses of one or two agents being maintained over the long term.

Further reading

Abrarnowicz D, De Pauw L, Le Moine A et al. 1996: Prevention of OKT3 nephrotoxicity after kidney transplantation. *Kidney International* **49** (**Supplement 53**) S39–43. This is an interesting paper which describes approaches to minimizing the cytokine release syndrome, which can induce substantial morbidity after initiation of OKT3 therapy.

Allison AC, Eugui EM and **Sollinger HW.** 1993: Mycophenolate mofetil (RS-61443): mechanisms of action in effects in transplantation. *Transplantation Reviews* **7**, 129–39. This review is an in-depth discussion of purine metabolism in lymphocytes, and the importance of this new chemical compound in inhibiting the immune response through a specific block of the inosine monophosphate dehydrogenase enzyme.

Burke JF Jr, Pirsch JD, Ramos EL *et al.* 1994: Long-term efficacy and safety of cyclosporine in renaltransplant recipients. *New England Journal of Medicine* **331**, 358–63. This paper describes the long-term experience of cyclosporine therapy without evidence of progressive toxic nephropathy. These authors note that graft failure is most often due to rejection.

Campana C, Regazzi MB, Buggia I *et al.* 1996: Clinically significant drug interactions with cyclosporine. *Clinical Pharmacokinetics* **30**, 141–79. This is an excellent review outlining all of the various drug interactions that occur with cyclosporine in clinical practice.

Fryer JP, Granger DK, Leventhal JR *et al.* 1994: Steroid-related complications in the cyclosporine era. *Clinical Transplantation* **8**, 224–29. This review also outlines many of the problems related to long-term corticosteroid use in clinical transplantation. Despite cyclosporine and the use of lower doses of steroids, many complications still persist.

Halloran PF. 1997: Immunosuppressive agents in clinical trials in transplantation. *American Journal of Medical Sciences* **313**, 283–8. A recent overview of current approaches to immunosuppression, including some discussion of new modalities in clinical trials.

Helderman JH, Van Buren DH, Amend WJ Jr and **Pirsch JD.** 1994: Chronic immunosuppression of the renal transplant patient. *Journal of the American Society of Nephrology* **4** (**Supplement 8**), S2–9. This review outlines clinical approaches to transplant patients using predominantly prednisone- and cyclosporine-based immunosuppression.

Hricik DE, Almawi WY and **Strom TB.** 1994: Trends in the use of glucocorticoids in renal transplantation. *Transplantation* **57**, 979–89. This review outlines our progress in using lower doses of glucocorticoids in kidney transplantation in order to avoid both short- and long-term adverse effects.

Kahan BD, Dunn J, Fitts C *et al.* 1994: The Neoral formulation: improved correlation between cyclosporine trough levels and exposure in stable renal transplant recipients. *Transplantation Proceedings* **26**, 2940–43. This review describes the rationale behind the new micro-emulsification formulation of cyclosporine in clinical practice, which provides more reliable and stable drug levels.

Malinow L, Walker J, Klassen D *et al.* 1996: Antilymphocyte induction immunosuppression in the post-Minnesota antilymphocyte globulin era: incidence of renal dysfunction and delayed graft function. A single center experience. *Clinical Transplantation* **10**, 237–42. This review outlines the experience of a single transplant center in using polyclonal and monoclonal antilymphocyte induction therapy in kidney transplant patients. **Manez R, Jain A, Marino IR** and **Thomson AW.** 1995: Comparative evaluation of tacrolimus and cyclosporine as immunosuppressive agents. *Transplantation Reviews* **9**, 63. This review outlines some of the comparative clinical characteristics of cyclosporine and tacrolimus in clinical transplantation. It discusses clinical efficacy and toxicity in a variety of forms of solid organ transplantation, as well as pharmacokinetic properties and drug interactions.

Montagnino G, Tarantino A, Banfi G *et al.* 1994: A randomized trial comparing triple-drug and double-drug therapy in renal transplantation. *Transplantation* **58**, 149–54. This paper compares cyclosporine–prednisone therapy either alone or with azathioprine in kidney transplant recipients, and it demonstrates no substantial difference in overall outcome.

Morris RE. 1992: Rapamycins: antifungal, antitumor, antiproliferative and immunosuppressive macrolides. *Transplantation Reviews* **6**, 39–87. This extensive review outlines what is known about the various chemical and clinical properties of the rapamycin class of immunosuppressive macrolides. An extensive background is provided with regard to experimental and clinical trial data.

Paul LC, Zaltzman JS and **Cardella CJ.** 1995: Prophylactic antilymphocyte therapy in kidney transplantation: quo vadis? *Transplantation Reviews* **9**, 200–6. This review outlines our understanding of induction antilymphocyte antibody therapy in kidney transplantation. It also contrasts the use of polyclonal vs. monoclonal antibody preparations with clinical response and incidence of adverse events.

Schroeder TJ, Brunson ME, Pesce AJ *et al.* 1989: A comparison of the clinical utility of the radioimmunoassay, high-performance liquid chromatography and TDX cyclosporine assays in outpatient renal transplant recipients. *Transplantation* **47**, 262–66. This paper describes all of the known cyclosporine determination assays and outlines important issues related to reliability, reproducibility and rapidity of turnaround times with the various assays.

Sollinger HW for the US Renal Transplant Mycophenolate Mofetil Study Group. 1995: Mycophenolate mofetil for the prevention of acute rejection in primary cadaveric renal allograft recipients. *Transplantation* **60**, 225–32. This important study outlines the initial experience with mycophenolate mofetil for prophylaxis against the development of acute rejection in the first 6 months post-transplantation. It demonstrates a 50% reduction in the incidence of rejection compared to azathioprine together with cyclosporine- and prednisone-based immunosuppression.

Tornatore KM, Biocevich DM, Reed K *et al.* 1995: Methylprednisolone pharmacokinetics, cortisol response, and adverse effects in black and white renal transplant recipients. *Transplantation* **59**, 729–36. This review is an excellent discussion of corticosteroid pharmacokinetics, adrenal responses, and adverse events in renal transplant recipients.

Weir MR, Anderson L, Fink JK *et al.* 1997: A novel approach to the treatment of chronic allograft nephropathy. *Transplantation* **64**, 1706–10. This paper describes a new approach to altering immunosuppression in patients with biopsy-proven chronic allograft nephropathy and worsening renal function. Although only a 6-month follow-up is reported, its observations are encouraging, and they suggest that manipulation of immunosuppression may delay progressive renal dysfunction.

The role of histocompatibility in transplantation

3

Sandra Rosen-Bronson

Overview of histocompatibility antigens

Histocompatibility antigens

By definition, histocompatibility antigens are molecules that play a major role in determining whether transplanted tissue will be accepted as self (histocompatible) or rejected as foreign (histo-incompatible). Relevant histocompatibility antigens include red blood cell ABO antigens, minor histocompatibility antigens and, most importantly, major histocompatibility antigens.

ABO antigens are glycoproteins that are present on red cell membranes as well as endothelial cells and some types of epithelial cells. It is because of their expression on endothelial cells, and therefore their expression on the lining of blood vessels, that ABO antigens are prime targets for graft rejection in solid organ transplantation. Minor histocompatibility antigens are peptides that are generated during the normal catabolism of cellular proteins that demonstrate allelic variation from one individual to another. Polymorphic donor self-peptides act as minor histocompatibility antigens when they are bound to recipient human leukocyte antigen molecules and are recognized by recipient T-cell receptors. Although minor histocompatibility antigens play an important role in bone-marrow transplantation, their contribution in solid organ transplantation has not been clearly established. However, it is thought that minor histocompatibility antigens may play an important role in the development of chronic graft rejection.

Human leukocyte antigens (HLA)

In humans, the major histocompatibility antigens are referred to as human leukocyte antigens (HLA). HLA molecules are encoded by a cluster of genes located on chromosome six in a region called the major histocompatibility complex (MHC). Two classes of HLA molecules that are important in transplantation are encoded within the MHC, namely class I molecules (which include HLA-A, HLA-B and HLA-C molecules) and class II molecules (which include HLA-DR, HLA-DQ and HLA-DP molecules). Both types of HLA molecules are transmembrane glycoproteins that are expressed on the cell surface. HLA class I molecules are heterodimers consisting of a heavy chain encoded by polymorphic genes found within the MHC, and a non-polymorphic chain, β_2-microglobulin, that is encoded on chromosome 15. HLA class II molecules are heterodimers consisting of an α-chain and a β-chain, both of which are encoded by genes within the MHC on chromosome 6. Genes encoding the three different isotypes of HLA class II molecules (HLA-DR, HLA-DQ and HLA-DP) are found in subregions within the MHC. The genes for the class II chains are designated A and B for the respective α- and β-chains. The HLA-DR subregion contains a single α-chain gene (DRA) and, depending on which HLA haplotype is present, one or two expressed β-chain genes (DRB1 and DRB3, DRB4 or DRB5). Each of the β-chains is capable of forming a heterodimer with the DR α-chain to make a DR molecule. The HLA-DQ subregion contains a single expressed polymorphic α-chain gene, DQA1, and a single expressed polymorphic β-chain gene, DQB1. The HLA-DP subregion also contains a single expressed polymorphic α-chain gene, DPA1, and a single expressed polymorphic β-chain gene, DPB1.

The genes encoding the HLA molecules are highly polymorphic. Although the polymorphism of HLA alleles is complex, there is also extensive homology among all alleles and, in particular, among alleles of a single locus. Based on the extent of this homology, alleles of a given locus are divided into broad subgroups or antigen groups. The number of different alleles within an antigen group currently ranges from as few as one to more than 30. The nature of the allelic variation can be a single nucleotide difference or, more commonly, alleles appear to include a patchwork of short sequences which are mixed in different combinations in various alleles. The extensive sequence-sharing among different alleles and antigen groups is reflected in the specificity of antibodies formed against HLA antigens. That is, antibodies formed through sensitization to a single HLA antigen often react with multiple HLA antigens that share similar stretches of amino-acid sequence encoded by the shared nucleotide sequences.

HLA genes are inherited as a set on a chromosome, and therefore individuals inherit one set of HLA genes from each parent. Because of their close physical linkage on the chromosome, HLA genes are normally inherited in a block from the parents, unless a recombination event has occurred. The term *haplotype* (half of the genome typing) refers to the combination of linked genes transmitted on a single parental chromosome. Thus there are normally only four genotypes transmitted from parents to offspring, and the probability of siblings being HLA identical is 25%.

HLA genes are expressed co-dominantly – that is, each individual expresses both parentally transmitted HLA molecules. A typical HLA phenotype would include two types (different alleles) of each HLA encoded molecule, unless the individual is homozygous for one or more inherited HLA genes. The distribution and frequency of HLA genes and specific HLA haplotypes varies between different ethnic and racial groups. Some HLA genes are present in all populations, but are found in frequencies that vary from one population to another. Other HLA genes are restricted to specific populations, and certain haplotypes appear to be population restricted.

Sometimes combinations of genes occur within the population more frequently than would be expected on the basis of gene frequencies. This phenomenon is referred to as linkage disequilibrium, and it is quite common in the HLA system. For example, if the HLA-A1 and HLA-B8 genes were in equilibrium within the population, the expected occurrence of an HLA haplotype bearing both A1 and B8 would be 1.6%. However, in certain Caucasian populations the actual incidence of this haplotype is as high as 8%, which is far in excess of the expected frequency. Linkage disequilibrium is seen throughout an entire haplotype, and is especially prominent among the HLA class I molecules. Linkage disequilibrium is clinically important in donor selection for transplantation. Donors for patients with certain HLA phenotpes, such as A1, B8 or A3, B7, are more common because these antigens are in strong linkage disequilibrium in Caucasian populations. By contrast, donors for patients with HLA phenotypes that do not show linkage disequilibrium are proportionately more difficult to find.

Structure and antigenicity of HLA molecules

Structurally, the HLA class I and class II molecules are members of the immunoglobulin family, and HLA class I and class II molecules are structurally similar enough to be nearly superimposed. HLA class I antigens, HLA-A, HLA-B and HLA-C are constitutively expressed on all nucleated cells. The density of surface expression varies in different cells and tissues, but class I molecules are found in high concentrations on antigen-presenting cells and lymphocytes.

HLA class II antigens, HLA-DR, HLA-DQ and HLA-DP, are constitutively expressed only on B-lymphocytes, monocytes and macrophages. In addition, HLA-DR is expressed on activated T-lymphocytes, and class II molecules can be induced on various cells by cytokines such as the interferons produced during inflammation.

The minimum structural unit that can be recognized by a B- or T-cell is called an antigenic determinant or epitope. Individual epitopes may be as small as 6 to 10 amino acids, and HLA molecules, which are composed of more than 200 amino acids, contain multiple alloepitopes that are capable of inducing humoral or cellular responses following alloimmunization. Two types of HLA epitopes have been defined serologically, namely private epitopes, which occur only on a single gene product, and public epitopes, which are common to more than one gene product. Public epitopes can either be shared among a limited number of HLA molecules or can be widely distributed among HLA molecules. Antibodies to public epitopes have been used to categorize HLA gene products into major cross-reactive groups (CREGs). Some public epitopes appear to be highly immunogenic and are present at high frequency. Two examples of high-frequency public epitopes are the Bw4 and Bw6 epitopes present on all HLA-B molecules as well as a few HLA-A and HLA-C molecules. The Bw4 and Bw6 epitopes have been identified as two different amino-acid-sequence patterns in positions 79 to 83 of the $\alpha 1$ domain of HLA class I molecules. All HLA-B molecules have either the Bw4 or the Bw6 sequence pattern at these positions, and therefore all individuals type positive for either Bw4, Bw6, or both Bw4 and Bw6. In the transplant setting, the Bw4 and Bw6 public epitopes have significant clinical relevance in that patients who are homozygous for the Bw4 epitope frequently develop antibody directed at the Bw6 epitope, and conversely patients who are homozygous for the Bw6 epitope frequently develop antibody directed at the Bw4 epitope. This results in a single alloantibody directed against a single public epitope that has reactivity directed against as many as 80–90% of HLA molecules.

Histocompatibility nomenclature

HLA nomenclature has become more complicated during the last decade as DNA-based molecular HLA typing methods have become commonplace. In most cases the serologic HLA type is easily derived from the HLA genes. However, the serologic equivalents of all alleles are not yet known and the serologic specificity

Table 3.1 HLA nomenclature

HLA locus	Examples of serologic designation of HLA molecules	Examples of HLA DNA designations (low resolution or antigen level)	Examples of HLA DNA designations (high resolution or allele level)
A	A1, A2, etc.	A*01, A*02, etc.	A*0101, A*0201, A*0202, etc.
B	B7, B8, etc.	B*07, B*08, etc.	B*0702, B*0801, B*0802, etc.
C	Cw1, Cw2, etc.	Cw*01, Cw*02, etc.	Cw*0101, Cw*0201, etc.
DRB1	DR1, DR15(2), etc.	DRB1*01, DRB1*15, etc.	DRB1*0101, DRB1*0102, DRB1*1501, DRB1*1502, etc.
DRB3	DR52	DRB3*01, DRB3*02, etc.	DRB3*0101, DRB3*0102, DRB3*0201, DRB3*0202, etc.
DRB4	DR53	DRB4*01, DRB4*02, etc.	DRB4*0101, DRB4*0102, DRB4*0201, DRB4*0201, etc.
DRB5	DR51	DRB5*01, DRB5*02, etc.	DRB5*0101, DRB5*0102, DRB5*0201, DRB5*0202, etc.
DQB1	DQ2, DQ3, etc.	DQB1*02, DQB1*03, etc.	DQB1*0201, DQB1*0202, DQB1*0301, DQB1*0302, etc.

of some alleles is not necessarily that which would be predicted on the basis of the overall DNA sequence of the allele. For example, the molecule encoded by the HLA-B*4005 allele reacts serologically like HLA-B50, and the molecule encoded by the HLA-B*1522 allele reacts serologically like HLA-B35. Table 3.1 provides examples of serologic HLA specificities and the nomenclature for the corresponding HLA genes.

There are two basic ways of referring to the level or degree of HLA matching in transplantation. In solid organ transplantation, where it is only critical that the recipient shares the donor's antigens because the immune response involved in rejection is only in one direction (from recipient towards donor), the level of matching is typically referred to as the number of mismatches between the recipient and the donor. Table 3.2 shows an example of a 0 antigen mismatch. On the other hand, in bone-marrow transplantation where one is transplanting an intact immune system, and the immune response generated is recipient against donor and also donor against recipient, it is equally important that the donor shares all of the recipient HLA antigens. Thus in bone-marrow transplantation the degree or level of matching is referred to as the number of matches. For example, Table 3.2, shows an example of a 3/6 antigen match. The six antigens referred to in matching

Table 3.2 HLA matching nomenclature

	HLA type								
	A		**B**		**C**		**DR**		**DQ**
Recipient	1	2	7	8	1	7	2	3	1	2
Donor	1	1	8	8	2	4	3	3	2	2

Solid organ transplant = 0 mismatch
Bone-marrow transplant = 3/6 antigen match

nomenclature are the two antigens encoded by the HLA-A, HLA-B and HLA-DR loci.

Role of HLA in solid organ transplantation

Significance of HLA matching in solid organ transplantation

The benefits of donor–recipient HLA matching have been debated ever since the development of effective pharmacological immunosuppression. While it is true that the introduction of both cyclosporine as a maintenance immunosuppressive drug and anti-T-cell monoclonal antibodies (particularly OKT3) for the reversal of severe acute rejection episodes has improved overall 1-year graft survival, none the less the HLA effect is still apparent, and studies based on information from large databases continue consistently to demonstrate a linear relationship between long-term graft survival and decreasing degree of HLA mismatch or increasing degree of match. In 1997, the United Network for Organ Sharing (UNOS) reported the results of a multivariate analysis of the effect of HLA matching on cadaveric renal graft survival. The results of the analysis showed that whether donor/recipient match level was counted as the total number of mismatches (e.g. 5 mismatches) or as the number of mismatches at each locus (e.g. 1A, 1B, 2DR mismatches), HLA mismatch level was a good predictor of graft survival. The analysis indicated that different HLA risks affected graft survival in the short and long term. HLA-B locus mismatches and HLA-DR mismatches accounted for virtually all of the HLA effect seen in the first year post-transplant. Although the number of A locus mismatches did not predict graft survival during the first post-transplant year, in the long term such mismatches were more important for predicting graft survival than HLA-B or HLA-DR mismatches. Overall, the results of this study confirmed that in the recipient of cadaveric renal transplant there is a significant role of HLA matching in allograft loss, and that this effect is independent of other variables.

In recent years alternative strategies for identifying histocompatible organs for transplantation have been proposed based on the knowledge that each HLA molecule bears a number of alloantigenic epitopes. As discussed above, epitopes that are unique to a given HLA molecule are referred to as 'private determinants', while those that are shared among two or more different HLA molecules are referred to as 'public determinants'. A group of antigens that share one or more epitopes is said to be a cross-reactive group (CREG), defined empirically by antibody cross-reactivity. Since public epitopes are more common than private ones, matching CREGs rather than individual antigens might provide an opportunity for more patients to receive donor organs with some epitopes matched. The UNOS study described above also looked at the effect of CREG and amino-acid residue (epitope) matching on transplant outcome. The results of this study showed that matching HLA-A and HLA-B locus antigens according to CREGs or epitopes increased the number of zero-mismatched patients by 71–74%. In general, it was found that when recipients who are conventionally mismatched for A- or B-locus antigens are CREG/epitope matched, graft survival is almost always higher than for patients who are CREG mismatched.

The immune response involved in transplant rejection

The immune response involved in transplant rejection is referred to as an allospecific response and is triggered as a result of the recognition by recipient T-cells of non-self histocompatibility antigens. There are two types of alloimmune responses that are thought to play a significant role in transplant survival. Direct allospecific immune responses involve recognition of intact donor HLA molecules by recipient T-cell receptors. Indirect allospecific immune responses involve recipient T-cell recognition of peptides derived from donor HLA molecules bound to recipient HLA molecules. Although the direct alloimmune response is thought to play a primary role in acute transplant rejection, indirect allospecific interactions have been shown to play a significant role in chronic rejection.

Like all immune responses, allospecific immunity demonstrates both specificity and memory, and therefore patients who have been previously sensitized to HLA antigens are at greater risk of developing rapid and severe graft rejection. Sensitization to HLA antigens can occur through transfusion, pregnancy or a previous transplant. HLA antibody production by a sensitized patient can be restimulated through re-exposure to non-self HLA antigens, or by unrelated immune events such as a viral infection or an inflammatory process. Although uncommon, antibodies with specificity for HLA antigens have been reportedly generated through stimulation by certain bacterial antigens in the phenomenon referred to as molecular mimicry.

Transplant rejection is primarily caused by a cell-mediated immune response to HLA antigens expressed on graft cells or on donor antigen-presenting cells (passenger leukocytes) that migrate to regional lymph nodes. The process of graft rejection can be divided into a sensitization phase, in which antigen-reactive recipient lymphocytes proliferate in response to alloantigens on the graft, and an effector stage, in which immune destruction of the graft occurs. For initial sensitization to take place, CD4+ and CD8+ T-cells must proliferate as a result of the recognition of non-self HLA antigens. The response to major histocompatibility antigens involves recognition of both the HLA molecule and an associated peptide ligand in the cleft of the HLA molecule.

Activation of host T-helper cells requires interaction with an antigen-presenting cell (APC) expressing an appropriate peptide–HLA molecule complex together with a requisite co-stimulatory signal. Recognition of donor HLA antigens on the cells of the graft induces vigorous T-cell proliferation in the recipient. Both dendritic cells and vascular endothelial cells from the donor organ induce vigorous proliferation of recipient T-cells in this reaction. The major proliferating cell is the CD4+ T-cell, which recognizes HLA class II antigens directly, or HLA peptides presented by host APC. This amplified population of activated T-helper cells plays a central role in the induction of the various effector mechanisms involved in graft rejection.

A variety of effector mechanisms participate in allograft rejection. The most common of these are cell-mediated reactions involving delayed-type hypersensitivity and CTL-mediated cytotoxicity. In addition, complement–dependent antibody lysis and destruction by antibody-dependent cell-mediated cytotoxicity (ADCC) can occur. The hallmark of cell-mediated graft rejection is an influx of T-cells and macrophages into the graft. Histologically, the infiltration often resembles that seen during a delayed-type hypersensitive response in which cytokines produced by T-cells promote macrophage infiltration. Recognition of donor HLA class I antigens on the graft by recipient CD8+ cells can lead to CTL-mediated killing. In some cases graft rejection can also be mediated by CD4+ T-cells that function as HLA class II restricted cytotoxic cells.

In each of the effector mechanisms, cytokines secreted by T-helper cells play a central role. For example, IL2, INFγ, and TNFβ have each been shown to be important mediators of graft rejection.

IL2 promotes T-cell proliferation and is generally necessary for the generation of effector CTL. INFγ is central to the development of the delayed-type hypersensitivity response and promotion of the influx of macrophages into the graft with their subsequent activation into more destructive cells. TNFβ has been shown to have direct cytotoxic activity on cells of a graft. In addition, a number of cytokines promote graft rejection by inducing expression of HLA class I or class II molecules on graft cells.

HLA antibody and graft survival

Prior sensitization to HLA antigens and, in particular, the presence of circulating HLA antibodies in transplant patients represents a significant risk factor. The presence of HLA antibodies not only makes it more difficult to identify a compatible, cross-match-negative donor, but also studies have shown that in first cadaver-donor transplants, one-year survival rates are lower for sensitized patients than for unsensitized patients. Similarly, retransplants have also been found to have lower first-year survival for sensitized than for non-sensitized recipients. The percentage of panel-reactive antibody (PRA) is one of the main factors influencing first-year survival, and it has been documented that graft survival declines with increasing PRA level. An individual awaiting a renal allograft with a PRA of > 10% is at higher risk for rejection than a comparable recipient with a PRA < 10%.

The nature of HLA antibodies

The mixture of extensive polymorphism combined with the unique intermixing of shared nucleotide motifs present in HLA alleles is reflected in the HLA proteins expressed on cell surfaces as well as in the antibodies that are formed against them. When individuals are sensitized to HLA antigens through pregnancy, blood transfusion or transplantation, they are exposed to a large number of HLA epitopes. As each HLA molecule contains an average of 4–5 distinct epitopes, it is possible that an individual immunized by a single 6 antigen-mismatched donor could develop as many as 30 different HLA antibodies. In reality, however, this does not occur, and it is far more common for individuals to develop antibodies directed at different epitopes on one or two of the immunizing HLA molecules. The antibody can be directed against either private epitopes or, more often, against public epitopes shared among several different HLA molecules. Common public antibody specificities

Table 3.3 Common public antibody specificities

CREG designation pattern	Broadest antibody patterns	Common subset
1C	A1, 3, 11, 23, 24, 25, 26, 28, 29, 30, 31, 32, 33, 34	A1, 11, 25, 26; 1, 3, 11; 1, 3, 11, 23, 24; 11, 25, 26
2C	A2, 28, 23, 24, B57, 58	A2,28; 2, 28, 23, 24; A2, B57, 58
5C	B51, 52, 35, 53, 15, 57, 58, 18	B51, 52, 35, 53; B51, 52, 35, 53, 15; B51, 52, 35, 53, 15, 49; B51, 52, 35, 53, 57, 58
7C	B7, 42, 54, 55, 56, 27, 60, 61, 13, 41, 47, 48	B7, 42, 54, 55, 56, 27; 7, 42, 60, 61, 13, 41, 48; 7, 27, 13, 60, 61, 47
8C	B8, 64, 65, 38, 39, 18, 55	B8, 64, 65; 64, 65, 38, 39
12C	B44, 45, 49, 59, 13, 60, 61, 41, 48	B44, 45, 49, 50; 44, 45, 49, 50, 60, 61
4C	A23, 24, 25, 32 and all Bw4 positive HLA-B antigens	Bw4
6C	All Bw6 positive HLA B antigens and Cw 3, 7	Bw6

generated through sensitization to public epitopes shared within cross-reactive groups (CREGs) are listed in Table 3.3. In general, when patients make HLA antibodies, the initial antibody reactivity is weak and it appears to have a very narrow reactivity pattern. As the antibodies evolve, they become stronger and their reactivity pattern becomes broader.

Among the most immunogenic HLA epitopes are the Bw4 and Bw6 epitopes found in HLA-B locus antigens. Although most individuals express both Bw4 and Bw6 epitopes, individuals who are homozygous for Bw4 or Bw6 are highly likely to develop an antibody directed at the epitope (Bw4 or Bw6) that they lack. This is important in transplantation because an individual with a single antibody directed at the Bw4 epitope will react with approximately 80% of all potential donors tested. Likewise, an individual with a single antibody directed at the Bw6 epitope will react with approximately 85% of all potential donors tested.

IgM antibody

IgM antibodies directed to non-HLA antigens are common, react often with B-cells and less frequently with T-cells, and are harmless to the graft. Their clinical significance lies in the fact that they can cause a positive cross-match and inappropriately deny the patient a kidney transplant. Therefore histocompatibility laboratories must be able to distinguish between anti-donor IgM antibodies, which are almost always non-HLA and harmless, and IgG antibodies, which are almost always directed at HLA antigens and can be very harmful to the graft. The interpretation of the results has to take into account the infrequent possibility that the patient may have IgM anti-HLA antibodies. These antibodies can be detected shortly after transfusions or transplants. IgM anti-HLA antibodies are suspected of being harmful, but there is little evidence in the literature to that effect (probably due to the rarity of these situations).

Role of the histocompatibility laboratory in clinical management of the transplant patient

HLA typing methods

HLA typing is accomplished using either serologic typing methods or DNA-based methods. Although allele-level typing is critical for successful bone-marrow tranplantation, accurate serologic or antigen-level typing appears to be adequate for solid organ transplantation. However, DNA-based typing methods have been clearly shown to be more reliable and accurate than serologic typing methods for both HLA class I and class II antigens. For this reason, most HLA typing laboratories have either switched or are in the process of converting from serologic typing to DNA-based typing methods for HLA-A, HLA-B and HLA-C typing, as well as for HLA-DR and HLA-DQ typing.

Serologic methods

Serologic HLA typing is a standard microlymphocytotoxicity assay, and it is used to determine the HLA antigen profile on an individual's lymphocytes using a panel of well-characterized HLA antisera. The microlymphocytotoxicity assay is a two-stage, complement-dependent reaction in which lymphocytes are first incubated with antisera and then with fresh-frozen rabbit serum as a source of complement. The binding of antibody to specific HLA antigens on the lymphocyte surface activates complement, leading to membrane damage and eventually cell death. The membrane damage is visualized microscopically as uptake of a dye by the injured cells. When more than 50% of the cells in a test well have membrane damage, it is assumed that the cells express the HLA antigen targeted by the HLA antisera contained in the test well. Commercially available HLA class I typing trays contain panels of antisera for the identification of the HLA-A, HLA-B and HLA-C antigens. HLA class II typing trays contain panels of antisera with specificity for HLA-DR and HLA-DQ antigens. Typically HLA class I typing is carried out using unseparated lymphocytes or purified T-lymphocytes, and HLA class II typing is performed using purified B-lymphocytes.

DNA-based methods

There are currently three common variations of DNA-based HLA typing methods, namely sequence-specific oligonucleotide probe typing (SSOP), sequence-specific primer PCR amplification (SSP-PCR) and sequence-based typing (SBT). All three methodologies use genomic DNA as the starting material.

SSP-PCR

For SSP-PCR typing, PCR primer pairs are designed to anneal only to a specific allele or set of alleles. The HLA type of the target gene is determined by analyzing with which sequence-specific primer pairs amplification occurs. This technique is very rapid, since typing involves only SSP-PCR amplification of purified genomic DNA followed by visualization of the amplified products on an agarose gel stained with ethidium bromide. Typically a positive (amplification) control primer pair is included with each specific primer pair in order to monitor for amplification failures that can result in mistypings.

SSOP

This method of HLA DNA typing involves an initial PCR amplification of the gene of interest (e.g. HLA-A or HLA-B) using a locus-specific primer set designed to amplify the relevant polymorphic sequences of the gene of interest (e.g. exon 2 of HLA-A). The resulting amplified target DNA is subsequently spotted onto replica membranes. Each membrane is then probed using a different labeled antigen group or allele-specific oligonucleotide probe. Following hybridization of the specific probes, the HLA type is determined by analyzing the pattern of specific hybridization obtained with the panel of probes designed to detect different polymorphic sequences within the target gene. One variation of SSOP typing, often referred to as the reverse blot approach, involves linking a panel of specific probes to a membrane or to different wells of a microtiter plate. Thus for a reverse blot HLA DNA typing, the amplified target DNA from one person is tested with a single 'probe-strip' or microtiter tray.

SBT

Sequence-based typing involves the direct DNA sequencing of HLA genes. As in SSOP typing, SBT involves an initial PCR amplification of the gene of interest, followed by direct DNA sequencing using specific nested sequencing primer.

Detection and characterization of HLA antibodies

Donor-specific sensitization has long been a cause for concern in organ transplantation because of the potential for hyperacute rejection of renal allografts when donor-specific HLA antibodies are present in the transplant recipient's serum. The T-cell (or unseparated lymphocyte) cross-match has played an important role in renal transplantation. Nevertheless, several areas of controversy have emerged in recent years, including such considerations as what cell is relevant as the target (T-cells, B-cells, monocytes, endothelial cells), the sensitivity of the cross-match assay, the timing of the serum sample (historic vs. current), and which class of immunoglobulin predicts graft failure. One point that has become clear is that the antibody characteristic which most strongly correlates with adverse transplant outcome is specificity for HLA antigens. Studies in kidney, heart and liver transplantation have shown that the presence of antibody specific for donor HLA antigens is strongly correlated with early acute rejection and reduced graft survival, while graft survival and organ function are good when a positive cross-match is due to antibodies that are not HLA-specific. Thus the most important role of the histocompatibility laboratory in solid organ transplantation remains the detection, surveillance and characterization of HLA-specific antibodies in the transplant patient. Although the cross-match is the final diagnostic tool used to detect incompatibility, antibody screening is essential for prior characterization of the recipient sera and efficient recipient management.

Histocompatibility laboratories use an assay referred to as the panel-reactive antibody (PRA) test to monitor and characterize HLA antibodies. The name of the test is derived from the fact that the patient's serum is tested with a panel of HLA-typed cells. The percentage PRA reflects the number of different cells with which the cell reacts. Thus the percentage PRA is not a reflection of antibody titer, but rather it reflects the nature of the antibody specificity. Therefore, a patient with an antibody directed at a private epitope on a single HLA antigen could have a PRA of approximately 15%. On the other hand, a patient with an antibody directed at a public epitope such as Bw4 or Bw6 will have a PRA of > 80%. Both patients would be equally likely to experience hyperacute rejection if they were transplanted with an incompatible organ.

The selection of the PRA screening procedure and the frequency of the screening are decisions made by the histocompatibility laboratory based on the clinical needs and immunologic profile of the individual recipient. Highly sensitized individuals require more extensive and frequent screening than those who are not sensitized. Samples following potentially sensitizing events such as transfusion, pregnancy or graft rejection must also be screened. The window for detection of an anti-HLA antibody, when present, may be as short as 3–6 months.

The purpose of antibody screening is to determine the immune profile of the recipient in terms of previous HLA exposure. The goals of the PRA screen are (1) to ensure a true negative crossmatch with the intended donor by accounting for all relevant lymphocytotoxic antibodies, (2) to avoid false-positive crossmatches with intended donors by detection and characterization of irrelevant antibodies, (3) to predict the likelihood of finding a suitable cadaveric donor at random based on the level of sensitization and (4) to predict antigens to be avoided when donors are selected. Prior knowledge of which HLA antigens are unacceptable to a recipient allows for more efficient inclusion or exclusion of that recipient in final compatibility allocation of the donor organ.

The length of time for which an individual will be on the waiting-list can be predicted on the basis of the PRA level. Points used in the UNOS kidney allocation algorithm are also assigned based on the level or percentage PRA of the recipient. The level or percentage of reactivity with the random population as well as identification of the antigens for which an individual is presensitized enables efficient management of the recipient. By the periodic and routine screening of serum samples, alterations in an individual's immune profile can be noted and catalogued, providing further information that is useful in donor selection.

Methods for detection of HLA antibodies

The histocompatibility laboratory monitors for preformed HLA antibodies through periodic antibody screening assays referred to as panel-reactive antibody (PRA) assays, and by performing cross-matches between patients and prospective donors. HLA antibodies are detected by testing patient serum either with cells that express HLA antigens or with purified HLA antigens that are immobilized on a solid support such as a microtiter plate or microbead. When patient serum is tested directly with cells, purified lymphocytes obtained from peripheral blood, lymph nodes or spleen are typically used as the cell target. For complement-dependent lymphocytotoxicity assays, lymphocytes are often further purified into T-cell and B-cell subsets for cross-matches or antibody specificity testing.

The serum used for HLA antibody screening is typically a monthly sample sent to the laboratory for routine antibody monitoring. For final cross-matching prior to transplantation, the laboratory must use a serum sample that is less than 7 days old for patients with no history of prior sensitization, or a serum sample that is less than 48 h old for patients who are known to have been previously sensitized to HLA antigens. In addition, most histocompatibility laboratories include one or more historic samples together with the current serum sample.

Prior to 1980, a positive CDC cross-match with any past specimen was considered to be a contraindication for transplantation on the assumption that a prior response to donor antigens represented a risk for graft loss. Although a number of more recent reports have shown that good graft survival can be achieved under these circumstances, other studies report a higher probability of graft loss in these patients. The significance of a past positive, current negative cross-match may be related to the nature of the alloantigen exposures of individual patients. Patients who developed transient antibodies after blood transfusions may represent a group with a good prognosis, whereas previously transplanted or longstanding sensitized patients may represent a high-risk group. Some centers have established time limits (months or years before the date of cross-match) to determine when positive results with a past specimen can be disregarded, but there are few data to provide objective support for any particular cut-off time.

There are currently three general methods that are used for detection of HLA antibody. In order of increasing sensitivity these are complement-dependent lymphocytotoxicity (CDC), ELISA and flow cytometry assays. Although each method has advantages and disadvantages, the flow cytometric assays are rapidly emerging as the method of choice for HLA antibody detection, especially for patients with a history of prior sensitization to HLA antigens.

Complement-dependent lymphocytotoxicity assays (CDC)

The original CDC antibody screening and cross-match methods were essentially identical to that described above for serologic HLA typing by the microlymphocytotoxicity method. That is, the basic principle of the CDC assay is complement-mediated lympho- cyte membrane injury initiated by antibody bound to its specific antigen. For a CDC cross-match, donor lymphocytes are incubated with diluted and undiluted recipient serum prior to the addition of complement. The original or standard CDC assay has undergone various modifications to increase test sensitivity and specificity. Universally accepted modifications have included the addition of wash steps (Amos modified technique), prolonged incubation times, and the addition of antihuman globulin reagent (AHG).

Antihuman globulin-augmented cytotoxicity technique (AHG)

The antiglobulin variation of the basic microcytotoxicity tests is used for the detection of preformed HLA antibody using a PRA assay or a donor and recipient cross-match. Antihuman immunoglobulin is used in a manner similar to the Coombs reagent in red-cell serology. In this assay, diluted antiglobulin is added to the PRA or cross-match trays immediately before the addition of complement. It is thought that the binding of the antiglobulin to the antibody previously attached to the HLA anti- gens gives the complement a greater number of binding sites and can enhance the strength of reactions. This enhancement increases the sensitivity of the assay and therefore lowers the amount of anti- body necessary in a sample for cytotoxic detection.

PRA analysis by CDC

PRA screening using complement-dependent lymphocytotoxicity (CDC) assays is accomplished by reacting a given individual's sera with lymphocytes isolated from a selected panel of HLA-typed individuals. This cytotoxicity assay involves the activation of the complement cascade when antibodies in the serum react with their corresponding antigen on the surface of the lymphocytes. The end- point of the assay is a determination of cell viability. The size of the panel (the number of different cells tested) and the methods used to increase sensitivity vary from one laboratory to another. Panels may have cells from as few as 30 individuals, or they may represent more than 100 individuals. The construction of the panel reflects the need to detect antibodies to the highly polymorphic HLA system, as well as providing a statistically significant number of positive and negative cells to enable identification of the antibody specificity. The panel cells are typically either frozen or from freshly isolated lymphocytes. The standard complement-dependent cytotoxicity (CDC) method of PRA screening involves the incubation of the cells and sera for 30 min at room temperature prior to the addition of complement, and a subsequent 60-min incubation at room temperature. Modifications of this procedure include extension of the incubation times, incorporation of washes and also the addition of antihuman globulin. These variations are performed to enhance the sensitivity of the assay. HLA class I antibody is distinguished from class II antibody on the basis of differential reactivity with panels of isolated T-lymphocytes or panels of purified B-lymphocytes.

The CDC assay has been used for many years for the detection of HLA antibody. However, this test is limited by the requirement for viable lymphocytes, by the high variability of the test's complement component, and the inability to detect all HLA-specific antibodies (i.e. non-complement-fixing antibodies). Another disadvantage of CDC antibody analysis is that HLA antibodies are not the only antibodies detected in a CDC assay. Non-HLA autoantibodies can also be cytotoxic and are therefore detected in a complement-dependent lymphocytotoxic assay. These autoantibodies are not clinically relevant, as they do not impact on graft survival. In addition, CDC assays that are designed to be more sensitive to HLA antibodies are also often more sensitive to non-HLA autoantibodies. Fortunately, irrelevant autoantibodies are most often IgM class immunoglobulins, and their reactivity can be minimized by dithiothreitol (DTT) or by heat treatment of the serum prior to its use in a cross-match or PRA screen. HLA specificity can be confirmed by platelet absorption, inhibition by purified HLA antigens or inhibition by monoclonal antibodies. However, these techniques may be difficult to apply within the time constraints of a cross-match with a cadaver donor.

ELISA-based cross-match and PRA

Although it is not used extensively, SangStat Medical Corporation (Menlo Park, CA) markets an ELISA cross-match kit. This consists of a 96-well plate coated with the anti-HLA class I monoclonal antibody. For the cross-match, donor HLA antigens are isolated and prepared using manufacturer-provided reagents. Donor-soluble HLA antigens are subsequently captured on the cross-match plate by the monoclonal antibody during a 1-h incubation at room temperature. Unbound material is then removed by washing, and the plates are incubated for 1 h at room temperature with recipient serum. Subsequently, bound anti-HLA IgG is detected using peroxidase-conjugated antihuman IgG antibody. Each donor/recipient cross-match includes a test well that contains donor antigen and a corresponding well without donor antigen. The presence of specifically bound human IgG is determined by calculating the ratio of the absorbance obtained with donor HLA antigen divided by the absorbance obtained without donor HLA antigen. The ratio obtained from the donor/recipient cross-match wells is compared to a 'cut-off' value which is determined on the basis of the absorbance of positive and negative control wells. Ratios higher than the 'cut-off' value indicate the presence of specific anti-donor HLA class I IgG antibody in a patient specimen. Ratios lower than the 'cut-off' value indicate the absence of detectable antidonor HLA class I IgG antibody.

There are currently several commercial ELISA PRA assay kits available for the specific detection of HLA class I and HLA class II antibody. ELISA-based PRA analysis involves testing the patient's serum in microtiter plates that have been preloaded with soluble HLA antigens. The HLA antigens immobilized on the microtiter plates are affinity purified either from platelets or from EBV-transformed B-cell lines. ELISA PRA kits designed to determine the specificity of the HLA antibodies detected utilize microtiter plates in which each well contains purified HLA antigens from a single cell. HLA specificity is determined by analyzing the reactivity pattern of a given serum with the purified HLA antigens isolated from a panel of 30 cells. After the incubation with patient serum, the plates are washed with buffer, peroxidase-conjugated goat antihuman IgG is added to each well and the plates are incubated again. Following incubation with antihuman IgG, the plates are washed and a chromogenic substrate is added. After color development, the optical density of each well is measured using a standard ELISA plate reader. The results are determined by comparing the optical density obtained in test wells with the optical density from replicate positive and negative reference wells.

ELISA PRA assays have several advantages over CDC assays, including significant labor and cost savings. In addition, because the test utilizes immobilized purified HLA antigens, unlike a CDC assay, positive results will only be obtained when HLA-specific antibodies are present in the test serum. The method is also thought to be slightly more sensitive than AHG CDC testing, and it can clearly distinguish between IgG and IgM antibodies. When used in conjunction with other PRA test methods, ELISA PRA can also be very useful for determining HLA antibody specificity. At present the ELISA cross-match kit is not widely used by histocompatibility laboratories, and therefore sufficient data for reliability, sensitivity and specificity have not yet been accumulated. The fact that the kit is only designed to detect HLA class I antibody is also a significant disadvantage.

Flow cytometric cross-match and PRA assays

The flow cytometric cross-match (FCXM) was initially described in 1983. Since that time, a negative FCXM test has been shown to have important clinical relevance to kidney graft outcome as measured by improvement in early graft function and survival.

A flow cytometric cross-match, like a CDC cross-match, begins with the incubation of donor cells with patient serum. Subsequently, the method uses a combination of direct and indirect immunofluorescence to detect patient antibody binding and to distinguish between T-cell and B-cell binding. Patient antibody binding is detected indirectly using a secondary antibody such as an FITC-conjugated goat antihuman IgG. Simultaneously, T-cells and B-cells are distinguished by differential direct immunofluorescent staining with fluorescently labeled CD3 and CD19 or CD20, respectively. The flow cytometer – a microscope with a memory – provides an electronic histogram of increased fluorescence intensity on donor T-cells and B-cells in the presence of test serum that contains putative HLA antibodies compared with HLA antibody-negative control serum. Fluorescence intensity results that are logarithmically acquired are most often expressed as the difference in channel shift values found with a positive test serum vs. the value found with negative control serum. A positive T-cell FCXM is often reported to be a channel shift value of > 10 on a 256-channel log scale and $\geq$ 40 on a 1024-channel log scale. The precise cut-off value for determining a positive or negative cross-match is determined by the individual laboratory. In order to establish the cut-off value for a positive cross-match, approximately 20 cross-matches are carried out using normal human serum that is known not to contain antibody reactivity and representative cells, including peripheral blood lymphocytes and lymphocytes isolated from lymph nodes and spleen. The mean and standard deviation are calculated for the series of cross-matches and the cut-off point

selected for a positive cross-match is usually three standard devia-
tions higher than the mean channel shift of the 20 negative cross-
matches. Separate cut-off values are established for T-cells and for
B-cell cross-matches. In recent years the flow cytometric cross-
match has become much more standardized between different
laboratories. Intra-laboratory test reproducibility is satisfactory on
the basis of replicate testing in formal proficiency programs, and
false-positive results are rare.

Flow cytometry can unambiguously determine whether a positive T-cell cross-match is due to IgG antibodies, and it is also useful
for detecting IgG anti-B cell antibodies, although sometimes the
results can be inconclusive due to the higher IgG background of B-
cells. IgM antibodies directed to T-cells can also be detected by
flow cytometry if a FITC-conjugated goat antihuman IgM is substituted in the assay. However, the clinical usefulness of this test has
not been established, and IgM antibodies to B-cells cannot be
measured due to the cells' high level of surface IgM.

Early on, the flow cytometric cross-match was thought by some
to be too sensitive, and there was concern that flow cross-match
results would not be clinically relevant. However, the majority of
published international studies have found that a positive FCXM
(i.e. negative CDC) is associated with unfavorable kidney graft
outcome. Higher levels of early graft loss have been shown in
FCXM-positive regraft recipients, regraft recipients with identifi-
able HLA antibodies and primary kidney graft recipients,
compared with FCXM-negative patients. A positive FCXM has also
been shown to be associated with postoperative complications,
including primary non-function, increased rejection episodes, a
need for higher levels of immunosuppression, and longer hospitalization times. Although most positive FCXMs are T-cell positive
(CDC negative), there are some reports in which FCXM T-negative,
FCXM B-positive kidney graft recipients experienced poor graft
outcome.

Flow cytometric PRA analysis

There are currently two methods for detection of HLA antibodies
using flow cytometric techniques. A cellular flow PRA can be
performed using a panel of HLA types cells similar to the panels
used for the CDC PRA assay. This approach is useful because it can
allow definition of HLA antibody specificity. However, as in a CDC
PRA, it is not possible to distinguish definitively between HLA-
specific antibody and lymphocyte-specific autoantibody.

Recently, a flow cytometric method of simultaneously screening for both HLA class I and class II specific antibody using a panel of microbeads, called FlowPRA beads, has been described. For this assay a panel of microbeads is coated with either affinity-purified HLA class I or purified HLA class II antigens. A pool of 30 different class I and 30 different class II microbeads is used for screening for the presence of HLA antibody in a patient's serum sample. The percentage PRA in a given serum sample can be determined by measuring the percentage of microbeads that react positively to the serum. The assay involves incubation of patient serum with a mixture of non-fluorescent FlowPRA beads coated with HLA class I antigens and FlowPRA beads coated with HLA class II antigens. At the end of this incubation the beads are washed and subsequently incubated with FITC-conjugated goat antihuman IgG. Following this incubation, the beads are once again washed and a fixing solution is added prior to analysis on a flow cytometer. As in a flow cytometric cross-match, FITC-conjugated goat antihuman IgM can be substituted and HLA-specific IgM antibody detected. Recent improvements in the FlowPRA assay method have included the ability to determine the HLA antigen specificity of antibody contained in patient samples.

In addition to being faster and less expensive than most other assays, the advantages of this approach to HLA antibody analysis are that FlowPRA beads enable more precise conclusions, as they avoid the detection of autoantibody and they clearly distinguish between the presence of HLA class I (T-cell) antibody and HLA class II (B-cell) antibody. Previously, class II antibodies were often defined indirectly by B-cell-positive and T-cell-negative reactions. Therefore class II antibodies could not be clearly defined if the serum contained both class I and class II antibody. In addition to detecting only HLA-specific antibody, like the flow cytometric cross-match, the FlowPRA bead assay is more sensitive than the AHG-CDC and ELISA methods. When used in conjunction with a flow cytometric cross-match, the FlowPRA bead assay is extremely useful for predicting a negative cross-match as well as for confirming the validity and clinical significance of a positive cross-match by facilitating the distinction between a positive flow cross-match caused by the presence of HLA-specific antibody and a positive flow cross-match caused by irrelevant IgG autoantibody.

Management of the highly sensitized patient and identification of highly responsive patients

Among the most difficult patients to transplant successfully are those who have been previously sensitized to HLA antigens and who have antibodies that are reactive with a large percentage of all HLA antigens (i.e. have a high PRA). The identification of a compatible transplant donor for such highly sensitized patients can be very difficult. In some cases, compatible donors can be successfully identified using a computerized matching algorithm which not only takes into account the patient's and donor's HLA types, but also enables the development of an efficient strategy for donor selection based on the computer assignment of acceptable HLA-A and HLA-B mismatches for each patient. The computer program is based on a standard 2×2 table analysis of correlations between serum reactivity with an HLA-typed cell panel, but in addition it incorporates the concept of public HLA determinants based on the serologic cross-reactivity among class I antigens.

Alternative strategies for successfully transplanting the highly sensitized patient include attempts to lower the HLA-specific antibody levels in the patient serum temporarily or even permanently. Sequential plasma pheresis to reduce patient antibody titers temporarily is sometimes used to create a window of opportunity for transplantation in highly sensitized patients. In such cases, a critical role of the histocompatibility laboratory is to monitor carefully further reductions in HLA antibody titers and to evaluate the efficacy and the end-point of this therapeutic approach. It has been reported that a more permanent reduction in antibody titer can be achieved in some highly sensitized patients after a course of treatment using intravenous gammaglobulin (IVIG). In the laboratory, IVIG has been shown to be useful for reducing panel-reactive antibodies *in vitro*, thus facilitating the identification of the HLA specificity of the antibodies. It also has been reported that, for individual patients, successful *in-vitro* antibody reduction by IVIG treatment of patient serum is predictive of a favorable outcome *in vivo* if the patient is treated with a course of IVIG pre-transplant and, if necessary, at the time of antibody resurgence. Although the precise mechanisms are unclear, it has been suggested that the IgG fraction of IVIG induces IgM anti-idiotypic blocking antibody in high-PRA patients. IVIG treatment may therefore have the potential to be able to induce blocking antibodies in some patients 'at will', rather than waiting for their serendipitous appearance.

Further reading

Bjorkman PJ, Saper MA, Samraoui B, Bennett WS, Strominger JL and Wiley DC. 1987: The foreign antigen binding site and T-cell recognition regions of class I histocompatibility antigens. *Nature* **329**, 512–18.

Brown JH, Jardetzky TS, Gorga JC *et al.* 1993: Three-dimensional structure of the human class II histocompatibility antigen HLA-DR1. *Nature* **364**, 33–9.

Chapman JR, Taylor CJ, Ting A and Morris PJ. 1986: Immunoglobulin class and specificity of antibodies causing positive T-cell crossmatches: relationship to renal transplant outcome. *Transplantation* **42**, 608–13.

Garovoy MR, Rheinschmidt MA and Bigos M. 1983: Flow cytometry analysis: a high-technology crossmatch technique facilitating transplantation. *Transplantation Proceedings* **15**, 1939.

Halloran PF, Wadgymar A, Ritchie S, Falk J, Solez K and Srinivasa NS. 1990: The significance of the anti-class I antibody response. I. Clinical and pathologic features of anti-class I-mediated rejection. *Transplantation* **49**, 85–91.

Olerup O and Zetterquist H. 1992: HLA-DR typing by PCR amplification with sequence-specific primers (PCR-SSP) in 2 hours. *Tissue Antigens* **39**, 225–35.

Talbot D, Givan AL and Shenton BK. 1990: The prospective value of the preoperative flow cytometric crossmatch assay in renal transplantation. *Transplantation* **49**, 809–10.

4 Kidney transplantation

James B. Whiting and David K. Klassen

Introduction

Animal experiments in organ transplantation began in the early 1900s with Alexis Carrel's pioneering research on vascular surgery and transplantation. Carrel began his work in France, where he developed modern techniques of vascular suturing from which he was able to embark on a series of experiments in transplantation. He demonstrated that transplanted organs could function in recipient animals for varying periods of time. The difference in survival between autografts and allografts was recognized, but the nature of graft rejection was not. Carrel left France in 1904, continued his work at the University of Chicago and the Rockefeller Institute in New York, and received the Nobel Prize in 1912. Experiments in organ transplantation continued throughout the early 1900s, including a series of unsuccessful human cadaveric transplants attempted by Hugh Voranoy in the Soviet Union in 1933.

Beginning in the 1940s, Peter Medawar, working in London, conducted a series of experiments that proved to have made a major contribution to the understanding of transplantation. These experiments included a series of skin grafts in rabbits that demonstrated the immunological basis of graft rejection. He went on to show that this immunologic process could be overcome if allograft cells were introduced to the host during fetal or neonatal development. Medawar received the Nobel Prize in 1960 for this work.

Successful clinical kidney transplantation was achieved in 1954 when Joseph Murray, working at the Peter Bent Brigman Hospital in Boston, performed the first successful identical-twin transplant. This had been preceded by a series of cadaveric transplants performed by David Hume at the same hospital. Some of these cadaveric transplants in non-immunosuppressed recipients were able to function for a significant period of time. The Nobel Prize was awarded to Murray in 1990 for his pioneering efforts. Cadaveric transplantation was made feasible by the introduction of non-lethal pharmacologic immunosuppression, which was first demonstrated in 1959 by Schwartz and Damashek using 6-mercaptopurine, and then in 1961 by Roy Calne using azathioprine, a 6-mercaptopurine analog.

The next major milestone in transplantation in the USA was political rather than medical. The Medicare End-Stage Renal Disease Program, passed by Congress in 1973, provided financial support for dialysis and transplantation, and extended therapy for end-stage renal disease (ESRD) to many patients. The development of cyclosporine in the late 1970s and its clinical introduction in 1983 resulted in a marked improvement in the survival of allografts. This also allowed the expansion of non-renal transplantation such as liver or heart transplants to larger numbers of patients. Since that time, kidney transplant results have continued to improve. The projected half-life for living donor transplants performed between 1995 and 1996 is 16.7 years. The projected half-life for cadaveric transplants performed during the same period is 10.4 years. One-year graft survival rates for living donor kidneys have reached approximately 92%, and the rate for cadaveric kidneys is 84%, based on national data.

In 1999, there were over 20 000 solid organ transplants performed in the USA. Of these, over 12 000 were kidney transplants. Approximately two-thirds of these kidney transplants were from cadaveric donors. With the expansion of organ donation to living non-related donors and the demonstration of their superior outcomes compared to cadaveric transplantation, living donor transplantation is increasing significantly. This situation has been further increased by the recent development of laparoscopic donor nephrectomy, a development that was stimulated by the severe shortage of cadaveric organs for donation. At the end of 1997 there were over 36 000 patients awaiting kidney transplantation. However, the number of cadaveric organ donors has failed to keep pace with growing transplant waiting-lists. In 1999, the time period for which the most recent data are available, there were slightly more than 5000 cadaveric donors available for kidney transplantation in the USA.

Recipient evaluation

One of the most difficult issues for a patient with chronic renal insufficiency who is facing the prospect of transplantation is appropriate timing of the transplant procedure. Most nephrologists and transplant surgeons agree that pre-emptive transplantation – that is, before initiation of chronic dialysis – offers patients the best prospect of maintaining good health and quality of life. Pre-emptive transplantation with a living donor transplant is seldom a problem. Evaluation of both the donor and the recipient can be done relatively rapidly, and the elective nature of the procedure allows it to be scheduled to the best advantage of both the recipient and the donor. However, pre-emptive transplantation in the setting of cadaveric kidney donation is becoming increasingly difficult. In this setting, it is essential to know the average waiting times on the cadaveric transplant list within the Organ Procurement Organization serving the transplant center where the procedure is to be performed. Local waiting times can vary widely across the country, and are significantly influenced by the recipient's ABO blood group status, as well as the percentage panel-reactive antibody (PRA). The increasing numbers of patients who are waiting for cadaveric transplants, coupled with the relatively slow growth in the availability of suitable cadaveric transplant donors, has resulted in progressively longer waiting periods. On a national basis, the median waiting time to kidney transplantation has more than doubled between 1990 and 1997. Patients entering the transplant waiting-list in 1997 have had a median waiting time of 3.0 years to cadaveric kidney transplantation. Given the variability in the rates of progression of kidney disease, it has become extremely difficult to match predictably a patient's need for cadaveric transplantation with the availability of an organ prior to the initiation of chronic dialysis. The intense demand for transplantable organs and the issue of equal access to this limited resource by all patients has resulted in pressure for the creation of standard kidney transplant recipient listing criteria. As a result, the United Network for Organ Sharing has developed mandatory guidelines for the accumulation of waiting time on the kidney transplant list. These guidelines, which were developed in 1997, allow a patient to be placed on the list at any time at the discretion of the transplant surgeon and nephrologist. However, the accumulation of waiting time does not begin until the patient's measured glomerular filtration rate reaches 20 mL/min or less. This allows a patient with relatively higher glomerular filtration rates to be transplanted if a zero (0) antigen-mismatched kidney becomes available. Currently, zero antigen-mismatched cadaveric transplants account for approximately 15% of all cadaveric transplants performed in the USA.

Early in the evaluation process for kidney transplantation, it is important to assess the possibilities for living donor transplants. Most transplant programs agree that living donor transplantation is advantageous because it avoids the logistical problems associated with waiting on the cadaveric transplant list, and it has clearly documented superiority over cadaveric transplants in both short- and long-term graft survival. Live donors have traditionally been first-degree relatives of the recipient who, in addition to being ABO-compatible, have good tissue matches with the recipient. At this time there is strong evidence to support the use of organs from donors who are less well matched or who are not biologically related but rather emotionally committed, (e.g. a spouse or close companion). Kidney transplants from living non-related donors have a significantly better long-term graft survival than do cadaveric kidney transplants.

The medical evaluation of transplant candidates should focus on those factors which will maximize safety and outcome for the recipient and ensure the best possible utilization of the donor organ. Although the evaluation must be individualized for each patient, a number of factors are common to the assessment of all candidates. Contraindications to transplantation include active or recent malignancy, active infection, severe uncorrectable non-renal diseases, and psychiatric disease or substance abuse that may adversely affect patient compliance and outcome (see Box 4.1).

Immunosuppressive therapy may promote the growth of some forms of malignancy, and it is important to assess the likelihood of recurrence of malignancy after the transplant. The Cincinnati Transplant Tumor Registry, an international registry for malignancies in solid organ transplant recipients, has data on thousands of patients which allows the assessment of the risk of tumor recurrence in a variety of clinical situations (see Table 4.1). There are a number of malignancies in which little or no waiting time is required to ensure a low risk of recurrence following transplantation. After local therapy, patients with *in-situ* bladder carcinoma have a very low risk of recurrence and do not require a waiting period. Similarly, the Registry data show that the vast majority of patients with *in-situ* cervical cancers do not develop recurrence after appropriate therapy, and thus require no waiting time prior to transplantation. Patients with the *in-situ* lobular breast carcinoma have a relatively favorable prognosis and do not warrant prolonged waiting prior to transplantation. The good prognosis of patients with Duke's A colon cancer suggests that no waiting time

---

Box 4.1 Absolute contraindications to transplantation

Active or recent malignancy
Active infection
Severe uncorrectable non-renal disease
Active substance abuse

Table 4.1 Recommended tumor-free waiting periods prior to transplantation

Malignancy	Time
Basal cell	None
In-situ bladder	None
In-situ cervical	None
Incidental renal cell	None
Clark's level 1 melanoma	None
Duke's A colon	None
In-situ lobular breast	None
Uterine	2 years
Prostate	2 years
Lymphoma	2 years
Squamous-cell skin	2 years
Breast	2–5 years
Melanoma	2–5 years
Invasive cervical	2–5 years
Colorectal	2–5 years

is required. Basal-cell skin carcinomas and Clark's level I melanomas also have a good prognosis, and patients with these conditions can be transplanted with little or no waiting time. Similarly, the incidental finding of a small renal-cell carcinoma does not impact on the post-transplant course, and these patients can also be transplanted early.

Other cancers require a longer period prior to transplantation. Patients with more advanced stages of breast cancer have a relatively low rate of recurrence if the transplant is delayed for at least 2 years and possibly 5 years following the therapy for these malignancies. A similar waiting time is recommended for colorectal cancers and more advanced stages of melanoma.

Cardiovascular disease remains one of the leading causes of death in both dialysis and transplant patients. Knowledge of a patient's cardiovascular disease status and risks prior to transplantation can minimize surgical risk. The recipient's evaluation should focus on identifying known risks for coronary artery disease, including diabetes mellitus, hypertension, smoking, hyperlipidemia, a family history of premature coronary artery disease, and age greater than 45 years in men and greater than 55 years in women. It is clear that these risk factors are more common in the dialysis population than in the general population. Risk factors for perioperative morbidity and mortality include a myocardial infarction in the 6 months preceding surgery, unstable angina, congestive heart failure, ventricular arrhythmias, and EKG abnormalities such as ST-segment changes or left bundle branch block. The history and physical examination of the patient should focus on finding signs and symptoms suggestive of diffuse vascular disease, including careful examination of peripheral pulses, auscultation for bruits, or evidence of claudication. The role of stress testing and angiography in transplant recipients prior to surgery remains controversial and must be individualized. Diabetic patients are a subgroup at particular risk. Studies have shown that one-quarter to one-third of asymptomatic diabetic patients who present for possible kidney transplantation will have significant coronary artery lesions. All patients require a preoperative EKG, and diabetic patients should also have an exercise stress test or thallium scintigraphy or dobutamine cardiac echo. Patients who are found to have significant abnormalities are referred for cardiac catheterization. Those patients who have documented coronary artery disease or severe peripheral vascular disease are referred for possible surgical correction prior to transplantation.

Active bacterial infection is generally a contraindication to renal transplantation. The history and physical examination should concentrate on areas of occult infection that may be overlooked if they are not actively sought, including infections related to dental caries. Other sources of occult infections include dialysis access grafts and peritoneal dialysis catheters. Patients should have a urine culture if they still produce significant amounts of urine. Patients with a history of recurrent urinary tract infections should be evaluated for possible structural abnormalities in the urinary collecting system. This may require renal ultrasound, intravenous pyelography or cystoscopy. Urologic consultation is often of benefit in these situations. Serologic studies to search for evidence of previous infections with viral pathogens that are known to be important in the post-transplant period are sent. Both IgG and IgM titers for a cytomegalovirus (CMV), Epstein–Barr virus (EBV) and herpes simplex type I and type II should be sent. Screening is also undertaken for human immunodeficiency virus (HIV) and human T-lymphocyte virus I (HTLV I), as is screening for varicella and rubella. Patients who test positive for HIV are not considered further for transplantation.

The issue of hepatitis B and hepatitis C remains controversial. Hepatic cirrhosis is a contraindication to kidney transplantation, although those with both ESRD and advanced liver disease may be candidates for combined kidney/liver transplantation. Patients with chronic hepatitis B have been reported in some studies to have a high incidence of post-transplant cirrhosis and hepatic failure, although other studies have shown a relatively benign course. Renal transplantation is not contraindicated for hepatitis B surface-antigen-positive patients, although they should be screened for serologic evidence of active viral replication with hepatitis B e antigen or hepatitis B DNA. These patients are at high risk for disease progression after transplantation. In addition, patients with elevated liver enzymes should have a liver biopsy to assess hepatic histology. Patients with hepatitis C are also at increased risk for progression of liver disease after transplantation, but the findings of outcome studies are not conclusive. Patients with hepatitis C and elevated liver enzymes should undergo liver biopsy.

In cases where the cause of end-stage renal disease is known to be primary (see Table 4.2), the nature of the glomerulopathy may have an impact on the post-transplant outcome. For example, focal segmental glomerular sclerosis has a recurrence rate of 20–30%. Patients at highest risk are younger individuals who originally presented with aggressive disease, or who developed rapid recurrence following a previous transplant. In this setting, graft loss may occur in up to 30–40% of cases. Membranous nephropathy has a recurrence rate that is relatively low (3–7%). It typically presents with nephrotic syndrome 6 months to 2 years after transplant,

Table 4.2 Primary renal disease recurrence after transplantation

	Recurrence rate (%)	Graft loss with recurrence (%)	Comments
Membranous transplants Nephropathy	3–20	Minimal	HLA identical May have increased risk
IgA nephropathy living	40–60	< 10	More common in related transplants
Focal segmental glomerulosclerosis disease	20–30	30–40	Younger patients with previously aggressive disease are at high risk
Type I membranoproliferative glomerulopathy Glomerulonephritis	20–30	30–40	Difficult to distinguish transplant
Type II membranoproliferative glomerulosclerosis	80–90	10–20	May have long course Graft failure
Anti-GBM disease	5–10	Unusual	Delay transplant for 6 months after documentation of negative antibody titers

Table 4.3 Secondary renal disease recurrence after transplantation

	Recurrence rate (%)	Graft loss with recurrence (%)	Comments
Lupus nephritis	Rare	0	
Wegener's granulomatosis	Low	0–40	Can be treated with cyclophosphamide
Hemolytic–uremic syndrome	10–25	10–40	Avoid LRD in familial hemolytic–uremic syndome
Diabetic nephropathy	100	5	Graft loss isolate
Amyloidosis	5–20	30	
Henoch–Schonlein purpura	10–15	10–20	Delay transplantation for 6–12 months after loss of purpura

LRD, living related donor.

but graft losses are relatively rare. Recipients of grafts from HLA-identical siblings may be at increased risk for recurrence. Type I membranoproliferative glomerular nephritis has a recurrence rate of 20–30%, although this may be somewhat decreased since the introduction of cyclosporine. Histologically this lesion can be difficult to distinguish from transplant glomerulopathy, presenting with proteinuria, hematuria or both. Among patients with recurrent disease, graft loss may occur in 30–40% of cases. IgA nephropathy recurs in up to 50% of cases, presenting with microscopic hematuria and proteinuria. Patients with HLA, B35 and DR4 may be at increased risk. Graft loss occurs in approximately 10% of patients with recurrent disease. Anti-GBM disease has a recurrence rate of near zero (0) if a 6- to 12-month interval with documented negative anti-GBM antibody levels is achieved.

Among secondary glomerulopathies (see Table 4.3), Henoch–Schonlein purpura has a recurrence rate of approximately 10–15%. It presents at 8 to 18 months post-transplant and may be associated with skin lesions. These patients have a rate of graft loss of approximately 10–20%. The available data suggest that a 6- to 12-month waiting period after the loss of purpura is appropriate prior to transplantation. Patients with systemic lupus erythematosus (SLE) have a very low rate of recurrence (less than 1%). Hemolytic–uremic syndrome (HUS) has a recurrence rate in the range 13–25%. Interestingly, both cyclosporine and tacrolimus are associated with *de-novo* HUS. HUS patients with recurrence have a graft loss rate of approximately 10%. Patients with diabetic nephropathy have a recurrence rate close to 100%, as indicated by glomerular-based membrane thickening and mesangial expansion at 2 years post-transplant. However, graft loss is uncommon.

Several non-glomerular disorders can recur in the renal allograft. Of particular note is oxalosis, which has a very high recurrence rate. Consideration should be given to combined liver and kidney transplantation to correct the underlying metabolic defect. Early transplantation and aggressive dialysis may minimize the risk of recurrence. The recurrence rate of cystinosis is about 10%, with a minimal impact on graft function. Recurrences in Fabry's disease, sickle-cell nephropathy and scleroderma are all rare, although few data are available. It is important to note that patients with Alport's syndrome may develop anti-GBM disease post-transplant. This diagnosis needs to be considered, as therapy with plasmapheresis can be of benefit.

Bladder dysfunction is frequently difficult to diagnose in dialysis patients. Elderly men should be screened for prostate disease by a digital rectal examination, and may benefit from a screening prostate-specific antigen determination, although the value of this is not proven. Routine evaluation with a voiding cystourethrogram is not required. Prostatic hypertrophy in anuric patients is best managed post-transplant. Diabetic patients frequently have neurogenic bladder dysfunction, but this is not a contraindication to transplantation, and is generally easily managed medically post-operatively. Children and adults with congenital structural urinary tract abnormalities may benefit from evaluation with cystoscopy and retrograde pyelograms. Patients with chronic pyelonephritis secondary to ureteral reflux may require pre-transplant nephrectomy.

An important component of recipient evaluation is an assessment of any psychological issues or substance abuse issues which may affect the outcome of the transplant. An evaluation by a social worker affiliated to the Transplant Program is requested prior to transplantation, with particular attention being paid to issues of medical non-compliance. Patients with a history of multiple episodes of non-compliance with medical therapy should be considered high-risk transplant cases. However, compliance issues can differ between dialysis and transplant patients, and multiple opinions should be sought prior to making the decision not to list a patient with a history of non-compliance. Patients with a history of drug or alcohol abuse are required to document participation in a rehabilitation program for a minimum of 6 months. Random drug screens can be obtained to document abstinence. Psychiatric

---

Box 4.2 Pre-transplant recipient check-list

All patients
Electrocardiogram (within 6 months)
Chest radiograph (within 6 months)
Dental evaluation
Gallbladder sonogram
Pap smear
Mammogram (over 50 years of age)
PPD
Psychosocial evaluation by social worker

As indicated
Dobutamine stress echocardiography, adenosine thallium perfusion or
   exercise stress test
Voiding cystourethrogram
Endoscopy
Arterial Doppler examination of carotid arteries and/or lower
   extremities
Toxicology screens for substance abuse
Aortogram
Echocardiogram
Pulmonary function testing

---

illness and mental retardation are not contraindications to transplantation. Patients who are well controlled under medical supervision may be considered. A check-list of commonly used medical screening tests for transplant recipients is shown in Box 4.2.

Tissue typing and the cross-match

Compatibility between potential renal donors and recipients is determined by the ABO blood group and the human leukocyte antigen (HLA) system. Rules governing compatibility *vis-à-vis* the ABO system are essentially the same as for blood transfusion. There have been anecdotal descriptions of successful ABO-incompatible kidney transplantation, but these have generally been in special situations where either the target antigen density or the recipient pre-transplant antibody concentration was particularly low. The role of the HLA system in determining compatibility is more complicated and, at times, more controversial. The genes that code for HLA antigens are located on the short arm of chromosome 6. There are six loci with extensive gene-product expression, namely A, B, C, DR, DQ and DP. The antigens coded by A, B and C are collectively known as class I and appear on all somatic cells.

The antigens coded by DR, DQ and DP are known as class II and are found predominantly on cells of lymphoid origin. HLA typing can be achieved by a variety of methods, both molecular and serological, with molecular methods now being most common because of their increased sensitivity and reliability. It is critically important that all recipients are screened for the presence of preformed anti-donor HLA antibodies, as transplantation in the face of these antibodies will usually result in hyperacute rejection and graft loss. This is achieved by the use of a cross-match. Several different methods have been described, and technical considerations can greatly affect the sensitivity and specificity of the test. In general, the tests involve screening for both IgG and IgM antibodies directed against T- and/or B-lymphocytes using cell washes, anti-human globulin augmentation, incubation with complement and/or flow cytometry. With the exception of the above screening of preformed anti-donor HLA antibodies, the impact of HLA histocompatibility on outcomes after renal transplantation and its proper role in allocation are controversial. Clearly there is a beneficial biologic effect of better HLA donor/recipient matches, and currently 0 antigen-mismatched kidneys are shared on a national basis in the USA. The magnitude of the biologic effect of lesser HLA matches and the consequences of imposing wider sharing for lesser matches form the core of the debate. It requires enormous numbers of patients, and some would argue inadequate immunosuppression to demonstrate statistically an outcome benefit for lesser degrees of HLA matching. At the same time, the additional cold ischemic time and logistical barriers imposed if nationalized sharing of all kidneys was established would probably be considerable. Newer typing techniques and the interest in 'public' antigens and cross-reactive groups have only muddied the waters further, and the debate continues.

Donor evaluation

The standard surgical approach for living donor nephrectomy has utilized a flank incision through the retroperitoneum. The procedure is remarkably safe, produces a graft of excellent quality, and allows easy exposure in the case of anomalous anatomy. Modern studies suggest a mortality of 0.03% and a complication rate of 2–10%. None the less, the procedure results in significant morbidity mostly in terms of postoperative pain and lost employment and function. The recent development of laparoscopic techniques of donor nephrectomy has been well accepted by patients, and in multiple small series these techniques appear to produce similar recipient results, with equivalent donor mortality and morbidity and significantly less pain. Although long-term results are not yet available, the procedure has become the standard approach at many transplant centers across the country. The majority of donor kidneys in transplantation come from individuals who have suffered irreversible brain death following a catastrophic intracranial event. Cerebrovascular accidents are the most common etiology of brain death, followed by trauma. Patients who are in irreversible comas but who are not suffering brain death have only been considered as potential organ donors after the cessation of cardiac function and respiratory standstill. These donors have been termed 'non-heartbeating' donors. A number of donor clinical characteristics have been linked to a higher likelihood of recipient graft dysfunction as well as increased resource utilization. These include advanced donor age, non-heartbeating status, pre-existing donor hypertension or diabetes mellitus, and donor instability around the time of brain death or procurement. Collectively, donors with one or more of these criteria have been described as 'expanded criteria donors'. Exactly which characteristics or combinations of factors are most important in determining eventual graft function remains controversial. However, there are over 50 000 patients awaiting kidney transplants in the USA, and as long as donor demand far outstrips donor supply, there will be interest in all possible mechanisms for expanding the donor pool. Currently, 25–35% of all transplanted kidneys come from living donors, while a further 20–25% of kidneys come from expanded criteria donors.

Donor and recipient surgery

The standard surgical approach for renal implantation has been placement of the renal allograft in the iliac fossa. This avoids contamination of the peritoneal space in the event of complications, provides for proximity to the recipient bladder and ureter for re-establishment of urinary continuity, and allows for a safe approach for percutaneous renal biopsy when necessary. Although many technical nuances have been described, it is clear that the kidney can be safely implanted in either fossa and in multiple orientations. Vascular continuity is usually re-established by anastomosing the renal vein and artery to the external iliac vein and artery, respectively, with a fine monofilament vascular suture, but again a vast array of technical modifications has been described. Multiple renal arteries can occur in approximately 20% of kidneys, and these must be perfused because of the end-artery nature of renal vasculature and the lack of intrarenal collateralization. Multiple renal veins do not necessarily need to be reconstructed because of the rich intrarenal network of venous collaterals. In general, the most important principle is to provide a secure conduit for unobstructed inflow and outflow, while keeping the warm ischemic time to a minimum. Once the kidney is reperfused, urinary continuity is re-established, generally through direct ureteroneocystostomy with an absorbable suture. Alternatively, a ureteroureterostomy can be used at the discretion of the operating surgeon. In either case, the most important technical consideration is to ensure that the ureter is well vascularized throughout, and especially at the level of the ureteral anastomosis. A stent can be used across the anastomosis if this is so desired, and can later be removed cystoscopically. Gravity drainage of the bladder through a Foley catheter is commonly utilized for the first 48 h.

Various attempts have been made to ameliorate the vasospasm and reperfusion injury that can accompany the re-establishment of blood flow after a period of cold ischemia. Calcium-channel blockers, loop and osmotic diuretics as well as various α- and β-adrenergic agents have all been utilized, although no clear standard exists.

Great care should be taken to optimize the physiologic condition of the patient before, during and immediately after the operation. Attention should be given to maintaining adequate intravascular volume, especially in view of the fact that many patients may be relatively hypovolemic following recent dialysis. Central venous or pulmonary artery monitoring is not necessary unless the recipient has significant pre-existing cardiopulmonary disease. Postoperatively, an adequate intravascular volume must be maintained to provide for renal perfusion. Postoperative hypovolemia can lead to hypotension, renal hypoperfusion and exacerbation of any tubular injury sustained at the time of donor harvest or implantation. This is particularly important as most patients will develop a brisk post-transplant diuresis. Serum electrolyte abnormalities (especially potassium) and acid–base balance should be corrected prior to induction of anesthesia and monitored throughout the perioperative period. In most cases there should be sufficient time to perform dialysis preoperatively if the patient's physiologic condition so dictates.

The choice of anesthetic techniques and agents will be determined by the patient's underlying physiology, but anesthesia in the patient with end-stage renal disease requires an anesthesia team with significant experience of the metabolic perturbations that are common in end-stage renal disease.

Postoperative management

Since the very earliest days of solid organ transplantation, the attempt to abrogate or ameliorate the specific immune response to a transplanted organ has provided much fascination and frustration in the field of transplantation. Clinical immunosuppression is an empiric practice with no clearly dominant strategy. Immunosuppressive regimens are based on combination therapy, and monotherapy with any one agent is not consistently achievable in transplant patients at this time.

Steroids

The use of adjunctive corticosteroids, particularly in the early postoperative period, is critical for graft success due to a variety of immunologic actions that affect both cellular and humoral immunity. One of the primary modes of action of corticosteroids appears to be the inhibition of IL-1 production by activated antigen-presenting macrophages. In this way, steroids indirectly inhibit cytokine-driven T-cell proliferation. Methylprednisolone (Solu-Medrol) is the preferred intravenous form, with conversion to prednisone when the patient is tolerating oral inake. Steroids have a number of well-known adverse effects, including impairment of wound healing, predisposition to infection, fluid retention, gastrointestinal complications and psychiatric symptoms. Some centers have pursued complete cessation of steroids with the goal of eliminating their considerable side-effects, especially in children, in whom growth is severely affected. However, the results have been equivocal.

Cyclosporine and tacrolimus (FK506)

Discovered in 1972, the clinical introduction of the fungal metabolite cyclosporine A in the early 1980s revolutionized the field of transplantation. Its primary mechanism of action is inhibition of gene transcription of several cytokines, most notably IL-2, thereby blocking early T-cell activation. Its efficacy has been well documented both anecdotally and in large, multicenter, randomized trials, and currently cyclosporine or tacrolimus (another fungal metabolite with a similar mechanism of action) form the backbone of the vast majority of clinical immunosuppressive regimens. Both drugs have many adverse effects, most notably nephrotoxicity, which may or may not be dose related. They are associated with the development of hypertension, hyperlipidemia, hyperkalemia, headaches and other neurologic symptoms. Nephrotoxicity may require discontinuation of the drugs. Immunosuppression is generally monitored by a combination of trough blood levels and clinical effect, rather than precise dosing. Importantly, although the side-effect profile of tacrolimus is similar to that of cyclosporine, an adverse effect that occurs with one drug will not necessarily occur with the other. Tacrolimus has also been successfully used to treat chronic rejection and even OKT3-resistant rejection ('salvage therapy') in liver, kidney, and pancreas grafts.

Azathioprine and mycophenolate mofetil (MMF)

Azathioprine was first used in clinical renal transplantation in 1961. It is an antimetabolite that inhibits purine nucleotide synthesis, thus in turn inhibiting the multiplication of effector lymphocytes during the immune response, although its efficacy has never been clearly defined in any prospective randomized trial. The drug is inexpensive, equivalent as an IV or oral preparation, and generally well tolerated. The most common adverse effect is leukopenia through bone-marrow suppression, although jaundice, alopecia, anemia and gastrointestinal upset have also been reported. Mycophenolate mofetil (MMF) is another purine synthesis inhibitor, which was approved for use in the USA in 1995. Large prospective trials comparing it with azathioprine have demonstrated the efficacy of MMF, with significant decreases in acute rejection. The drug is very well tolerated, but may cause gastrointestinal upset or diarrhea as well as leukopenia or thrombocytopenia. Both azathioprine and MMF exploit the deficiency of the purine salvage pathway in lymphocytes. Thus inhibition of de-novo purine synthesis can produce a relatively specific effect.

Antilymphocyte globulins (ATGAM and OKT3)

Antilymphocyte globulins were first developed in the 1960s in an attempt to develop specific immunosuppressive agents to augment the broad non-specific effect of steroids and azathioprine, the only agents available at the time. ATGAM, a polyclonal antilymphocyte preparation, is made by immunizing horses to a human thymocyte preparation, then purifying the IgG antihuman thymocyte fraction from the animals' serum. The exact mechanism of immunosuppression involves more than simple clearance of lymphocytes, and inhibition of T-cell proliferation is probably important.

Nevertheless, clinical efficacy can be measured by monitoring the levels of CD3-positive lymphocytes. ATGAM is administered centrally, and it often causes fever, chills and thrombocytopenia. In addition, because the product is derived from animals, there is a small but measurable incidence of hypersensitivity reactions. The dosage is 10–20 mg/kg/day, and it may be titrated according to the desired response.

Thymoglobulin is a polyclonal anti-rabbit preparation approved for use in the USA in 1999. It has been demonstrated to be effective both as a treatment of established rejection and as induction therapy to decrease the rate of acute rejection. It also usually requires a central access, it has adverse reactions similar to those of ATGAM, and its efficacy can be monitored by following peripheral CD3-positive lymphocyte counts. The dosage is 1–2 mg/kg.

OKT3 is a murine monoclonal antibody directed against the CD3 complex of the human T-lymphocyte. It has dramatic immunosuppressive effects, with circulating T-cells becoming virtually undetectable within minutes after administration. The usual adult dose of the drug is 5 mg. It is administered intravenously as a bolus, and the adequacy of the clinical response is gauged by measuring the absolute numbers of CD3-positive lymphocytes in the circulating blood. OKT3 levels are principally useful in cases where the drug is not producing the desired clinical effect. Since OKT3 is a murine antibody, recipients can develop human antimurine antibodies (HAMA) that will neutralize the drug. Nearly all patients develop an acute symptom complex, consisting of fever and chills, following the first dose of the drug. Repeat dosing is associated with nausea, vomiting, dyspnea, wheezing, diarrhea and rash. These symptoms are decreased by premedication with steroids as well as antihistamines and other agents. Pulmonary edema and cardiac arrest have also been reported, and these appear to be more likely to occur if the patient is hypervolemic at the time of administration. OKT3 was first used as a treatment for steroid-resistant rejection in both kidney and liver transplants, and it is extraordinarily effective, reversing established rejection in over 95% of patients.

Anti-IL-2 receptor antibodies

Two new monoclonal antibodies directed against the T-cell IL-2 receptor have recently been approved. The antibodies are considered to be chimeric or humanized in that the variable region is at least partly composed of mouse sequences, while the constant region is human. As a result, the antibodies have long half-lives, are not immunogenic and can have long-lasting effects. Clinical studies have indicated that the agents may be useful in induction therapy after kidney transplantation.

There is no clear consensus on the exact role of antilymphocyte antibody therapy in renal transplantation. Clearly there is a role for treatment of severe or resistant rejection, but whether the agents should be used immediately after transplantation in order to spare patients the nephrotoxicity of cyclosporine and tacrolimus is subject to controversy.

Early complications

Early graft dysfunction

Graft dysfunction in the first few months postoperatively can be divided into three broad categories, namely mechanical, immunologic and medical. Successful treatment and ultimate long-term graft function depend on the timely diagnosis of the mode of dysfunction.

Mechanical dysfunction

Venous thrombosis is a relatively rare occurrence post-transplant (0.5–1.5% of cases), but has catastrophic results. The diagnosis is confirmed by ultrasound or radionuclide imaging and appears early (during the first 30 days) in the post-transplant course. Angiography is rarely necessary. Clinical presentation consists of pain over the allograft and hematuria. A number of associated factors have been reported, including technical error, kinking of the renal vein, retransplantation and postoperative hypotension. The prognosis is poor and transplant nephrectomy is usually required, although there are a few anecdotal reports of effective thrombolytic therapy. Renal artery thrombosis is also rare, presenting as an acute decrease in urine output without pain or other symptoms. It is associated with the same causative factors as venous thrombosis. The prognosis is poor and the result is usually graft loss.

Urologic complications occur in 2–4% of transplant recipients. No good comparison of complication rates exists that uses different techniques of ureteral anastomoses, although most studies suggest a lower incidence of urinary leak and stenosis using an extravesicular neocystostomy. It remains controversial whether internal ureteral stenting at the time of transplantation affects the overall rate of urological complications.

Urinary leaks occur early and are associated with technical

errors or distal necrosis of the transplanted ureter. A leak may present as graft dysfunction, drainage from the surgical wound, increased drainage from a closed suction drain around the graft, or pain in the region of the graft. The diagnosis is made by analysis of drainage, radionuclide scanning or percutaneous nephrostogram. Therapy is usually surgical, although stenting can be used as a temporizing measure or in cases of minor leaks.

Ureteral stenosis usually occurs several weeks to several months post-transplant, and is thought to be secondary to ischemia or infection, but it has also been associated with rejection. Stenosis usually presents as steadily declining graft function and hydronephrosis evident on ultrasound examination. The diagnosis is complicated by the mild dilation of the collecting system that is commonly seen in up to 30% of normal transplanted kidneys. Balloon ureteroplasty is successful in up to 50% of selected patients, and is most successful with short segment strictures. Repair can be achieved by reimplantation of a shortened ureteral segment into the bladder, or by ureteroureterostomy to the native ureter. In extreme situations, direct anastomoses between the allograft pelvis and the urinary bladder have been performed. Even more creative solutions, using Fallopian tubes as conduits, have also been used.

Urinary obstruction can also be caused by a lymphocele (a collection of lymphatic fluid leaking into the retroperitoneal space). Lymphoceles are generally associated with inadequate ligation of lymphatics at the time of transplant, and they present as declining renal function associated with a perinephric collection and often hydronephrosis. Fluid analysis from percutaneous sampling may be necessary to differentiate lymph from urine or blood, and the treatment is usually surgical, by either open or laparoscopic marsupialization of the collection into the peritoneal cavity. Limited success has been described with percutaneous drainage or ablative caustic therapy.

Various other miscellaneous causes of mechanical dysfunction (e.g. clot retention, ureteral edema) have been described and diligent diagnosis of postoperative graft dysfunction must be undertaken in order to ensure both the survival of the graft and the well-being of the patient.

Immunologic dysfunction – acute rejection

Although a detailed description of the immune response to a renal allograft is beyond the scope of this chapter, rejection is clearly one of the best-studied causes of early graft dysfunction.

Hyperacute rejection is an intense antibody-mediated reaction of the host against an allograft caused by the presence of preformed antidonor antibodies, usually of the anti-ABO or anti-HLA type. Grossly, the kidney appears flaccid and blue and remains so after reperfusion as the process develops over the first few minutes to hours post-transplant. Histologically, it is characterized by small-vessel engorgement of glomerular and peritubular capillaries, with neutrophilic infiltration and progression to frank tubular necrosis, vascular thrombosis and fibrinoid necrosis. The occurrence of hyperacute rejection has been largely eliminated by sensitive cross-matching of recipient serum to detect the presence of antidonor antibody.

Accelerated acute rejection is a poorly defined process that is thought to represent a combination of antibody-mediated and cell-mediated events. It commonly occurs in the first 2 to 4 days post-transplant, and it generally carries a poor prognosis, although grafts can be salvaged with aggressive therapy.

Acute rejection is a cell-mediated process that generally occurs at any time from 2 days to several years post-tranplant. Clinically it is heralded by a sharp deterioration in renal function, and if left unchecked it will progress to graft failure. Histologically, cellular rejection is characterized by an interstitial cellular infiltrate of lymphocytes, lymphoblasts, monocytes and/or macrophages. There is interstitial edema and tubular injury, with lymphocytes invading the tubules (tubulitis). The changes associated with vascular rejection consist of intimal damage and vasculitis. In the past a variety of grading systems for rejection have been used. Recently, the 'Banff criteria' were developed and refined by transplant professionals through a consensus process, and these are rapidly becoming the most commonly used criteria in both clinical practice and trials.

Although there has been much interest and research directed at non-invasive, serologic or cytologic methods for diagnosing rejection, percutaneous renal biopsy remains the gold standard. Treatment of acute rejection is achieved through augmentation of immunosuppression. Increased corticosteroids are considered to be first-line therapy, with antilymphocyte-antibody therapy reserved for steroid-resistant cases. Various other immunologic manipulations may be successful, including changing calcineurin inhibitors or the addition of new agents. Graft loss from acute rejection is now extremely rare, although an episode of acute rejection seems to put patients at risk for subsequent development of chronic graft dysfunction. Furthermore, additional immunosuppression used to treat rejection puts recipients at increased risk for infection, thus further increasing morbidity. Historically, rates of rejection following renal transplantation have been as high as 70%.

However, with the advent of more effective immunosuppressive agents, rates as low as 10% have been reported in 'low'-risk patients. Various risk factors for the occurrence of rejection have been reported, which include but are not limited to donor age, duration of cold ischemic time, donor–recipient HLA match, ethnicity, age, and the occurrence of acute tubular necrosis post-transplant.

Medical dysfunction

A significant degree of renal impairment resulting from acute tubular necrosis (ATN) occurs in up to 40% of cadaver recipients post-transplant. This is a result of a multitude of factors, most commonly causing decreased renal perfusion. Donor factors (e.g. age, method of death, need for vasopressors), recipient factors (e.g. age, cardiac output, vascular insufficiency) and ischemic insults incurred during retrieval, cold storage and reimplantation all contribute to such impairment. The diagnosis of ATN post-transplant in an oliguric or anuric patient is in many ways a diagnosis of exclusion. Radionuclide scanning and/or ultrasonography can be helpful, although ultimately differentiation between ATN and rejection or drug toxicity relies on histology. The long-term consequences of ATN and its impact on graft survival are controversial. Graft survival is decreased in patients who experience ATN, but the actual magnitude of this decrease, and the relative contribution of the ATN itself compared to that of conditions such as acute rejection, remains undefined.

Drug nephrotoxicity can occur in conjunction with a host of agents, but is most uniquely associated with the use of calcineurin inhibitors following renal transplantation. There are three common clinical scenarios of calcineurin toxicity. The first is acute, seen with intravenous dosing or very high levels of the drugs. This is thought to be mediated primarily through afferent arteriolar vasoconstriction, and can readily be treated by dose reduction or cessation of the drug. The second scenario is a form of toxicity that may be seen at any time after several weeks post-transplant. This is associated with gradually deteriorating renal function and can be very difficult to differentiate from other forms of graft dysfunction without invasive testing. Serum trough levels may be within the therapeutic range. Histology often demonstrates tubular vacuolization and glomerular capillary thrombosis. The treatment is either severe dose reduction or, if feasible, complete withdrawal of the drug. Calcineurin inhibitors can also be responsible for a progressive chronic deterioration in renal function that occurs months to years after transplantation. Histologic studies demonstrate interstitial fibrosis and arteriolar changes, and there is little response to dose reduction. The mechanism of this chronic toxicity has not been elucidated.

Infectious complications

One of the most prevalent and troublesome complications that has been seen in transplant recipients is infection. A truism in transplantation has been that any therapeutic manipulation that increases the degree of immunosuppression will also increase the predilection for infection. Although improved modes of diagnosis and more powerful antibiotics may influence this relationship, the reality remains unchanged. Serious infections in transplant patients can present insidiously, and a high index of suspicion must be maintained in any patient with low-grade fever and/or malaise. Aggressive diagnostic workup and therapy should be pursued in most cases in order to gain an early foothold against common infections, and to identify unusual opportunistic organisms that might not be adequately treated with standard empiric therapy.

Bacterial infections, both Gram-negative and Gram-positive, are most prevalent in the first weeks to months post-transplant. Urinary tract infections are the commonest source of bacterial infection after renal transplantation, followed by surgical infections.

Fungal infections are common in transplant recipients, primarily because of defects in cell-mediated immunity related to chronic immunosuppression. Opportunistic organisms such as cryptococcus, aspergillus and even rhizopus can occur, and often account for significant morbidity. Antifungal prophylaxis has not generally been employed after renal transplants, although it has been shown to be of benefit in the management of patients after other abdominal organ transplantation.

Viral infections are also important sources of morbidity in transplant recipients, cytomegalovirus (CMV) being the most important viral pathogen. CMV infections are common in the general population, and approximately 60% of patients have been infected in the past. With the initiation of immunosuppression, these latent infections can reactivate in patients who had been infected prior to transplantation. In addition, CMV-naive patients who receive an organ from a CMV-exposed donor can develop primary CMV infections that are more virulent and difficult to treat than an infection which is due to reactivation. Clinically, CMV infections appear from 4 to 10 weeks post-transplant, or after an increase in immunosuppression therapy used to treat rejection. Symptoms can be diverse, ranging from low-grade fever and malaise to invasive hepatitis, esophagitis, retinitis, gastritis, colitis or life-threatening pneumonitis. Diagnosis is difficult, sometimes requiring pathologic confirmation, although either immunohistochemical techniques for locating CMV antigens in infected cell cultures or molecular techniques can speed up diagnosis.

Until the development of the guanine analog, ganciclovir, in the late 1980s, there was no effective treatment available. The occurrence of invasive CMV disease usually meant the loss of the graft in the case of kidney patients, as immunosuppression had to be drastically reduced or completely withdrawn. Most mild infections are now easily treated, and even severe infections rarely result in graft loss. None the less, CMV remains an important source of morbidity and increased resource utilization. Most programs now employ some type of prophylaxis for CMV infection, depending on the immunosuppressive protocol employed and the donor–recipient CMV status.

In addition, CMV infection itself can affect the immune response. There is an association between increased incidence of rejection and increased episodes of CMV disease that may be due to more than just increasing or decreasing levels of therapeutic immunosuppression. CMV can cause an immunosuppressive effect through reduced production of interleukin-1, or conversely it can be immunostimulatory, causing increased expression of cell-surface antigens. At present its precise role remains difficult to define.

Outcomes

After years of justifying renal transplantation primarily through its improved quality of life and decreased expense as compared to dialysis, recent evidence has emerged that unequivocally demonstrates a life-extending benefit for transplantation. It is apparent that the cumulative risk of dying while awaiting renal transplant is significantly higher than after receiving a transplant. The United Network for Organ Sharing (UNOS) has reported that 1-year patient survival after kidney transplantation was over 95% as of 1997, while the overall 4-year survival rate is approximately 87%. The primary causes of mortality are accelerated cardiovascular and cerebrovascular disease, infections and malignancy.

Graft survival has improved significantly during the last

decade. One-year graft survival for recipients of living donor kidneys was 94% in 1997, while recipients of cadaveric kidneys showed a graft survival rate of 89%. There are expectations that the recent improvements in short-term graft survival as well as improvements in other aspects of post-transplant care will finally make an impact on long-term graft survival. For the period from 1987 to 1997, the 4-year graft survival rates for living donor and cadaveric donor kidneys were 81% and 67%, respectively.

Chronic graft dysfunction

Although the outcomes of renal transplantation have improved greatly in recent years, chronic graft dysfunction remains a major problem. One-year graft survival has improved from an average of 50% in the 1970s to almost 90% in the late 1990s, but the half-life of an initially successful renal allograft has remained at approximately 7–8 years. The main reasons for this are deaths due to cardiovascular disease, malignancy and chronic graft dysfunction.

There are a number of causes of chronic graft dysfunction. Cyclosporine toxicity has already been discussed. In addition, the diseases that were initially responsible for renal failure can recur in the transplanted kidney. Various systemic diseases (e.g. diabetes mellitus, amyloidosis and hemolytic uremic syndrome) can recur in the allograft, while others (e.g. lupus) recur rarely. Focal segmental glomerulosclerosis can reappear quite rapidly in renal allografts, with a frequency of 20–100%. Recently, serologic markers have been developed which can help to predict the likelihood of recurrence of this disease. Most other forms of chronic glomerulonephritis will not recur post-transplant with any significant frequency, but of these, type II membranoproliferative glomerulonephritis and IgA nephropathy have the highest recurrence rate. Several other diseases, such as anti-glomerular basement membrane disease or oxalosis, also have significant recurrence rates.

The commonest form of chronic graft dysfunction and the commonest cause of graft loss in otherwise healthy patients is chronic allograft nephropathy, previously known as 'chronic rejection'. Chronic allograft nephropathy is manifested clinically by an insidious, progressive deterioration in allograft function without a clear precipitating cause. It can occur at any time from months to years post-transplant, even after years of stable renal function. Histologically, it is typified by mesangial interposition and an increased mesangial matrix in the glomeruli, intense interstitial fibrosis and tubular atrophy and fibrous intimal thickening and disruptions of the internal elastica of the renal vessels, resulting in severe luminal narrowing.

Renal artery stenosis is a late-occurring vascular complication. It is also rare (2–10% incidence) and is clinically heralded by graft dysfunction and hypertension. Percutaneous balloon angioplasty is generally the treatment of first choice, and tends to be most successful in early and proximal lesions, with surgical correction reserved for angiographic failures.

The change in terminology from 'chronic rejection' to 'chronic allograft nephropathy' has come about as research has suggested that there may be several different etiologies of this condition, some of which are not related to alloimmunity and are therefore 'antigen-independent'. In experimental models a bewildering array of insults can result in the histologic picture of chronic allograft nephropathy, including but not limited to multiple acute rejection episodes, inadequate immunosuppression, initial ischemic injury to the graft, various forms of infection, and provision of inadequate nephron mass. In clinical transplantation, early acute rejection has been linked to a higher incidence of chronic allograft nephropathy, as has CMV infection and advanced donor age. Cadaveric transplant recipients have a higher incidence of chronic nephropathy than do living donor recipients, and the role of nephron mass may be important, as smaller kidneys transplanted into larger recipients seem to experience more chronic allograft nephropathy than vice versa. Increased or altered immunosuppression can often stabilize renal function for a period of time, but significant improvement in long-term (> 10 years) graft survivals will probably require a more detailed understanding of this condition.

Long-term morbidity and rehabilitation

As short-term graft survival has improved, attention has shifted to complications that beset the transplant recipient as a result of chronic immunosuppression. The incidence of malignancy in immunosupressed patients increases with time, and it exceeds that of the general population by several orders of magnitude. It has been estimated that a transplant recipient living in an area of high sunlight exposure has a 60% chance of contracting some type of malignancy after 20 years of immunosuppression. The most common cancers are squamous and basal cell carcinomas of the skin, followed by those of the lymphoreticular system. Population-based reports of cancer rates from countries with national health systems and more complete reporting of malignancy indicate an increased risk of virtually every type of malignancy in transplant recipients. Furthermore, tumors in transplant recipients tend to be more aggressive that those in the general population. Several hypotheses have been proposed, including impaired immune surveillance, chronic antigenic stimulation, reactivation of latent oncogenic viruses, and the direct oncogenic effects of immunosuppressive drugs.

Cardiovascular morbidity and mortality occur with a prevalence that is three- to fivefold higher than in age-matched controls. Indeed, death with a functioning graft is the primary cause of graft loss in many series. The accelerated course of cardiovascular disease in transplant recipients is believed to be related to hypertension, diabetes and hyperlipidemia which develop as a consequence of chronic immunosuppression.

Metabolic bone disease is a common finding in long-term transplant recipients. Avascular necrosis of the femoral head, vertebral fractures and severe bone and joint pain are all manifestations of osteomalacia and osteopenia seen after transplantation, largely due to the use of corticosteroids.

Despite these problems, longitudinal studies of quality of life in transplant recipients demonstrate a significant improvement compared to the situation pre-transplant. However, health status scores rarely reach the levels seen in the age-matched general population. Vocational rehabilitation is markedly superior in transplant recipients compared to those on dialysis, with almost twice as many transplant patients being actively employed.

Transplantation is known to be an expensive endeavor. Approximately $1.2 billion of a $13 billion ESRD budget is allocated to transplantation. Nevertheless, multiple analyses have established transplantation as a cost-effective therapy for ESRD, compared to dialysis. Despite the success of renal transplantation, significant financial hurdles remain which impede the long-term rehabilitation of patients. Immunosuppressive coverage under Medicare, the primary payer for renal transplantation in the USA, is discontinued after 3 years, leaving many patients in financial difficulties. The economic burden of post-transplant morbidities remains poorly defined.

Living donor evaluation

Living donor transplantation is becoming increasingly common. It has a number of major advantages, including prolonged short-term graft and patient survival. However, long-term graft survival with living donor transplantation is dramatically superior to that obtained with utilization of cadaveric organs. A two-haplotype living donor transplant has an expected half-life of nearly 25 years, compared with 9 years for cadaveric organ transplants. This improved long-term graft survival is seen with living related transplants as well as living unrelated transplants. The improvement in graft survival with completely HLA-mismatched living unrelated transplants compared to similarly mismatched cadaveric transplants highlights the fact that non-immunologic factors such as renal ischemia may be more important than tissue matching in long-term graft outcome. Due to the limited supply of available cadaveric organs, many transplant patients are requesting living donor transplantation. In addition, there are other significant benefits. Although the average waiting time for cadaveric transplantation varies across the USA, in many areas the typical waiting period exceeds 3 years, and it increases each year. Living donor transplantation often allows the transplant to be performed on a relatively elective basis, and it allows the complete avoidance of dialysis. This may also enable the recipient to return to work sooner, and to enjoy a more satisfying lifestyle.

The major ethical problem with living donor transplantation is that the donor assumes a degree of medical risk without clear benefit to him- or herself. Specifically, this includes not just the risk of surgery and anesthesia, but also the potential long-term risk of living with a solitary kidney. The focus of the donor transplant evaluation is to minimize any risk to the donor (see Box 4.3). Contraindications to living kidney donation are listed in Box 4.4. Surgical mortality from donor nephrectomy has been studied and has been found to be extremely low (0.03%). Morbidity appears to be approximately 2.5% or less. The recent development of laparoscopic donor nephrectomy has significantly decreased patient morbidity, and at some select centers, it is now considered to be the standard approach to donor nephrectomy. Hospital stays have been significantly reduced as a result, and the donors return to work more quickly, with less time and income lost.

The long-term medical risks of unilateral nephrectomy have been extensively studied. The results of a large meta-analysis indicate that unilateral nephrectomy does not lead to a progressive decline in renal function. The lifespan of donors has been shown to be the same as that of controls. Small increases in systolic and diastolic blood pressure have been noted, but these increases are not clinically significant and are not predictive of an increased risk of developing hypertension.

One goal of the medical evaluation of a prospective donor is to screen for the presence of hereditary renal disease. When the

Box 4.3 Medical evaluation of potential living donor candidates

ABO typing
Tissue typing (HLA)
Chest radiograph
Electrocardiography
Physical examination
Complete chemistry screen
Complete blood count and coagulation studies
Urinalysis and urine culture
Spot urine for protein-to-creatinine ratio
Glomerular filtration rate, calculated by Cockroft–Gault method
Hepatitis A, B and C serologies
IgG and IgM titers for CMV, EBV and HSV I and II
FTA, RPR, HIV and HTLV 1
Toxoplasmosis titer
Varicella zoster titer
Sickle-cell screen
Renal sonogram (with history of polycystic kidney disease)
Glucose tolerance test (if positive family history)
Mammogram (if over 50 years of age)
Pap smear
Renal arteriogram/spiral CT angiogram/magnetic resonance
     angiography
Final cross-match

Box 4.4 Exclusion criteria for living donations

Diabetes
Hypertension
Proteinuria
Glomerular filtration rate < 80 mL/min
Nephrolithiasis
Sickle-cell trait
Transmissible infectious disease
Malignancy
Psychiatric or social contraindications

primary renal disease of the recipient is unknown, it is important
to screen a donor for diseases that have a hereditary component,
such as diabetes and hypertension, in addition to the obvious
familial conditions such as Alport's syndrome or polycystic kidney
disease. All donors are screened for diabetes by simple blood
glucose determination. However, potential donors for recipients
with diabetes must be screened more carefully. Type II diabetes has
a clear familial component, and for this reason all potential related

donors for patients with type II diabetes undergo an oral glucose tolerance test. In families with a strong history of type I diabetes mellitus a glucose tolerance test should also be performed. In younger potential donors, it may be necessary to screen further for anti-islet cell antibodies or anti-GAD antibodies.

The screening of adult donors for possible polycystic kidney disease is relatively simple. Renal ultrasound in patients who are over 30 years of age rules out polycystic kidney disease with nearly 100% sensitivity. In patients between the ages of 20 and 30 years, renal ultrasound is less sensitive. In this setting a computed tomographic scan with small cuts through the kidney can exclude the possibility of occult polycystic kidney disease. Hereditary nephritis is easily ruled out by standard chemistry screening and urinalysis. Although systemic lupus erythematosus can run in families, a careful history and physical examination is adequate to exclude this diagnosis. Serologic testing for lupus can be utilized if there is concern based on the history and physical findings.

Blood pressure should be carefully evaluated for any evidence of hypertension. Special caution should be noted in the case of a young adult donor who exhibits borderline hypertension. These patients are at increased risk of developing hypertension later in life.

An important component of the donor evaluation is an assessment of the risk of transmission of infectious diseases. Donors are screened by physical examination for the presence of any signs suggestive of active bacterial infection. It is essential that donors are screened for evidence of chronic viral infection. Serologic screening is obtained for hepatitis A, B and C. Screening for HIV infection is mandatory for all donors, as is an analysis of HIV risk factors. Serology should also be obtained for CMV and EBV. A history of malignancy in a potential donor requires careful assessment. A disease-free interval of 5 years is a conservative waiting period that reasonably ensures a low risk of transmission of malignancy to the recipient.

Adequacy of renal function is obviously important. Most programs agree that a glomerular filtration rate of 80 mL/min or greater is adequate to ensure safe kidney donation. A renal sonogram is used to ensure that there are two kidneys present, and to rule out gross structural abnormalities and the presence of kidney stones. Traditionally, arteriography has been used to define the renal artery anatomy prior to the donor procedure. However, more recent experience with spiral CT scanning and magnetic resonance angiography has shown good sensitivity in detecting multiple renal arteries, and these techniques have gained wider acceptance as an alternative to highly invasive angiography.

An evaluation of the psychosocial context in which donation takes place is also important. It is the responsibility of the Transplant Center to ensure that the autonomy of the donor is protected and that donation is truly voluntary. Screening by a social worker in the Transplant Center is most useful in this regard. Detailed psychological evaluations can be performed when indicated to determine the motivation of the donor. It has become evident that donation is often associated with positive psychological benefits for the donor. Studies of donors have revealed that in many cases there is improved self-esteem associated with the donation.

Further reading

Churchill BM, Steckler RF, McKenna PH *et al*. 1993: Renal transplantation and the abnormal urinary tract. *Transplantation Reviews* 7, 21–34. A comprehensive review of the structural abnormalities of the urinary drainage system and how they are best approached during transplant surgery.

Flowers JL, Jacobs S, Cho E *et al*. 1997: Comparison of open and laparoscopic live donor nephrectomy. *Annals of Surgery* 226, 483–90. A description of the most recent technique for donor nephrectomy and the results of the largest series in the literature.

Johnson EM, Remucal MJ, Gillingham KJ *et al*. 1997: Complications and risks of living donor nephrectomy. *Transplantation* 64, 1124–8. An account of an extensive single-center analysis of the risks of living kidney donation.

Kasiske BL and Bia MJ. 1995: The evaluation and selection of living kidney donors. *American Journal of Kidney Diseases* 26, 387–98. A complete discussion of the clinical issues encountered when assessing prospective kidney donors.

Kasiske BL, Ramos EL, Gaston RS *et al*. 1995: The evaluation of renal transplant candidates: clinical practice guidelines. *Journal of the American Society of Nephrology* 6, 1–34. An extensive article on clinical algorithms developed by the American Society of Transplant Physicians for the evaluation of renal transplant candidates.

Kotanko P, Pusey CD and Levy JB. 1997: Recurrent glomerulonephritis following renal transplantation. *Transplantation* 63, 1045–52. The most recent review article on the subject of recurrent glomerular disease following transplantation.

Lee A, Wilson R, Douek K *et al*. 1994: Prospective risk stratification in renal transplant candidates for cardiac death. *American Journal of Kidney Diseases* 24, 65–71. An article which analyzes the cardiac risk factors prior to transplantation.

Morris, PJ (ed.) 1994: *Kidney transplantation: principles and practice*, 4th edn. Philadelphia, PA: W.B. Saunders Co.

Penn I. 1993: The effect of immunosuppression on pre-existing cancers. *Transplantation* **55**, 742–47. A review of the recurrence rate of different cancers using data from the Cincinnati Transplant Tumor Registry.

Racusen LC, Solez K and **Burdick JR** (eds) 1998: *Kidney transplant rejection: diagnosis and treatment*, 3rd edn. New York: Marcel Dekker.

Ramos EL. 1991: Recurrent diseases in the renal allograft. *Journal of the American Society Nephrology* **2**, 109–21. An excellent comprehensive review of the rates of recurrence of all forms of glomerular disease following renal transplant.

Ramos EL, Kasiske BL, Alexander SR *et al.* 1994: The evaluation of candidates for renal transplantation. *Transplantation* **57**, 490–97. A comprehensive review of the clinical issues relating to transplant recipient evaluation.

Sells RA. 1997: Cardiovascular complications following renal transplantation. *Transplantation Reviews* **11**, 111–26. An extensive review of the predisposing factors for cardiovascular complications after renal transplantation and the preoperative evaluation.

Sesso R, Klag MJ, Ancao MS *et al.* 1992: Kidney transplantation from living unrelated donors. *Annals of Internal Medicine* **117**, 983–89. A presentation of data from the Brazilian Transplant Registry documenting the excellent results obtained from living non-related kidney donors.

Starzl TE, Shapiro R and **Simmons RI** (eds) 1992: *Atlas of organ transplantation*. Philadelphia, PA: J. P. Lippincott Co.

Terasaki PI (ed.) 1991: *History of transplantation: thirty-five recollections*. Los Angeles, CA: UCLA Tissue Typing Laboratory. This volume documents extensively the early days of clinical transplantation as experienced by the people directly involved.

Terasaki PI, Cecka JM, Gjertson DW *et al.* 1995: High survival rates of kidney transplants from spousal and living unrelated donors. *New England Journal of Medicine* **333**, 333–6. An analysis of the results of living unrelated kidney transplants from the UNOS database.

United Network for Organ Sharing (UNOS) 1998: *UNOS 1998 Annual Report*. Washington, DC: US Department of Health and Human Services.

5 Liver transplantation

Lynt B. Johnson, Jeffrey S. Plotkin, Paul C. Kuo, Jacqueline C. Lauren and Vinod K. Rustgi

Introduction

The clinical application of liver transplantation grew from experimental techniques employed in dogs by Moore in Boston and Starzl in Chicago and Denver in 1956. Starzl first attempted replacement of a diseased liver in a patient with biliary atresia in 1963. Despite extensive laboratory successes, this attempt in a small child with multiple prior operations and significant portal hypertension resulted in the intraoperative death of the recipient due to massive hemorrhage. During the ensuing years, isolated attempts at liver transplantation were made at several institutions. However, these efforts did not result in any long-term survivors, and an unofficial moratorium on clinical liver transplantation resulted. The development of antilymphocyte serum in 1966 improved graft survival, and Starzl performed the first successful long-term liver transplant procedure in 1967. Barriers to solid organ transplantation included the lack of social and legal reform measures allowing use of organs for transplantation from donors after declaration of brain death. The Harvard Ad-Hoc Committee Report on Brain Death in 1968 gained public support, and soon afterwards the courts provided a legal definition of the concept of death and cessation of brain function. However, consistent long-term success had to await the evolution of more refined immunosuppression techniques.

With the introduction of cyclosporine A in 1979, liver and other solid organ transplantation began to emerge as a viable treatment for end-stage organ disease. The National Institutes of Health Consensus Development Conference on Liver Transplantation in 1983 further validated the field of liver transplantation as a therapeutic option for patients with end-stage liver disease. New liver transplant centers began to develop worldwide, and successful liver transplantation became the expectation. Other significant advances included the development of University of Wisconsin (UW) solution by Belzer for preservation of hepatic allografts, which safely extended preservation times and allowed sharing of organs from great distances, thus relaxing logistical constraints. Refinement of anesthetic and perioperative management of the liver transplant recipient further improved the operative results. Shaw and colleagues introduced a venovenous bypass circuit which allowed a smoother hemodynamic course during interruption of the venous return circulation to the heart, enabling the operation to proceed in a more controlled fashion. Other innovations included the development of the 'piggyback' technique, which allows preservation of the recipient vena cava, and the development of the immunosuppressive agent tacrolimus in 1986. The most recent development in liver transplantation has been the practical application of living donor liver transplantation to children and adults awaiting liver transplantation.

Recipient evaluation

Potential candidates

Patients with acute or chronic end-stage liver disease who show signs of continued hepatic decompensation despite medical management, and patients with certain inherited metabolic diseases that are reversible by liver replacement, may be considered for liver transplantation. Patient selection is paramount to the overall success of liver transplantation. Thus the procedure is contraindicated in individuals who would not be expected to gain a long-term benefit. The most common indications for liver transplantation for treatment of end-stage liver disease include hepatic parenchymal diseases such as post-necrotic cirrhosis from viral and non–viral causes, including hepatitis C and hepatitis B as well as certain medications or toxins, cryptogenic cirrhosis or autoimmune hepatitis. Patients with alcoholic cirrhosis are considered if there is substantial evidence of reform and a low risk of recidivism. Most transplant centers require patients to refrain from all substance use for 6 months, and to participate in a substance recovery program prior to qualifying for transplantation (see Box 5.1). Acute hepatic necrosis in which there is global destruction of hepatic parenchyma requires urgent transplantation. In this setting patients will generally die within 7–10 days if a transplant is not performed. In most cases the etiology of death is cerebral edema and/or multisystem organ failure. Causes of acute hepatic necrosis (fulminant hepatic failure) include hepatitis A, B, C or delta,

---

Box 5.1 Common indications for liver transplantation

Cirrhosis
Viral, cryptogenic, autoimmune, medication, toxin

Cirrhosis (viral)
Hepatitis BsAg+, hepatitis C, hepatitis delta

Cirrhosis (alcohol)
Patients with alcoholic cirrhosis are considered for transplant if they meet current criteria for abstinence and reform:
• abstinence from alcohol for 6 months;
• ongoing participation in a formal substance abuse treatment program;
• presence of adequate psychosocial supports as determined by social service and psychiatry consultants.

Cirrhosis (cholestatic)
Primary sclerosing cholangitis, primary biliary cirrhosis, secondary biliary cirrhosis, biliary atresia (most common indication in children)

Metabolic diseases
Hemachromatosis, Wilson's disease, alpha-1-antitrypsin deficiency, glycogen storage disease, tyrosinemia, familial amyloidotic polyneuropathy, other metabolic disorders treatable by liver replacement

Acute hepatic necrosis
Viral (hepatitis A, B, C, delta), drug, toxin, Wilson's disease, cryptogenic

---

Wilson's disease, and drug exposure or toxin ingestion. Hepatic necrosis due to acetaminophen poisoning is a major etiology of fulminant hepatic failure in many countries. Generally, ingestion of more than 5 g of acetaminophen in less than 24 h is necessary to induce hepatic failure, although in combination with other toxins, especially alcohol, far less acetaminophen is required to induce significant injury.

Exclusion criteria

Conditions that would probably result in graft failure or patient death should be excluded by the formal evaluation process. Patients with active substance abuse are poor candidates for liver transplantation due to the risk of recurrent hepatic injury, as well as the ethical issues of allocation of a limited resource. The outcome of hepatic transplantation in patients with active systemic sepsis most often involves early postoperative demise due to multisystem organ failure and hemodynamic insufficiency. Some patients with combined liver and other end-stage organ disease may have a satisfactory outcome after combined transplantation (e.g. of a liver and a kidney for concomitant liver and renal failure). However, each patient should be evaluated on the basis of the likelihood of long-term success following the combined transplant. In general, patients who require a thoracic transplant (heart or lung) in combination with a liver transplant have fared extremely poorly and should be viewed as poor candidates. Patients with advanced primary hepatocellular carcinoma (stage 3 or 4), as well as those with metastatic disease from other primary cancers, are also poor candidates. Older patients (over 65 years of age) are evaluated on a case-by-case basis. Chronological age is not as important as the coexistence of other medical conditions or severe debilitation which may hamper satisfactory recovery. Screening for occult cancer in the older liver transplant candidate is paramount, as the presence of a malignancy outside the liver would be a contraindication to liver transplantation. Patients who are infected with the human immunodeficiency virus (HIV–1) are also poor candidates for liver transplantation, due to the risk of opportunistic infections in this population (see Box 5.2). Some patients who are treated with protease inhibitors have undetectable levels of HIV DNA in their serum. The risk of transplantation in this population is currently being investigated.

Box 5.2 Contraindications to liver transplantation

Absolute
Active substance abuse
Systemic sepsis
Life-limiting coexisting medical condition: advanced cardiac, pulmonary, renal, neurologic or other systemic disease
Uncontrolled psychiatric disorder
Presence of malignancy outside the liver
Inability to comply with immunosuppression regimen
Patients unable to participate in long-term adherence to a disciplined medical regimen

Relative
Patients with severe hemodynamic and multisystem organ compromise requiring substantial pressor, ventilatory and renal support should undergo daily evaluation of the appropriateness of liver transplantation while maximal medical supports are instituted
Primary hepatic malignancy (stage 3 or 4)
Age > 75 years
HIV positive
Stage IV coma

Each potential candidate is evaluated by a multidisciplinary group of consultants who comprise a liver transplant screening committee. Each member of the consultant group assesses patients from their unique perspective with regard to any pre-transplant concerns or postoperative management issues that may affect the outcome. These consultants include physician specialists in transplantation surgery, hepatology, anesthesiology and psychiatry. Additional consultants are involved when this is indicated by medical status or coexisting diseases, and their fields of expertise include infectious disease, cardiology, nephrology, pulmonary medicine or blood bank/hematology.

In addition to the consultant interviews, radiology and laboratory investigations are performed in order to elucidate the cause and nature of the patient's liver disease, assess their functional capacity, determine the patency of the hepatic vascular supply, exclude liver masses and identify coexisting medical conditions that would compromise patient or graft survival. A complete biochemical and liver profile, hepatitis serologies, virology studies (including cytomegalovirus, Epstein–Barr virus and HIV), complete blood count and coagulation profiles are obtained. An assessment of blood type and the presence of any special transfusion-related problems should be performed. Pulmonary and cardiac functional studies, as well as routine cancer screening, are also performed.

Care of the patient with chronic liver disease: management of common complications

Referral for transplant consideration is usually prompted by the development of one of the complications of end-stage liver disease. These include variceal hemorrhage, decreased hepatic synthetic function (jaundice, prolonged prothrombin time, hypoalbuminemia), encephalopathy, intractable ascites, spontaneous bacterial peritonitis, progressive fatigue or muscle wasting.

Variceal hemorrhage

Patients with upper gastrointestinal bleeding should be admitted to the intensive-care unit and undergo emergent endoscopy. If appropriate, sclerotherapy or banding is performed for the treatment of varices. For those patients who fail medical and endoscopic therapy, a transjugular intrahepatic portosystemic shunt (TIPS) is used to lower portal venous pressures and control variceal hemorrhage. Surgical shunts should be reserved for the patient with Child's class A cirrhosis with variceal bleeding that is refractory to endoscopic treatment. The treatment of refractory variceal bleeding has been dramatically changed by the introduction of TIPS in 1990 by Palmaz. Numerous reports have shown the efficacy of TIPS in the management of patients with variceal bleeding secondary to portal hypertension, as well as other indications such as refractory ascites, hepatic hydrothorax and Budd–Chiari syndrome.

The procedure is performed by puncturing the right internal jugular vein and advancing a curved needle into the superior vena cava through the right atrium and into the right or middle hepatic vein. The needle is advanced across the hepatic parenchyma until an intrahepatic branch of the portal vein is identified and punctured. The stent is a tubular wire mesh mounted on a balloon catheter that is dilated once it is in position in order to open the bridge of hepatic parenchymal tissue between the hepatic vein and the portal vein. This intrahepatic portal venous systemic shunt effectively reduces the portal pressure and the risk of further bleeding. The stent is generally 8 to 12 mm in diameter and is dilated to achieve a portal pressure gradient of less than 12 mmHg in order to eliminate variceal perfusion.

Technical success with TIPS placement can generally be achieved in more than 90% of patients. However, the procedure can result in catastrophic complications in inexperienced hands. Major immediate complications of TIPS placement include intra-abdominal hemorrhage from capsular puncture through the hepatic parenchyma or outside the portal vein. Anecdotally, the procedure is more difficult in those patients whose livers are significantly small and shrunken. Hemobilia and subcapsular bleeding can also occur. Shunt stenosis or thrombosis may occur and must be treated by thrombolysis, balloon dilation or placement of an additional internal stent. In one series, rebleeding occurred in 8% of patients at 6 months and in 18% by 1 year, and the 30-day mortality rate was 3%. Encephalopathy can also be a challenging complication following TIPS placement. The incidence of hepatic encephalopathy depends on several factors, including Child's classification, shunt diameter, history of encephalopathy and age above 65 years. Treatment of post-TIPS encephalopathy should include oral lactulose therapy and, if the condition is severe, occlusion of the stent may be necessary. Hepatic decompensation following TIPS can be a devastating complication that requires urgent transplantation.

Management of TIPS stents should include periodic imaging to diagnose and treat occult dysfunction caused by stent stenosis or thrombosis. Clinical presentation of stenosis or thrombosis of the shunt is often subtle. Duplex ultrasonography is the screening test most often performed. Depending on the method of investigation and the length of follow-up, the incidence of shunt dysfunction is in the range 20–50% at 1 year. In one study, 50% of stents required revision by 1 year for stenotic segments. In general, patients should be screened every 6 months while the stent is in place. Sonographic examination should include evaluation of the stent, portal vein and draining hepatic vein, with an assessment of flow, peak velocity and direction of flow. The detection of shunt stenosis requires a baseline examination to compare changes in peak velocities, as each individual will have different flow characteristics throughout the stent. In one study, temporal changes in peak flow velocity when correlated with angiographic findings showed 93% sensitivity and 77% specificity. However, the isolated peak flow velocities did not correlate. Recurrent variceal bleeding or refractory ascites in this setting should automatically prompt imaging of the TIPS stent to preclude shunt dysfunction. The most reliable examination for symptomatic patients is percutaneous hepatic venography. This test not only enables a direct visualization of stenosis, but also allows measurement of the portal vein-to-stent and stent-to-hepatic vein gradients in order to determine the significance of an apparent narrowing. Portal vein-to-stent gradients should be < 15 mmHg, while the hepatic vein-to-stent gradients should be 0 mmHg. Other angiographic signs of a significant stenosis include retrograde opacification of varices. Clinical presentation of TIPS stenosis may be occult, or it may present with variceal bleeding or ascites. Stenosis is corrected by balloon dilatation or insertion of a second stent within the lumen of the initial stent. Other causes of shunt dysfunction include acute angulation leading to kinking of the stent.

Ascites

All patients with newly diagnosed or worsening ascites should undergo a diagnostic paracentesis if one has not been performed previously. For evaluation, approximately 50 mL of ascitic fluid are withdrawn, and a note is made of the fluid's appearance and color. A laboratory analysis of cell count and differential, total protein, albumin, triglycerides and amylase is performed. Fluid samples are also sent for Gram staining, AFB staining, aerobic, anaerobic, tuberculin and fungal cultures and cytological study. At the time of paracentesis, blood samples are sent for liver biochemical tests, alphafetoprotein, amylase, lipase and thyroid function tests. Other tests that are included in the evaluation of newly diagnosed ascites are urinalysis and urinary electrolytes and protein, and ultrasound examination of the liver with Doppler examination and chest X-ray. Uncomplicated ascites secondary to portal hypertension and cirrhosis is initially treated with the aim of improving hepatic function. All hepatotoxic drugs, including alcohol, are discontinued and attempts are made to improve nutritional status. Sodium restriction to 0.5–1 g of sodium daily, fluid restriction to less than 1 L daily, and bed rest are prescribed. If these measures do not produce a spontaneous diuresis, diuretic therapy is initiated with the goal of fluid loss of 1 L or 1–2 pounds per day. Spironolactone is started at a dose of 100–200 mg PO per day given in a single dose. The diuresis is considered to be suboptimal if the urine sodium concentration is less than 10 mEq/L. The dose of spironolactone may be increased up to 400 mg per day, as long as the creatinine level remains less than 1.8 mg%. If diuresis is not successful with spironolactone, furosemide is added, starting at a dose of 40 mg per day. The dosage may be increased to 160 mg per day in patients with peripheral edema. Patients who are receiving diuretic therapy initially have their serum electrolytes measured every 2–3 days. After the patient has reached a therapeutic dose of diuretics, electrolytes are monitored weekly. Metolazone, 5–20 mg per day, is initiated if adequate diuresis with spironolactone or furosemide is not achieved. Alternative diuretics that can be used if the patient is intolerant of spironolactone, furosemide and metolazone include bumetanide or ethacrynic acid as loop diuretic alternatives, and amiloride as a spironolactone alternative. Spironolactone and amiloride are discontinued if the patient becomes hyperkalemic. Diuretic therapy is discontinued or reduced if the creatinine level exceeds 1.8 mg% or if the patient develops excessive weight loss, dehydration or severe encephalopathy. Hydration in the form of albumin or crystalloid solutions is administered to patients who become dehydrated, and nephrotoxic drugs are avoided.

The options for patients with refractory ascites include therapeutic paracentesis, TIPS and liver transplantation. Therapeutic paracentesis is the first-line therapy in refractory ascites. Between 4 and 10 L of ascitic fluid are removed with each paracentesis. The ascitic fluid is analyzed for cell count and differential. Following therapeutic paracentesis, 6–8 g of sodium-poor albumin are administered per liter of ascitic fluid removed, with a maximum of 75 g of albumin per procedure. In patients who have persistent refractory ascites despite compliance with diet and diuretic therapy, TIPS is considered.

Encephalopathy

Portosystemic encephalopathy (PSE) is characterized by mental status changes, fetor hepaticus or asterixis in a patient with end-stage liver disease. The arterial ammonia level can be measured at the initial diagnosis of hepatic encephalopathy. However, ammonia levels do not always correlate with the severity of encephalopathy. Treatment of PSE includes the identification and correction of any precipitating causes. Sedative drugs are discontinued. Active infection and dehydration are common precipitating factors. Adequate calories (1800–2400 Kcal/day), primarily in the form of glucose or carbohydrates, are provided, and protein intake is restricted to 40 g/day. Vitamins and minerals are replenished, and electrolyte and acid–base imbalances and prerenal azotemia are corrected. As encephalopathy improves, dietary protein intake is increased to 60–110 g/day as tolerated. Amino-acid mixtures which are rich in branched-chain amino acids and low in aromatic amino acids and methionine may be used as a protein source or supplement. Lactulose is administered at oral dosages of 60–120 mg/day to produce two to three soft bowel movements per day. If encephalopathy is refractory to lactulose therapy, neomycin is given orally in doses of 2–6 g/day. It is recognized that prolonged use of this agent may cause renal failure and cranial nerve VIII damage, and for this reason it is used only in selected patients. Both lactulose and neomycin may be administered in an enema form for patients who are unable to tolerate oral intake.

Hepatorenal syndrome

The diagnosis of hepatorenal syndrome is made in the cirrhotic patient if there is progressive azotemia, creatinine levels exceeding 2.5 mg%, oliguria with a urine-to-plasma osmolality ratio of > 0.1, a urinary sodium concentration of < 10 mEq/L and a normal urinalysis. Hepatorenal syndrome is distinct from other types of renal failure such as exposure to nephrotoxins, infection, acute tubular necrosis and obstructive uropathy.

Treatment includes correction of factors that precipitate renal failure. Diuretics are stopped and the intravascular volume loss due to bleeding or dehydration is replaced. Serum electrolytes are corrected and infections are immediately treated. A renal ultrasound examination should exclude obstruction. All patients undergo fluid challenge using sodium-poor albumin or plasma to increase the circulating blood volume. Fluid challenge is best performed with a central venous pressure monitor in place. In patients who do not respond to fluid challenge, dialysis is considered. Continuous venovenous hemodialysis is particularly suitable for the cirrhotic patient, due to the low sytemic vascular resistance and hyperdynamic circulatory state that is characteristic of patients with chronic liver disease.

Spontaneous bacterial peritonitis

Patients with ascites and an ascitic fluid polymorphonuclear count of > 250 cells/mL and no other source of infection are presumed to have spontaneous bacterial peritonitis (SBP). Ascitic fluid and blood are sent for bacterial aerobic and anaerobic culture. Urinalysis and urine culture, chest X-ray and gynecological examination (in women) are performed. Antibiotic therapy is initiated with cefotaxime 1 g every 8 h for a period of 5 days. If multiple organisms are cultured from the ascitic fluid or blood, the patient may have secondary abdominal peritonitis. After intravenous therapy has been completed, patients are started on an oral quinolone as prophylaxis due to the high percentage of patients who develop recurrent SBP.

Donor evaluation

Donor organ allocation in the USA

In 1984, the United States Congress enacted the National Organ Transplant Act (NOTA), which established a national network for organ distribution. From this legislation was born the Organ Procurement and Transplant Network (OPTN). The government contract for the operation of the OPTN was granted to the United Network for Organ Sharing (UNOS) in 1986. The principle of liver allocation policy is equitable distribution based on medical utility and need, with current liver allocation modifications instituted in 1997. The modifications established minimum criteria that patients must meet in order to be listed for liver transplantation. Patients who have less than a 90% expectation of surviving for 1 year without transplantation are eligible for placement on waiting-lists. For patients with cirrhosis, a score of at least 7 as derived from the Child–Turcotte–Pugh Classification is required for listing (see Table 5.1). This would correlate with a Child's B or C classification. Cirrhotic patients with a single episode of gastrointestinal bleeding caused by portal hypertension or an episode of spontaneous

Table 5.1. Child–Turcotte–Pugh (CTP) scoring system

	Points		
	1	**2**	**3**
Encephalopathy	None	1–2	3–4
Ascites	Absent	Slight	Moderate
Bilirubin (mg/dL)	< 2.0	2–3	> 3.0
Bilirubin (mg/dL)*	< 4.0	4–10	> 10
Albumin (gm/dL)	> 3.5	2.8–3.5	< 2.8
Prothrombin time (s)	< 4.0	4–6	> 6.0
International normalized ratio (INR)	< 1.7	1.7–2.3	> 2.3

*In cases of primary biliary cirrhosis or primary sclerosing cholangitis.

bacterial peritonitis are exempt from the need to meet a minimum score, and can be listed independently of their Child's score. Disease-specific criteria for patients with cholestatic liver disease or fulminant hepatic failure were also established. For patients with fulminant hepatic failure, these criteria include the development of encephalopathy within 8 weeks of the onset of jaundice without prior liver disease. Regional Review Boards were established to petition for listing patients who did not meet these minimum criteria, and to monitor the integrity of the system.

Once patients are listed for transplantation with UNOS, organs are allocated using a local, regional and national priority system based on degree of medical urgency, blood-type similarity and weight stratification. Modifications to the geographically based allocation scheme are being developed to broaden the donor pool for potential recipients in an attempt to reduce the incidence of death while on the waiting-list.

Recipient surgery

A bilateral subcostal incision with a xiphoid midline extension is performed. Hepatectomy is begun by dividing the falciform ligament and coronary ligament to the level of the vena cava. The left and right coronary ligaments are divided. The hepatogastric ligament is then incised to permit further mobilization of the left lobe and assessment of the portal vein and hepatic artery. The common bile duct is identified and ligated high in the hilum. Dissection around the common hepatic duct is kept to a minimum in order to prevent disturbance of its blood supply. The hepatic artery and portal vein are skeletonized to their bifurcations, and the right lobe of the liver is then fully mobilized.

The liver is separated from the vena cava in order to anasta-mose the donor liver using the piggyback technique. This is achieved by dividing the small branches from the vena cava to the posterior right lobe and caudate lobe until the main hepatic veins are encountered. The right hepatic vein is divided between clamps and oversewn. Alternatively, a caval–caval anastamosis between the donor and recipient vena cava can be performed. In this case, the right adrenal vein is ligated and divided at its entry into the vena cava. The vena cava should now be freely mobile with the liver.

Vascular clamps are placed across the previously mobilized supra- and infrahepatic vena cava. For the piggyback technique, where the recipient vena cava is preserved, a clamp is placed across the common orifice of the middle and left hepatic veins. The middle and left hepatic veins are transected below their confluence with the vena cava, and the septum between the left and middle hepatic veins is divided to create a single opening. If a caval–caval technique is used, an incision is made in the liver overlying the vena cava, and the liver substance is bluntly dissected away from the hepatic veins. The vena cava is then tran-sected at this level. The liver is reflected cephalad and the infra-hepatic vena cava is transected where it enters the liver. The diseased liver is now removed.

The new donor liver is then sewn into place by completion of the caval anastomoses, followed by the portal venous and hepatic arterial anastomoses. The donor gallbladder is excised. The biliary anastomosis is created using an end-to-end choledocho–chole-dochostomy or a Roux-en-Y choledochojejunostomy. The latter technique is used if the recipient bile duct is unsuitable, or in cases of sclerosing cholangitis.

Donor surgery

The cadaver donor operation is performed through a midline inci-sion. The donor liver is visually inspected for mass lesions and degree of steatosis. The falciform, left and right triangular liga-ments are divided. The gastrohepatic omentum is divided, taking care to inspect the region for a replaced left hepatic artery. The dissection of the hepatoduodenal ligament then proceeds with identification of the hepatic artery and dissection proximally to the level of the celiac axis. Again the porta is inspected for the presence of a replaced right hepatic artery originating from the superior mesenteric artery. The common bile duct is divided and the portal vein is dissected free. Cannulae are inserted into the infrarenal aorta, inferior mesenteric vein and inferior vena cava. Following systemic heparinization, the abdominal organs are flushed with preservative solution and topically cooled with ice saline. The liver is excised and prepared for shipment.

Living donor liver transplantation

Between 1989 and 1999 over 1000 living donor liver transplant operations have been performed globally, with most of these being undertaken in Asia, the USA and Western Europe. The procedure was first accepted for pediatric liver transplantation, but was later applied to adult recipients awaiting liver transplantation. Live donor liver transplantation (LDLT) using a left lateral segment for pediatric recipients has become a routine and successful alternative to cadaveric transplantation, and has markedly reduced the waiting-list mortality rate. In addition, the safety of this technique for the living donor has been established. LDLT is an outgrowth of the techniques of reduced–size and split-liver transplantation from cadaveric donors. In reduced-size liver transplants, the cadaveric liver is cut down to match more closely the size of the recipient liver. In split-liver transplantation, the donor liver is divided between two recipients. Traditionally, in LDLT the donor contributes a portion of the right or left lobe for transplantation. In children weighing less than 30 kg this has generally been the left lateral segment. In larger children the left or right lobe is satisfactory, while in adults the best results from LDLT have been obtained from right lobe grafts. The donor liver subsequently regenerates, while the successfully transplanted liver will normalize its size to that of the recipient's body.

Postoperative management

Following completion of the operation, the patient is transferred to the intensive-care unit and extubated when standard extubation criteria are met. Blood analysis, including total bilirubin, aspartate aminotransferase (AST), alanine aminotransferase (ALT) and alkaline phosphatase, is obtained immediately after the operation, and every 4 h for 24 h and then daily for the uncomplicated patient. A Doppler ultrasound study is performed if there is not adequate graft function within 6–12 h of operation to allow evaluation of hepatic artery and portal vein patency.

Complications

Primary non-function

Primary non-function (PNF) is a devastating condition that develops immediately postoperatively when the graft fails to function. The syndrome is characterized by increasing prothrombin time, AST and ALT, poor bile production and neurologic or renal impairment, and it occurs in 5% of patients following transplant. The etiology of PNF is thought to be multifactorial. However, there is a marked association of the phenomenon with donor organs that are severely steatotic (fatty), and with prolonged use of high-dose pressors in donors prior to organ procurement. Urgent retransplantation is often necessary. The use of intravenous PGE1 (alprostadil), 10 µg/h → 40 µg/h, has provided some therapeutic benefits. Exclusion of other causes of early graft dysfunction, especially hepatic artery/portal vein thrombosis, must be documented (see Figure 5.1).

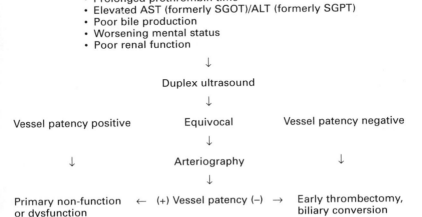

Primary graft non-function

- Prolonged prothrombin time
- Elevated AST (formerly SGOT)/ALT (formerly SGPT)
- Poor bile production
- Worsening mental status
- Poor renal function

↓

Duplex ultrasound

↓

Vessel patency positive   Equivocal   Vessel patency negative

↓

Arteriography

↓

Primary non-function   ←   (+) Vessel patency (−)   →   Early thrombectomy,
or dysfunction   biliary conversion

To hepaticojejunostomy

↓

PGE1, therapy (10–40 µg/h), urgent retransplant

Figure 5.1 Algorithm for evaluation of poor graft function. AST, aspartate aminotransferase; ALT, alanine aminotransferase

Hemorrhage

Bleeding in the immediate postoperative period is generally caused by inadequate hemostasis of raw peritoneal surfaces, or by early graft dysfunction with dysfibrogenemia. A primary fibrinolytic process can occur which may be responsive to Amicar (ε-aminocaproic acid) or aprotinin. Fibrinogen and platelet levels are monitored and replaced if necessary to keep fibrinogen levels at > 100 and platelet levels at > 70 000. Bloody drain output of > 500 mL/h × 2 h often necessitates re-exploration. Occasionally, no surgical bleeding points can be identified, in which case perihepatic packs are left around the liver until correction of coagulopathy is achieved medically.

Hepatic artery thrombosis/portal vein thrombosis

Early and late graft dysfunction can be caused by hepatic artery or portal vein thrombosis. Hepatic artery thrombosis is by far the more common occurrence. A high index of suspicion for this catastrophe allows early diagnosis and prompt intervention. The spectrum of presentation of vascular compromise is quite variable. The commonest biochemical abnormality is elevation of AST (SGOT). As the liver has a dual blood supply to hepatic parenchyma, thrombosis of a single vessel can be subtle. However, the bile ducts are solely dependent on the hepatic artery for perfusion. Thus hepatic artery thrombosis can result in leakage from the biliary anastomosis, biliary strictures or intrahepatic bile lakes and abscesses. Vascular thrombosis can easily be detected by duplex ultrasound scanning of the liver. If this scan is equivocal, then prompt arteriography can be used for confirmation, followed by urgent exploration. Early thrombosis necessitates an attempt at thrombectomy in order to restore patency. In addition, operative conversion of the biliary anastomosis to Roux-en-Y hepaticojejunostomy prevents inevitable disaster due to breakdown of the choledocho–choledochostomy. Late asymptomatic thrombosis usually requires cholangiography to exclude an occult stricture.

Acute rejection

Up to 60% of patients may experience an episode of acute rejection after liver transplantation. Early rejection episodes normally occur at 7 to 10 days post-transplant. The initial signs of rejection include an increase in bilirubin, low-grade fever, malaise and decreased bile production. Significant elevations in AST (SGOT) and ALT (SGPT) activity usually signal an aggressive rejection episode, and this can be confirmed by liver biopsy. Lymphocyte infiltration of the portal tract with bile duct injury, eosinophilia and endothelialitis is pathognomonic for acute rejection. Rejection episodes are treated with a 2-day methylprednisolone bolus (1 g) followed by a steroid recycle. OKT3 is utilized for biopsy-proven steroid-resistant rejection or aggressive rejection.

Infectious complications

The biliary tree remains the main source of early post-transplant bacterial infections. Leaks from the bile-duct anastomosis can result in intra-abdominal abscesses. Furthermore, cholangitis can occur, and is difficult to eradicate if an indwelling T-tube or biliary stent is present. Urinary tract infection, pneumonia and catheter-related infections can also complicate the early postoperative period, due to bacterial infection. Cytomegalovirus (CMV) is the commonest viral infection post-transplant. Patients at high risk for CMV include those treated with OKT3, retransplants and CMV-negative recipients who receive a liver allograft from a CMV-positive donor. The commonest presentation of CMV in this population is CMV hepatitis. Typically, elevation of liver function tests (LFTs) together with spiking fevers, arthralgia, myalgia and leukopenia is characteristic. Liver biopsy will often demonstrate intranuclear inclusion bodies and micro-abscesses. Other common sites of involvement include the gastrointestinal tract and lungs.

Prophylaxis of high-risk recipients with CMV immune globulin combined with gancyclovir is utilized. In addition, gancyclovir is used for treatment of active disease. Other members of the herpes virus family, particularly herpes simplex, varicella zoster and Epstein–Barr virus, can produce significant post-transplant morbidity. Treatment with oral or intravenous acyclovir is employed. Fungal infections post-transplant can also be a grave source of morbidity. The spectrum of involvement ranges from oral and esophageal involvement to fungal sepsis. *Candida*, *Cryptococcus* and *Aspergillus* are the commonest offending organisms. Protozoal infections are quite rare, since trimethoprim–sulfamethoxazole has been employed as prophylaxis for *Pneumocystis* infection. Trimethaprim–sulfamethoxazole is given once a day for 6 months or until the prednisone dose is ≤ 10 mg/day.

Immunosuppression

The liver is a more immunopermissive organ than the kidney, pancreas or heart. Thus the intensity of immunosuppression is generally less in recipients of liver allografts than in recipients of kidney, pancreas or heart allografts. The standard of maintenance immunosuppression is a balanced multi-drug regimen based on cyclosporine or tacrolimus. Both of these drugs have significant nephrotoxic properties, but tacrolimus appears to cause more renal dysfunction at therapeutic doses. Subsequently, renal function determines which regimen is utilized. Patients are routinely given methylprednisolone, 500 mg intraoperatively at the time of graft reperfusion. The specific maintenance regimen that is utilized is determined on the first postoperative morning depending on the assessment of early renal function.

Dosing guidelines

In patients who initially demonstrate good liver and renal function, common regimens involve a starting oral dose of 0.1–0.15 mg/kg/day tacrolimus in divided doses, starting 24 h after liver reperfusion. For patients with poor graft function (transaminases > 2500, international normalized ratio (INR) > 2 and/or inadequate bile output), it is advisable to start with a reduced dose of tacrolimus (0.05–0.075 mg/kg/day). Lower doses of tacrolimus are also warranted in patients who receive grafts of marginal quality (prolonged ischemia, older donors > 60 years of age, steatotic grafts). Reduced hepatic metabolism will result in higher circulating levels and possible toxicity. If toxicity occurs in recipients of older organs, the tacrolimus dosage should be decreased further. Patients with poor renal function may benefit from delaying tacrolimus therapy for 72 h, until the urine output exceeds 60 mL/h or the serum creatinine concentration decreases. Tacrolimus should also be delayed in comatose patients with acute or acute-on-chronic liver failure who demonstrate stage III to IV encephalopathy until awakening. Induction therapy with OKT3 may be appropriate for these patients or for those who manifest severe renal failure.

Prednisone tapering and monitoring

The concomitant use of steroids in tacrolimus-treated patients should follow a relatively rapid taper. On the first postoperative day, 100–200 mg/day IV is administered, divided into four doses. This is tapered by approximately 25% every 48 h until a dosage of 20 mg/day is reached by postoperative day 9. Thereafter, the steroid dose is tapered, with the target dose of oral prednisone being 10–15 mg/day by postoperative day 30, 7.5–10 mg/day by day 60, 5–7.5 mg/day by day 90, and 2.5–5 mg/day by day 180. After 1 year, it may be possible to discontinue steroids altogether in selected patients.

Outcome

Outcomes following liver transplantation are quite good. The national 1-year and 3-year graft survival rates are 80% and 70%, respectively. The corresponding patient survival rates are 86% and 76%, respectively. Recipients are able to return to work and contribute to society. By 5 years after the transplant, over 50% of patients are gainfully employed.

Further reading

American Medical Association. 1968: *Definition of irreversible coma. Report of the Ad Hoc Committee of the Harvard Medical School to Examine the Definition of Brain Death. Journal of the American Medical Association* **205**, 337–40.

Cosimi AB. 1991: Update in liver transplantation. *Transplantation Proceedings* **23**, 2083–90.

Haskal ZJ, Pentecost MJ, Soulen MC *et al*. 1994: Transjugular intrahepatic portosystemic shunt stenosis and revision: early and midterm results. *American Journal of Radiology* **163**, 439–44.

Kuo PC, Plotkin JS, Gaine S *et al*. 1999: Portopulmonary hypertension and the liver transplant candidate. *Transplantation* **67**, 1087–93.

Lucey MR, Brown KA, Everson GT *et al*. 1997: Minimal criteria for placement on the liver transplant waiting-list: a report of a national conference organized by the American Society of Transplant Physicians and the American Association for the Study of Liver Diseases. *Liver Transplantation and Surgery* **3**, 628–37.

Plotkin JS, Scott VL, Puma A *et al*. 1996: Morbidity and mortality in patients with coronary artery disease undergoing orthotopic liver transplantation. *Liver Transplantation and Surgery* **2**, 426–30.

Plotkin JS, Kuo PC, Rubin LJ *et al*. 1998: Successful use of chronic epoprostenol as a bridge to liver transplantation in severe portopulmonary hypertension. *Transplantation* **65**, 457–59.

Richter GM, Noeldge G, Palmaz JC *et al*. 1990: Transjugular intrahepatic portocaval stent shunt: preliminary clinical results. *Radiology* **174**, 1027–30.

Rossle M, Haag K, Ochs A *et al.* 1994: The transjugular intrahepatic portosystemic stent–shunt procedure for variceal bleeding. *New England Journal of Medicine* **330**, 165–71.

Starzl TE, Marcioro TL, Von Kaulla KN *et al.* 1963: Homo-transplantation of the liver in humans. *Surgery, Gynecology and Obstetrics* **117**, 659–76.

Pancreas transplantation

6

Eugene Schweitzer, Alan Farney and
Elsie Allen

Introduction

The modern era of diabetes management began in 1922 with the first clinical use of insulin. Before then, most insulinopenic diabetics had little hope of survival for more than a few years. Since then, the death rate among diabetics due to coma has been reduced to less than 1%. It is a miracle of modern medicine that the majority of diabetics can now expect a relatively normal lifespan.

Despite the recent advances in the treatment of diabetes, patients still experience a suboptimal quality of life because of dietary restrictions, as well as the need for glucose monitoring and insulin injections. Some cannot achieve glycemic stability despite their best efforts, and are then compelled to live with possibly fatal hypoglycemic reactions or accept the consequences of chronic hyperglycemia, including retinopathy, nephropathy, neuropathy and accelerated atherosclerosis. Many of these unfortunate patients helplessly resign themselves to progressive mixtures of dialysis, blindness, lower extremity pain and numbness, nausea, vomiting, diarrhea, constipation, stroke, heart attack and amputation.

Pancreas transplantation can vastly improve the diabetic's quality of life by normalizing the blood sugar, thereby reducing the risk of secondary complication progression.

Diabetes mellitus

Diabetes mellitus is defined as a group of metabolic diseases characterized by hyperglycemia resulting from defects in insulin secretion, insulin action, or both. There are many pathologic processes that lead to diabetes by either destruction of pancreatic β-cells or diminished tissue responses to insulin. These complex

---

Box 6.1 Criteria for the diagnosis of diabetes mellitus

Symptoms of diabetes (polyuria, polydipsia, unexplained weight loss) plus random plasma glucose concentration $\geq$ 200 mg/dL

or

Fasting plasma glucose concentration $\geq$ 126 mg/dL (7.0 mol/L)

or

Serum glucose concentration $\geq$ 200 mg/dL during an oral glucose tolerance test (75 g anhydrous glucose)

---

abnormalities result in the common clinical feature of hyperglycemia (see Box 6.1). There are currently over 50 heterogeneous etiologic classifications of diabetes, including autoimmune, genetic, polyendocrine, gestational, infectious and drug-related disorders. However, the vast majority of cases of diabetes fall into two broad categories.

The first category is type 1 diabetes, the cause of which is an absolute deficiency of insulin secretion. It is this group of diabetics that provides candidates for pancreas transplantation. There are between one and two million type 1 diabetics in the USA. Over 30 000 new cases are diagnosed each year, and the incidence is rising, the majority of these cases being due to β-cell destruction. These patients often have little or no endogenous production of insulin. Most but not all type 1 diabetics have serum antibodies to islet proteins, including cytoplasmic islet-cell autoantibodies (ICA), and autoantibodies reacting with insulin, such as GAD65 (glutamic acid decarboxylase, an islet neuroendocrine enzyme) and ICA512/IA-2 (an islet membrane granule protein). One or more of these autoantibodies are present in 85–90% of type 1 diabetics when hyperglycemia is initially detected. Association with particular HLA haplotypes indicates a genetic predisposition. In Western countries, approximately one in 300 individuals develops type 1 diabetes, compared with approximately one in 20 first degree relatives of affected individuals. However, the role of environmental factors is supported by the fact that the concordance rate of development of type 1 diabetes in monozygotic twins is less than 70%. Immune-mediated diabetes commonly occurs in childhood and adolescence, but can occur at any age, even into the eighth and ninth decades. Children and adolescents typically present with ketoacidosis as the first manifestation of the disease. Adults may retain sufficient β-cell function to prevent ketoacidosis for many years. Although patients are rarely obese when they develop type 1 diabetes, obesity is not incompatible with the diagnosis.

The second category is type 2 diabetes, which is much more prevalent than type 1. This term is used for patients who show insulin resistance, and who usually have a relative rather than absolute insulin deficiency. Patients with this form of diabetes may have insulin levels that appear normal or even elevated. However, high glucose levels in these patients should result in even higher insulin levels had their β-cell function been normal. Therefore insulin secretion is defective in these patients and insufficient to compensate for insulin resistance. Specific etiologies of this form of diabetes are unknown. Although the genetics of type 2 diabetes are complex, the genetic component is even stronger than in type 1. The risk of developing type 2 diabetes increases with increasing age, obesity, lack of physical activity, and history of gestational diabetes, and is higher in certain racial and ethnic groups. Most type 2 diabetics are obese, and obesity itself causes insulin resistance. In the absence of the stress of another illness, ketoacidosis is rare in this setting.

Whatever the cause of diabetes, treatment goals are similar, namely to prevent acute consequences and chronic complications of hyperglycemia. Acutely, untreated hyperglycemia can cause polyuria, polydipsia, weight loss, blurred vision, non-ketotic hyperosmolar syndrome and ketoacidosis. Chronic hyperglycemia, as manifested by an elevated glycoslyated hemoglobin (Hgb-A_{1C}) level, causes permanent tissue damage. The mechanisms by which glucose damages tissues include glycosylation of proteins and other macromolecules, and excess production of toxic polyol compounds. Patients with chronic hyperglycemia are at increased risk for secondary complications, the severity of which is proportional to the average degree of serum glucose elevation. Maintenance of euglycemia prevents complications, including impaired growth and increased susceptibility to infection, retinopathy with possible blindness, nephropathy with risk of renal failure, peripheral neuropathy with foot ulcers, amputations and Charcot joints, autonomic neuropathy with gastroparesis, constipation or diarrhea, urinary retention, orthostatic hypotension, sexual dysfunction, accelerated atherosclerosis with ischemia and amputation of extremities, stroke, and myocardial infarction.

Medical treatment currently available includes dietary restrictions, weight loss, exercise, administration of subcutaneous insulin by periodic injection or continuous infusion, and oral hypoglycemic agents which either stimulate insulin release from a functioning pancreas or sensitize tissues to the action of insulin. The choice of treatment depends on the capacity of the patient's pancreas to produce insulin and the degree of tissue resistance to its actions.

History of diabetes and pancreas transplantation

Descriptions of disease states resembling diabetes date back thousands of years (see Table 6.1). However, until the twentieth century, physicians had little idea what caused the disease and very few useful treatments to offer. Patients who are now classified

Table 6.1 Milestones in diabetes and pancreas transplantation

Year	Milestone
1550 BC	Beer's papyrus describes a polyuric state resembling diabetes
400 AD	Indian physicians Suzutan and Charka note that diabetic urine has a sweet taste
1776	Dobson demonstrates that the sweet substance in urine is sugar
1788	Crawley first implicates the pancreas in diabetes by finding a shrivelled pancreas with stones in a diabetic patient at autopsy
1869	Medical student Paul Langerhans identifies pancreatic islets, but does not understand their function
1889	Minkowski and von Mering demonstrate the importance of the pancreas in diabetes by showing that the urine of pancreatectomized dogs contains large amounts of glucose. They successfully treat the dogs with pancreatic material
1910	Jean de Meyer gives the name 'insulin' to the hypothetical glucose-lowering hormone that he believed was produced by the islets of Langerhans
1922	Banting, Best, McLeod and Collip isolate insulin and treat their first diabetic patient, Leonard Thompson
1923	Improved commercial extraction techniques make insulin widely available
1955	Sulfonylurea oral hypoglycemic agents become available, and the structure of insulin is delineated
1962	The first successful non-identical twin kidney transplants are performed using azathioprine and prednisone immunosuppression, ushering in the era of cadaver solid organ transplantation
1966	Lillehei and Kelly perform the first whole pancreas transplant in humans. Najarian demonstrates that kidney transplantation can be performed safely in diabetics, thereby making diabetics with renal failure acceptable candidates
1978	First successful islet transplant in humans
1982	Cyclosporine becomes available and dramatically improves the results of all types of solid organ transplants
1993	The Diabetes Control and Complications Trial reports that glucose control correlates inversely with the progression of diabetic complications
1995	Tacrolimus and mycophenolate mofetil enter clinical usage

as type 1 diabetics usually died prior to or shortly after diagnosis. Early physicians interpreted the polyuria as an indication that it was the kidneys that were diseased. In fact, the word 'diabetes' comes from the Greek root meaning 'to run through'. It had long been known that urine from these patients contained a sweet substance. 'Mellitus' is derived from the Greek root for 'honey.' It was not until the eighteenth century that elevated glucose levels were found in the serum, suggesting that diabetes was a systemic disorder. It was also noted that a temporary improvement could be achieved by starvation diets that were low in carbohydrates and high in protein and fat. However, this treatment produced patients who were literally living skeletons. Although a role for the pancreas in diabetes was suggested in the eighteenth century, it was not proven until the experiments of Minkowski and von Mering at the end of the nineteenth century.

Insulin was first identified and used clinically in 1922. With insulin, diabetics could now be kept alive for many years. Advances in understanding of the pathophysiology, epidemiology and molecular biology of diabetes, together with improvements in glucose monitoring, insulin formulations and the development of oral hypoglycemic agents, have drastically improved the survival of diabetic patients. At the same time, however, a completely new set of problems emerged for diabetic patients. The threat of imminent death was replaced by the threat of debilitating secondary complications. Although the role of chronic hyperglycemia in the development of these problems was debated for years, a large trial sponsored by the National Institutes of Health, published in 1993, finally proved the long-term benefits of maintaining normal blood glucose levels. Since then, efforts have been directed towards finding combinations of therapies that work best to achieve stable euglycemia for the individual diabetic patient.

The role of transplantation in the management of diabetics started with kidney transplants. Apart from those few cases that involved identical twins, kidney transplantation first became feasible in 1962 when azathioprine and prednisone were first used together clinically. Diabetics were initially considered too 'high-risk' to undergo transplantation. However, after Najarian and Simmons published acceptable results in these patients, kidney transplantation became the preferred renal replacement therapy. Diabetes now constitutes the leading cause of renal failure in the USA, and these patients have benefited from recent improvements, especially with regard to immunosuppression and antimicrobial agents.

The first human pancreas transplant was performed in 1966 at the University of Minnesota. The graft was a segmental transplant with exocrine drainage into the bowel and it functioned for 2 months. A total of 49 transplants were performed during the ensuing 10 years, but early enthusiasm was dampened by very low success rates, caused in part by suboptimal surgical techniques and inadequate immunosuppression. In contrast to kidney transplantation, in which the modern techniques had been worked out far in advance of the first clinical transplants, it was not until many years after the first clinical pancreas transplants that the surgical techniques matured.

A major problem during early transplantation was dealing with pancreatic exocrine secretions. In 1976, Dubemard attempted to obliterate the secretions of the pancreas by injecting the pancreatic duct with silicone. However, this technique resulted in pancreatitis, increasing the risk of thrombosis and infection, and causing extensive fibrosis involving both exocrine and endocrine tissue. Others simply left the duct open to allow the exocrine secretions to drain freely into the peritoneal cavity, which caused pancreatic ascites, and sometimes extensive peritoneal inflammation. In 1976, Gliedmann proposed the technique of suturing the pancreatic duct to the recipient's ureter. Although the first case was a success, most subsequent cases were not. However, this led to the modern techniques in which exocrine secretions are drained into the urinary bladder, an approach that was initially popularized by Sollinger. A button of duodenum surrounding the pancreatic duct was initially sutured to the dome of the urinary bladder. However, it later became evident that it was simpler to suture a segment of duodenum to the bladder as a conduit for secretions, and this is the technique most commonly used today.

Another technical obstacle to early pancreas transplantation was the fact that the liver and pancreas share both the celiac arterial trunk and the portal vein, posing the problem of how to procure a transplantable pancreas from a multiorgan donor. An early solution was to transplant only the tail of the pancreas, which contains the highest density of islets, although this technique was associated with a relatively high complication rate. The problem of vascular supply and venous drainage has since been resolved by reconstruction of the pancreatic arterial blood supply with an iliac artery Y-graft from the donor.

Acute rejection was another problem that plagued early transplant patients. The rate of acute rejection has always been higher and early diagnosis more difficult to make in pancreas transplants than in kidney transplants. This was especially true when only azathioprine and high-dose prednisone were available for maintenance immunosuppression, but the situation has improved with the advent of cyclosporine, tacrolimus and mycophenolate mofetil. In contrast to kidney transplantation, where serum creatinine is a sensitive indicator of acute rejection, no laboratory test is a reliable indicator of early pancreas rejection. By the time the plasma glucose level begins to rise, it has become almost irreversible. A significant advance occurred when it was recognized that simultaneous transplantation of a kidney with a pancreas in diabetics with renal failure resulted in better pancreas graft survival than when the pancreas was transplanted alone. This was partly due to the fact that rejection of the kidney, which could be detected by monitoring creatinine levels, correlated with the presence of pancreas rejection. In the early days it was also difficult to confirm rejection due to fear of bleeding complications and duct injury resulting from a biopsy. Transcystoscopic pancreas biopsy was useful because it allowed an injured duct to drain harmlessly into the urinary bladder. However, the yield of this technique was low. The modern method of ultrasound-guided percutaneous pancreas biopsy did not become standard until the 1990s.

A final technical issue that has yet to be resolved is the optimum location of the pancreas transplant. The standard location has been the pelvis, with vascular anastomoses made with the recipient iliac vessels. This approach has been challenged by Gaber, who has advocated transplantation to a central abdominal location, with venous drainage to the recipient portal vein. Although the latter technique is associated with lower systemic insulin levels, and possibly a lower risk for progression of atherosclerosis, the true risks and benefits of this technique are still being investigated.

During the 1980s, whole organ pancreas transplants became increasingly successful, such that it is now possible to achieve graft survival rates similar to those for other solid organ transplants. However, in contrast to other transplant recipients, up to 25% of pancreas transplant patients suffer significant postoperative morbidity due to coexisting morbid conditions. During the past few decades, islet cell transplantation has been attempted as an alternative to whole organ transplantation. Unfortunately, the success rate of islet transplants is low. There have been more than 300 allogeneic islet transplants in adults with type 1 diabetes since the 1970s, but fewer than 10% of them have been able to achieve insulin independence for any significant period. Currently, approximately 75% achieve some degree of function as demonstrated by C-peptide levels, but less than 10% develop long term (i.e. 1-year) insulin independence. Although there are numerous reasons for the lack of success with clinical islet transplantation, one important reason is irreversible acute rejection. Some researchers believe that if research developments allow greater success, islet transplants will become the treatment of choice for type 1 diabetics, even rendering pancreas transplants obsolete.

Indications and contraindications for pancreas transplantation

Indications

The indication for pancreas transplantation is inadequate glucose control by medical management. Medical treatment should not be considered a failure until the patient has made a diligent attempt to control the diabetes, including assistance from an endocrinologist, internist, primary care physician, dietitian or social worker. With sufficient support and motivation, most diabetics can successfully manage their diabetes medically.

Poor management is characterized by acute fluctuations in patients with 'brittle' diabetes, where extremely high or low blood glucose levels are apparently precipitated by only minor modifications of diet, activity or insulin dose. Attempts to maintain the blood sugar level in a range associated with a low risk of secondary complications often precipitates symptomatic hypoglycemia, which manifests as acute anxiety, diaphoresis and confusion in mild cases, or obtundation, seizures and coma when severe. When autonomic neuropathy masks the symptoms of early hypoglycemia, severe hypoglycemic reactions may occur without warning. Such patients are often unable to drive or perform other similar tasks. Some even need to have their partners wake them up in the middle of each night to ensure that they remain arousable. Uncontrollable glycemic hyperlability or inability to maintain acceptable glucose levels despite aggressive therapy is the primary indication for pancreas transplantation.

Contraindications

The few absolute contraindications to pancreas transplantation are similar to those for other solid organ transplants, namely uncontrolled malignancy or infection, inability to tolerate the surgical procedure, inability to understand the procedure or co-operate with the postoperative management, or an insurmountable technical barrier to the procedure.

On the other hand, significant insulin resistance, either alone or in combination with an absolute insulin deficiency, is a relative contraindication. Insulin resistance should be suspected in obese patients, those with late-onset diabetes, and those requiring over 40 units of exogenous insulin per day. Although it is possible to achieve an insulin-free state after pancreas transplantation in the face of insulin resistance, exogenous insulin might still be required, and glycemic control may remain suboptimal. Pancreas recipients who must administer even one unit of exogenous insulin per day are generally dissatisfied with the outcome. Furthermore, pancreas graft failure is often defined in statistical reports as the point at which the patient requires any amount of exogenous insulin.

Type 1 diabetics who are obese can pose formidable technical barriers to the transplant procedure, and are at increased risk for wound problems and other complications. Those with a body mass index (BMI) greater than 30 kg/m^2 are encouraged to lose weight before the operation.

Recipient evaluation

Renal evaluation

About 85% of the pancreas transplants performed in the USA are transplanted simultaneously with a kidney (SPK) for diabetics with end-stage renal disease (ESRD) for several reasons. First, there is no additional immunosuppressive 'penalty' in performing a pancreas transplant if the patient is already receiving a kidney, the treatment of choice for ESRD in diabetics. Second, graft survival rates of pancreas transplants performed simultaneously with kidney transplants have historically been 20–30% better than those transplanted as a solitary pancreas. This finding is at least partially explained by the difficulty of making the diagnosis of acute rejection in an isolated pancreas. Most biochemical markers of acute pancreatic rejection are neither sensitive nor specific. In a patient who receives a kidney transplant from the same donor, a rise in the serum creatinine concentration is a useful surrogate marker for pancreas rejection. Creatinine is a highly sensitive marker for early kidney rejection, and there is an 85–90% concordance rate of rejection in the two organs. Pancreas rejection can thus be detected and treated at an earlier stage when there is a kidney present to help to monitor rejection, thereby reducing the graft loss rate from irreversible rejection. Finally, it is sometimes more difficult to receive reimbursement for isolated pancreas transplants.

Since diabetic nephropathy is a prominent secondary complication of long-standing diabetes, the evaluation of any potential pancreas transplant recipient must include studies of renal function. In patients who are not yet on dialysis, this evaluation should include an estimate of the glomerular filtration rate (GFR) as well as quantification of proteinuria. The GFR can be estimated by a 24-h urine collection or by using the Cockroft–Galt formula. Patients with a creatinine clearance of less than 30–50 mL/min, or who have proteinuria in excess of 1 g/day before transplantation but are not yet on dialysis, should be considered for SPK rather than solitary pancreas transplantation. The immunosuppressive medications that are required to ensure survival of the allograft, including cyclosporine or tacrolimus, are nephrotoxic and likely to push a patient with marginal renal function to ESRD if a simultaneous kidney transplant is not performed. A better solution is to perform a pre-emptive kidney transplant from a living donor, followed by a PAK transplant approximately 3 to 6 months afterwards. This approach spares a kidney from the limited cadaver donor pool and allows a shorter waiting time for a pancreas, which is generally easier to obtain without an accompanying kidney. The recipient also benefits from longer graft survival after receiving a living donor kidney compared to a cadaveric kidney. Still better is the simultane- ous pancreas and live donor kidney transplant (SPLK), which requires only one transplant operation for the recipient. Patients with microalbuminuria alone can receive a solitary pancreas trans- plant, but should be placed on angiotensin-converting-enzyme inhibitors in order to slow the progression of diabetic nephropathy.

Cardiac evaluation

Diabetic kidney transplant recipients have an incidence of angio- graphically significant coronary artery disease (CAD) that approaches 25–50%. This, together with the fact that myocardial ischemia is often silent in diabetics, has prompted some centers to recommend routine coronary angiography before pancreas trans- plantation. Although myocardial perfusion imaging is relatively insensitive for detecting significant CAD in diabetics, it appears to be adequate for screening patients preoperatively for pancreas transplantation. Asymptomatic patients with negative stress tests can undergo pancreas transplantation with a negligible incidence of postoperative cardiac events. Symptomatic patients, or those with positive stress tests, should have coronary angiography. Significant lesions are then treated with percutaneous transluminal coronary angioplasty (PTCA) or coronary artery bypass grafting (CABG) prior to the transplant. The latter is associated with a better long-term outcome in diabetics. Patients who undergo pre- transplant coronary reconstruction also have negligible rates of adverse cardiac events during the post-transplant period. In patients with known coronary artery disease, perioperative management should include invasive cardiovascular monitoring, perioperative nitrates and beta-blockers.

Peripheral vascular evaluation

It has been said that the single most important aspect of the physical examination of a potential kidney or pancreas recipient is palpation of the femoral pulses. Atherosclerotic peripheral vascular disease is very common in patients with diabetes mellitus. Significant aorto-iliac occlusive disease, as evidenced by diminished or absent femoral pulses, is a relative contraindication to kidney and pancreas transplantation. These patients should undergo aortography with distal run-off in order to define the extent of the disease. If the aortogram indicates that the iliac arteries are inadequate, either aorto-iliac reconstruction is performed or the patient is eliminated from further consideration for transplantation.

Occasionally, patients present with distal ischemia, gangrene or infection, and this should be treated prior to transplantation. A history of transient ischemic attacks or stroke and the physical finding of a carotid bruit warrant preoperative carotid duplex scanning, and carotid endarterectomy when indicated.

Gastrointestinal evaluation

Patients with long-standing diabetes frequently develop autonomic neuropathy, which leads to debilitating problems such as gastroparesis and altered bowel function. These problems are not contraindications to transplantation, but the patient should be informed that pancreas transplantation may not result in a dramatic improvement. In addition, any suspicion of peptic ulcer disease should be followed by an upper endoscopy. Aggressive preoperative treatment of ulcers should reduce the likelihood that postoperative high-dose steroids will precipitate an exacerbation of ulcer disease. If blood serology is positive for hepatitis B surface antigen or for hepatitis C antibody, the patient should be evaluated by a gastroenterologist and a liver biopsy considered. Disease activity during evaluation may determine patient eligibility for transplantation, as any form of viral hepatitis may progress in an immunosuppressed patient. In addition, as cholecystitis carries a very high morbidity and mortality in the transplant recipient, potential candidates with cholelithiasis should undergo prophylactic cholecystectomy.

Donor evaluation

Donor risk factors for poor outcome

The ideal pancreas donor is a non-obese, hemodynamically stable, brain-dead patient between the ages of 15 and 45 years. The gross appearance of the gland during the procurement operation is often more important in determining suitability than historical or metabolic factors. The pancreas should be free of fatty infiltration, often visible as a subtle 'marbled' infiltration of fat, slightly more yellow in color than the pancreatic parenchyma. Fatty infiltration of the pancreas predisposes it to post-transplant peripancreatic infection, with a high risk of graft loss and generalized sepsis. The pancreas should also be soft in texture, without nodular or fibrotic areas suggestive of previous pancreatitis. Edema of the organ, as a consequence of the massive fluid resuscitation during care of the donor, is not a contraindication.

Use of a pancreas from donors over 45–50 years of age is associated with lower graft survival rates, and should only be used when the appearance of the gland and the Y-graft vessels are ideal. Organs from donors weighing less than 15 kg have small blood vessels that are technically difficult (but not always impossible) to reconstruct. However, these organs are at higher risk for postoperative thrombosis, especially if low flow through the small vessels is further reduced by swelling secondary to ischemic preservation injury.

Diabetes is an obvious contraindication to pancreas organ donation. Hypertension does not disqualify an organ, but may cause sufficient atherosclerotic disease in the iliac or superior mesenteric arteries to compromise arterial reconstruction. Furthermore, significant baseline atherosclerosis in a pancreatic allograft is of concern for the long-term outcome, since progressive arteritis and vascular occlusion may occur even in normal transplanted organs. In potential donors with significant risk factors for atherosclerosis, it is often useful to palpate the iliac arteries at an early stage of the procurement operation. Significantly diseased iliac arteries will contraindicate donation, unless the femoral or carotid arteries can be used, or other uncommon methods of pancreatic arterial reconstruction are possible.

Hyperglycemia in the donor is not a contraindication, since it is often a consequence of high-dose steroids given to reduce cerebral edema, or of high-volume administration of glucose-containing fluids. Similarly, hyperamylasemia is not a contraindication, but caution should be exercised in cases where it may have been caused by mesenteric ischemia secondary to hypoperfusion. These cases are identified by a history of significant, prolonged hypotension in the donor, and are often associated with markedly elevated transaminase levels indicating concurrent liver ischemia. In general, organs from unstable donors with long periods of hypotension, or the need for high-dose pressors to support the blood pressure, should be used cautiously.

Donor–recipient histocompatibility and cross-matching

Historically, the number of major histocompatibility antigens (HLA) that are mismatched between the donor and recipient has been an important determinant of long-term pancreas graft survival. Registry data have shown reduced graft survival rates for transplants performed when there are two or more HLA mismatches. While this is true for all pancreas transplants, it is especially relevant to solitary pancreas transplants. As a result, many centers will only transplant closely matched organs. However, more recent data indicate that new immunosuppressive medications and pancreas biopsy techniques have made HLA-matching less crucial. In patients who are treated with tacrolimus at transplant centers that are capable of performing percutaneous pancreas biopsies safely, any degree of donor–recipient mismatch can yield satisfactory results.

A donor–recipient cross-match is generally performed immediately before the transplant in order to identify recipient antibodies that would lead to early graft thrombosis. However, in cases where the organ has had a long cold preservation time before the cross-match is started, it may be preferable to forego the cross-match in order to reduce the risk of further ischemic injury. Such an approach is only acceptable if the recipient is known to have no circulating anti-HLA antibodies (i.e. a zero historical PRA), and has not had a recent sensitizing event such as a blood transfusion.

Recipient surgery

Pancreas recipients are treated with perioperative antibiotics, which are started preoperatively. Patients who are to undergo enteric drainage of pancreatic exocrine secretions should have whatever bowel preparation is possible in the time available. Our regimen includes a dose of oral erythromycin and neomycin on admission, and hourly thereafter for a total of three doses. A saline enema is also given to facilitate the postoperative return of bowel function.

Several techniques are currently considered acceptable for

Box 6.2 Advantages of surgical techniques

Exocrine secretion drainage

Bladder drainage
Can monitor for rejection by measuring the urinary content of pancreatic enzymes
Avoids potential peritoneal contamination by recipient's bowel contents, which can occur with enteric drainage
Anastomotic leak does not result in spillage of enteric contents, which can occur with enteric drainage

Enteric drainage
Avoids long-term complications related to bladder drainage, specifically recurrent urinary infections, systemic acidosis, dehydration, need for oral bicarbonate supplements, chemical cystitis and urethritis

Venous drainage

Systemic drainage
The pelvic position of the pancreas with this technique permits bladder exocrine drainage if desired
Allows transcystoscopic pancreatic biopsy
Percutaneous biopsy is easier than with portal-drained pancreas

Portal drainage
Avoids the hyperinsulinemia that is associated with systemic venous drainage

---

pancreas transplantation. The pancreas may be placed in the pelvis with the arterial anastomosis to the common or external iliac artery, and the venous outflow to the common or external iliac vein. In this case the head of the pancreas faces caudad. This location allows the exocrine secretions of the pancreas to be drained either into the bladder by a duodenocystostomy, or into the bowel by a duodenoenterostomy. The pancreas may also be placed on the small bowel mesentery, with the arterial anastomosis to the iliac artery or aorta, and the venous outflow to the portal vein. In this position the head of the pancreas faces cephalad. Exocrine secretions from a pancreas with portal venous drainage cannot be drained into the bladder, but must be drained into the bowel. Whenever a duodenoenterostomy is constructed, it can be a simple side-to-side anastomosis to a loop of jejunum, or to a Roux-en-Y limb. Each of these techniques has advantages and disadvantages (see Box 6.2). We currently use the portal venous technique almost exclusively. This technique has the advantage of being somewhat easier to perform, because it avoids the extensive mobilization of the iliac vein that is required when the pancreas is transplanted in the pelvis. It also has the theoretical advantage of lowering systemic insulin levels and has been associated with lower rejection rates at our center. In the case of a simultaneous pancreas–kidney transplant, the kidney is transplanted to the left iliac vessels, and is positioned comfortably in the left lower quadrant beneath the colon or in an extraperitoneal pocket.

Donor surgery

Pancreas organ procurement is usually part of a multiple organ procurement operation that includes removal of the heart, lungs, liver, pancreas and kidneys, in that order. Surgical teams from several different programs frequently participate, especially if the team performing the transplant of a particular organ is interested in doing its own procurement. Although this is still common practice, procurement techniques are becoming standardized, and there is now less likelihood that an organ procured by another team will suffer from utilization of an unconventional, suboptimal approach.

The pancreas dissection usually follows that of the liver team, who will generally have exposed the structures in the hepatoduodenal ligament from the common bile duct to the origin of the splenic artery. The inferior aspect of the common hepatic artery is dissected down as far as the splenic artery, and the origin of the splenic artery is encircled. The celiac artery need not be exposed until after the flush. The duodenum and head of the pancreas are mobilized medially as far as the aorta. The spleen and tail of the pancreas are also mobilized. The spleen is used as a handle for the tail of the pancreas. Dissection proceeds as far as the origin of the splenic artery superiorly, and as far as the inferior mesenteric vein inferiorly. The origin of the superior mesenteric artery is exposed by dissection through the dense neural tissue surrounding it in the area cephalad to the point where the left renal vein crosses the aorta. The inferior mesenteric vein is again identified below the tail of the pancreas lateral to the ligament of Treitz and medial to the descending colon. It can now be cannulated in preparation for the portal flush of the liver with preservation solution.

The standard preservation solution for the pancreas is the University of Wisconsin preservation solution, developed by Southard and Belzer. Its theoretical advantages for the pancreas over the older Eurocollins or silica gel solutions include reduced cell swelling, prolonged safe cold ischemic time, and better initial graft function. This solution is infused into the pancreas *in situ* via retrograde aortic perfusion, together with the other intra-abdominal organs. Ischemic injury to the pancreas, as with other solid organs, is a function of the duration of the preservation time.

Successful preservation of the pancreas for 3 days has been demonstrated in animal models of transplantation. However, in the clinical setting, preservation times of less than 12 h are considered to be optimal, and those of less than 24 h are common and acceptable. Preservation times between of 24 and 36 h are also acceptable, but they carry slightly more risk of ischemic injury. Organs that have been kept on ice for over 36 h are usually discarded.

Postoperative management and complications

Vascular complications

Acute thrombosis accounts for more than half of the pancreas grafts lost from technical failure. Thrombosis rates have been reported to be 5–10% for SPK transplants, and 10–20% for solitary pancreas transplants – higher than that of any other solid organ transplant. Factors that increase the risk of graft thrombosis include donor age > 45 years, cerebrovascular cause of donor death, use of a segmental pancreatic graft, reconstruction of the arterial inflow with a technique other than Y-graft, use of a portal vein extension graft, left-sided rather than right-sided graft placement, and prolonged graft pancreatitis after implantation. Thrombosis is thought to result from a combination of low blood flow caused by swelling, release of local and systemic procoagulant factors from postoperative pancreatitis, atherosclerosis of the pancreas or Y-graft, and mechanical kinking of the allograft portal vein.

Thrombosis of the pancreas usually occurs within the first 7–10 days. It is heralded by a continuous rise in the serum glucose levels and ever-increasing insulin requirements. The most accurate test for ruling out graft thrombosis is color-flow Doppler ultrasound. If the ultrasound scan shows thrombosis of the graft, urgent transplant pancreatectomy should be performed before systemic sepsis and adult respiratory distress syndrome (ARDS) develop. If the ultrasound scan shows partial thrombosis of a pancreatic vessel, or a high-resistance arterial signal suggestive of swelling secondary to preservation injury, anticoagulation with heparin should be considered. There are case reports in which thrombectomy of one of the graft vessels or resection of a partially infarcted graft resulted in salvage. However, the complication rate associated with heroic attempts to salvage partially thrombosed grafts is considerable. In an effort to reduce the thrombosis rate in solitary pancreas recipients, we have been using low-dose anticoagulation for the last several years. Postoperatively, patients are given a low-dose heparin infusion (300–500 U/h; keep partial thromboplastin time in the normal range). When patients begin to take oral medications, they are converted to coumadin, dosed to keep the INR around 1.8, which is stopped after 3 months.

Postoperative hemorrhage is the other major vascular complication following pancreas transplantation. The organ is surrounded by an abundance of small vessels that are divided during procurement. After reperfusion, some vessels remain in spasm and do not bleed until several hours postoperatively. The risk of postoperative hemorrhage is higher if anticoagulation is used to prevent graft thrombosis, and is reduced by meticulous hemostasis before the abdomen is closed. Surgical exploration should not be delayed by further imaging studies in a hypotensive patient with a falling hematocrit.

Duodenal anastomotic leak

Leakage from the duodenal anastomosis is a very serious complication that can lead to graft loss. A duodenal anastomotic leak is suspected in patients with signs of infection or peritonitis, including fever, leukocytosis, abdominal distension and pain. In bladder-drained pancreas transplants, the leak usually occurs shortly after the Foley catheter has been removed. Enteric-drained pancreas transplants usually leak between 3 days and 3 weeks postoperatively. Patients with suspected leaks are evaluated by computed tomography (CT) scan with oral and/or bladder contrast. The CT scan will often show a localized or generalized fluid collection and even extraluminal contrast and air.

Surgical repair of duodenal anastomotic leaks involves debridement of non-viable tissue and then suture closure, with appropriate culture and pathologic evaluation to exclude cytomegalovirus infection. Leaks of bladder-drained pancreas transplants should be decompressed for 10 days to 3 weeks with a Foley catheter. It is prudent to check the integrity of the repair with a cystogram prior to removal of the urinary catheter. Leaks from enteric-drained pancreas transplants should be decompressed by converting a jejunal loop to a Roux-en-Y type of anastomosis in order to divert the fecal stream away from the repair. Drains are usually placed in order to detect and control any recurrent leaks. Leaks that are totally controlled with drains in patients who show no signs of sepsis may close spontaneously or be more amenable to repair after several months of observation. Treatment with somatostatin may encourage healing by reducing pancreatic exocrine secretions.

Duodenal leaks are generally more difficult to control than the ureteric leaks that complicate kidney transplants, and they may necessitate transplant pancreatectomy. Repair of a duodenal leak is prone to breakdown due to local contamination with pancreatic contents that often contain activated pancreatic enzymes, enteric bacteria and fungi. Repeated attempts at repair are ill-advised, since recurrent spillage of infected pancreatic juice can cause peritonitis, abdominal abscess, life-threatening sepsis, and digestion of the abdominal wall, in which case wide debridement and extensive plastic surgical reconstruction may be required.

Abdominal abscess

Intra-abdominal infections complicate pancreas transplantation in 10–30% of recipients, a much higher incidence than that for other solid organs. The reasons for this are multiple. First, microbial contamination inevitably accompanies transplantation of the duodenal segment. Contamination can also result from asymptomatic, subclinical peritonitis in SPK recipients who are on peritoneal dialysis at the time of transplantation. Second, postreperfusion peripancreatitis, secondary to release of digestive enzymes from the surface of the pancreas, is not uncommon. Digestion of surrounding tissues, especially peripancreatic fat, produces necrotic debris and promotes microbial growth. Third, technical problems such as duodenal anastomotic leaks, especially with enteric-drained grafts, cause infectious complications. Peripancreatic infections are serious problems that necessitate graft removal in 10–15% of transplants in some series. Advanced infections that are not promptly treated can cause extensive necrosis of the abdominal wall, systemic sepsis and even death.

Intra-abdominal infection should be suspected in patients who develop fever, leukocytosis, hyperamylasemia, abdominal distention and/or ileus in the early postoperative period, and should be explored immediately, with meticulous debridement of necrotic tissue and lavage with antibiotic and antifungal solutions. Early postoperative infections are often diffuse and do not respond well to percutaneous catheter drainage. In fact, this approach often results in contamination of the abdomen with skin organisms, rather than successful treatment of an existing infection. Although exploration might seem to be a setback for the patient, it is actually the most expedient method of preventing development of sepsis.

After 2 weeks, peripancreatic collections tend to be more localized, and may be more amenable to percutaneous drainage. Subtle signs of sepsis should be evaluated by the usual routine diagnostic workup, and may include abdominal ultrasound, CT or magnetic resonance imaging (MRI). Although 3 weeks or more of intravenous antibiotics or antifungal agents may be required in cases of severe infection, prolonged courses may be associated with the emergence of resistant organisms. Even in the era of modern diagnostic techniques and antimicrobial agents, 1-year pancreas graft survival rates in patients with intra-abdominal infections are significantly lower than those in patients who do not develop infectious complications.

Rejection

In the recent past, nearly 90% of pancreas transplant recipients experienced at least one episode of acute rejection, an incidence more than two times higher than that of kidney transplant recipients. Modern immunosuppression has reduced the rejection rate to less than 50%. Rejection of a pancreatic graft is much more difficult to diagnose than that of a kidney. For kidney transplants, a rise in the serum creatinine level is a sensitive indicator of early acute rejection and, if closely monitored, most cases of acute kidney rejection are completely reversible. In contrast, the biochemical markers of acute pancreatic rejection are insensitive and non-specific. Therefore acute rejection is often diagnosed relatively late and is more likely to result in loss of the graft.

The most readily available method of detecting acute rejection is measurement of the serum amylase and lipase levels. These enzyme levels should be normal after pancreas transplantation. A rise in amylase or lipase after the 'normal' postoperative pancreatitis has resolved should raise suspicion of acute rejection. Serial measurement of urinary amylase levels in patients with bladder-drained pancreas transplants is another popular method of monitoring for rejection. A 50% decrease in urinary amylase concentration or the calculated hourly amylase excretion rate indicates the possibility of rejection. A surrogate marker for acute rejection in recipients of simultaneous pancreas kidney transplants is the serum creatinine level, since rejection occurs in both organs concurrently in 80–90% of cases. Other methods, which are used less frequently due to their insensitivity, unavailability or high cost, include measurement of urinary or serum anodal trypsinogen, insulin and pancreas-specific protein, urinary cytologic examination, and scans such as ^{99m}Tc-DTPA scintigraphy. On MRI scanning, the findings are non-specific, but include increased glandular size and parenchymal water content in T2-weighted images. However, MRI has the advantage of providing anatomic detail that cannot be visualized with other non-invasive imaging techniques. Some patients with acute rejection will present with normal biochemical indices, and only fever, graft

Table 6.2 Histologic grading of rejection in pancreas biopsies

Grade 0 (normal)	Unremarkable pancreatic parenchyma No inflammatory infiltrates
Grade 1 (inflammation of indeterminate significance)	Sparse septal mononuclear infiltrates No venous endotheliitis or acinar involvement
Grade 2 (minimal rejection)	Venous endotheliitis Mixed inflammatory cell septal infiltrates Acinar inflammation in up to two foci Ductal inflammation
Grade 3 (mild rejection)	Acinar inflammation in three or more foci Acinar cell drop-out or necrosis
Grade 4 (moderate rejection)	Grade 3 features plus arterial endotheliitis
Grade 5 (severe rejection)	Extensive mixed inflammatory infiltrates Confluent acinar cell necrosis

tenderness or other signs that are more classically associated with infection.

Bladder-drained pancreas recipients with elevated amylase or lipase levels should initially have a urinary catheter placed to decompress the bladder. If the problem is not rejection, but in fact reflux pancreatitis, enzyme levels will fall to normal after decompression. If the enzyme levels remain elevated, an ultrasound examination is performed to rule out a peripancreatic infection or vascular problem with the graft. However, most ultrasound scans performed in this setting are normal, and the workup proceeds to ultrasound-guided percutaneous needle biopsy. In experienced hands, this procedure is associated with a low complication rate, especially if ultrasound is used to identify the location of vascular structures. Histologic criteria for acute rejection include acinar inflammation, venous and arterial endotheleitis, mixed populations of small and large 'activated' lymphocytes and eosinophils, and areas of acinar cell necrosis. A grading system has recently been developed to guide treatment and predict outcome (see Table 6.2).

In contrast to acute rejection of renal grafts, which frequently responds to bolus corticosteroid treatment, most cases of acute pancreas rejection require 10 to 14 days of antilymphocyte antibody (thymoglobulin, ATGAM or OKT3) for successful resolution. The outcome depends primarily on the severity of rejection at the time of treatment.

Hyperglycemia

Hyperglycemia after pancreas transplantation requiring transient treatment with insulin has been reported in up to 70% of cases, and is often a consequence of ischemic injury to the pancreatic islets during organ preservation. It is associated with donor age over 45 years, but not with duration of cold ischemia. Since hyperglycemia in the immediate postoperative period may be caused by graft thrombosis, these patients should be followed with duplex ultrasound examinations of the pancreas every 2 to 3 days for the first 2 weeks. Hyperglycemia can be exacerbated by a number of factors. Recipient obesity and uremia increase insulin resistance, and administration of glucose-containing intravenous solutions increases the need for insulin. Immunosuppressive agents such as prednisone, cyclosporine and tacrolimus cause hyperglycemia by a variety of mechanisms, including inhibition of insulin secretion by islet cells. Postoperative infections and other stresses may also contribute.

If graft thrombosis is excluded, a continuous intravenous insulin infusion is given to maintain blood glucose levels near 150 mg/dL while the islets are recovering. In many patients the need for insulin can be reduced or eliminated by diet modification, elimination of glucose from intravenous fluids, weight reduction, adjustment of prednisone doses, or reducing the dose of tacrolimus by substituting cyclosporine or sirolimus.

Pancreatitis

Acute pancreatitis, characterized by elevated amylase and lipase levels, perhaps graft tenderness, and perhaps increased glandular size, is rejection until proven otherwise. If an allograft biopsy excludes rejection in this setting, then the differential includes biopsy sampling error, or an alternative cause of pancreatitis. Reflux pancreatitis in bladder-drained pancreas transplants can be diagnosed by normalization of enzymes with bladder decompressions as described above. Presentation of cytomegalovirus (CMV) infection of the pancreas is comparable with acute rejection, including similar histologic findings. Differentiation between the two conditions is crucial, as treatment for each of them is diametrically opposed to that of the other. Pancreatitis can also be caused by a variety of drugs, most notably sulfacontaining antibiotics and diuretics in transplant recipients.

Complications of bladder drainage

Hematuria of sufficient magnitude to necessitate cystoscopy occurs in 9–13% of bladder-drained pancreas transplants. The source is usually one of the bladder anastomoses, the duodenum, the transplant ureter or the bladder itself. Bleeding is probably exacerbated by fibrinolysis caused by activated trypsinogen and urokinase in the urine. Mild hematuria may be self-limited. However, brisk bleeding requires continuous bladder irrigation to prevent bladder distension and possibly even development of an anastomotic leak. If irrigation is necessary for more than 24–48 h, or if there is a decrease in hematocrit, cystoscopy should be performed. At that time, clots can be evacuated and small bleeding points can be coagulated. Open exploration is rarely necessary.

A number of factors contribute to development of recurrent urinary tract infections. For example, pancreatic secretions eliminate the urinary acidity that normally provides a natural defense against infection. Urinary retention secondary to a neuropathic bladder may be exacerbated by the bladder 'diverticulum' formed by the allograft duodenal cuff. Intermittent catheterization may be required to relieve distension. However, it may also allow the introduction of bacteria and iatrogenic infection. Moreover, retained sutures, staples or stones at the duodenocystostomy may harbor infection. Cystoscopy is indicated to rule out and possibly remove suture material at the anastomosis.

Periodic allograft pancreatitis occurs in some patients with a bladder-drained pancreas. This phenomenon is probably related to reflux of urine through an incompetent sphincter of Oddi, or to stagnation of exocrine secretions in the pancreatic duct due to chronic distension of a neurogenic bladder. The diagnosis is suspected if a patient presents with elevated serum amylase and lipase levels, but with a biopsy that fails to reveal acute rejection. In these patients, serum enzyme levels normalize after bladder decompression.

Non-anion-gap acidosis and dehydration may occur in patients with a bladder-drained pancreas because of sodium bicarbonate ($NaHCO_3$) wasting into the urine. Both the pancreatic acinar cells and duodenal Brunner's glands secrete $NaHCO_3$, and it has been hypothesized that excessive loss may occur when a long duodenal segment remains with the allograft. Some patients require more than 20 000 mg of $NaHCO_3$ per day (over 30 tablets) and/or acetazolamide to maintain normal serum HCO_3 levels. Patients with renal dysfunction are more prone to acidosis because the compensatory renal mechanisms of acid secretion and HCO_3 conservation are impaired. Most patients can be treated successfully with oral

HCO_3 supplementation, but some will require repeated admissions to hospital for intravenous repletion, especially if the prescribed amount of HCO_3 is intolerable.

Digestive enzymes secreted by the pancreas into the urine can cause distressing symptoms due to irritation of the genito-urinary tract. Dysuria, perineal pain, prostatitis, incontinence, urethritis and urethral perforation, as well as inflammation and peri-urethral ulceration of the glans penis, have all been described. Conversion from bladder to enteric drainage of pancreatic exocrine secretions due to intractable symptoms is necessary in about 7% of patients. Although surgical complications such as anastomotic leak or thrombosis of the pancreas occur in about 10% of conversions, this method is highly successful in eliminating the problems associated with bladder drainage.

Outcomes

Cost

Although successful pancreas transplantation can eliminate diabetes even in the most intractable cases, the broad applicability of the procedure has been limited by its financial expense as well as the risk of morbidity from the surgical procedure and immuno-suppressive medications. Although it seems that a detailed cost–benefit analysis should be able to address the concern that pancreas transplantation may be unjustified, several problems have limited these analyses to date. The actual costs of any medical intervention are notoriously difficult to measure, and reimbursements are frequently used as surrogate markers. Even so, charges for whole organ transplants vary widely. Recent studies indicate that total charges for SPK transplants, including 1 year of follow-up, range from $90 000 to $190 000.

Another factor that complicates any analysis of pancreas transplantation is that the cost should really be compared to the cost of poorly controlled diabetes, which is the state in which most candidates live prior to transplantation. Uncontrolled diabetes leads to metabolic derangements, blindness, kidney failure, amputation, heart disease and stroke. Care for any one of these complications requires huge financial expenditure. Furthermore, the costs of deterioration in individual quality of life and employment disability are enormous. The economic burden of diabetes in the USA in 1992 was estimated to be over $90 billion. When viewed in the context of the cumulative costs of care for debilitated diabetics, the cost of a pancreas transplant seems less formidable.

Patient and graft survival

Outcomes of pancreas transplant procedures are reported annually by the International Pancreas Transplant Registry. As of September 1999, nearly 13 000 pancreas transplants were reported to the registry, about 75% from the USA and 25% from outside the USA. Most cases (83%) were simultaneous pancreas–kidney transplants (SPK), with 12% pancreas after kidney (PAK), and 5% pancreas transplant alone (PTA). One-year patient survival was over 95% for all categories. Pancreas graft survival for those transplanted since 1996 was 85% for SPK transplants, and 91% for the kidneys. One-year graft survival for solitary pancreas transplants has continued to improve, but still lags behind the SPK transplants (PAK 76%, PTA 72%). From 1987 to 1993, most transplants were done with the bladder drainage technique. Since 1993 there has been a gradual rise in the proportion of enteric-drained pancreas transplants, which now comprise over 50% of the transplants reported most recently. Registry data indicated a lower graft survival rate for the enteric versus the bladder-drained transplants. The registry indicates significantly lower rates of graft loss due to acute rejection, which is less than 10% at 1 year. This is attributed to the new immunosuppressants, including tacrolimus and mycophenolate mofetil.

Benefits

Metabolic benefits

A functioning pancreatic allograft is the most reliable method for achieving normoglycemia in type 1 diabetics. Many groups have demonstrated normalization of fasting plasma glucose levels, intravenous glucose disappearance rates, acute insulin and c-peptide responses to intravenous glucose and arginine, and Hgb-A_{IC} levels in patients with functioning pancreas transplants. In patients who remain independent of exogenous insulin or oral hypoglycemic agents, pancreatic function remains strikingly stable over an extended period of time.

Secondary complications

The potential benefits of pancreas transplantation in preventing secondary complications of diabetes can be inferred from the results of the Diabetes Control and Complications Trial Research Group. This study demonstrated that a marked reduction in complications is obtained when good glycemic control is achieved by frequent insulin injections. Since successful pancreas transplantation achieves even better glycemic control than frequent insulin injections, and as it is hyperglycemia *per se* that causes the tissue damage which leads to complications, it is logical to conclude that pancreas transplants should reduce the risk of complications. However, relatively few studies have been conducted to explore this hypothesis, due to the relatively small number of pancreas transplants performed each year, and also because the techniques and results of pancreas transplantation are still in flux. None the less, the available data indicate that the secondary complications tend to stabilize or improve after transplantation.

Nephropathy

A number of studies have shown that successful pancreas transplantation in kidney transplant recipients prevents or slows the progression of diabetic nephropathy in the new kidney. In non-uremic patients, a pancreas transplant can reverse the early microscopic lesions of diabetic glomerulopathy.

Neuropathy

Indices of motor, sensory and autonomic neuropathy improve or stabilize in pancreas transplant recipients, in contrast to the deterioration that is observed in diabetics who are treated with exogenous insulin. This improvement is manifested as a dramatic improvement in strength and reflexes, and a reduction in neuropathic pain. Improvement in autonomic neuropathy after successful pancreas transplant was found to be correlated with improved survival in one study.

Retinopathy

Progression of advanced diabetic retinopathy is not altered in the first few years following a pancreas transplant. However, retinopathy in patients with long-functioning grafts tends to stabilize, in contrast to the deterioration that is observed in patients with failed grafts.

Quality of life

Patients with brittle diabetes, especially those with frequent hospital admissions or altered mental states due to labile blood sugar levels, experience an immediate improvement in their quality of life from the physiologic homeostasis afforded by the new pancreas. Several studies have shown that recipients of successful pancreas transplants perceive that their health, quality of life and expectations for the future are all improved by the procedure.

Beyond the improvement in quality of life afforded by regulation of previously labile blood sugar levels, and the reduction in the risk of complication progression afforded by normoglycemia, there are other benefits of pancreas transplantation that do not, in and of themselves, justify performing the procedure. Patients with functioning pancreatic allografts are no longer required to perform frequent fingerstick blood sugar tests and insulin injections. Those on an insulin pump are freed from the constant need for this device. Patients can take a normal diet for the first time in decades without fear of metabolic derangements. The cumulative improvement in quality of life that is experienced by these unfortunate patients is difficult for non-diabetics to appreciate fully, but is often quite remarkable.

Further reading

Bartlett ST, Schweitzer EJ, Johnson LB *et al*. 1996: Equivalent success of simultaneous pancreas–kidney and solitary pancreas transplantation. A prospective trial of tacrolimus immunosuppression with percutaneous biopsy. *Annals of Surgery* **224**, 440–52.

Benedetti E, Gruessner AC, Troppmann C *et al*. 1996: Intra-abdominal fungal infections after pancreatic transplantation: incidence, treatment and outcome. *Journal of the American College of Surgeons* **18**, 307–16.

Brayman KL, Najarian JS and **Sutherland DER**. 1993: Transplantation of the pancreas. In Cameron J (ed.), *Current surgical therapy*, 2nd edn. Baltimore, MD: Williams & Wilkins, 458–75.

Diabetes Control and Complications Trial Research Group. 1993: The effect of intensive treatment of diabetes on the development and progression of long-term complications of insulin-dependent diabetes mellitus. *New England Journal of Medicine* **329**, 977–86.

Drachenberg CB, Papadimitriou JC, Klassen DK *et al*. 1997: Evaluation of pancreas transplant needle biopsy. Reproducibility and revision of histologic grading system. *Transplantation* **63**, 1579–86.

Expert Committee on the Diagnosis and Classification of Diabetes Mellitus. 1997: Report of the expert committee on the diagnosis and classification of diabetes mellitus. *Diabetes Care* **20**, 1183–97.

Gaber AO, Shokouh-Amiri H, Grewal HP and **Britt LG**. 1993: A technique for portal pancreatic transplantation with enteric drainage. *Surgery, Gynecology and Obstetrics* **177**, 417–19.

Gruessner A and **Sutherland DER**. 1996: Pancreas transplantation in the United States (US) and non-US as reported to the United Network for Organ Sharing (UNOS) and the International Pancreas Transplant Registry (IPTR). In Cecka JM and Teriyaki PI (eds), *Clinical transplants*. Los Angeles, CA: UCLA Tissue Typing Laboratory, 47–68.

Gruessner RW, Sutherland DER, Troppmann C *et al*. 1997: The surgical risk of pancreas transplantation in the cyclosporine era. An overview. *Journal of the American College of Surgeons* **185**, 128–44.

Kennedy WR, Xavier N, Goetz FC, Sutherland DER and Najarian JS. 1990: Effects of pancreatic transplantation on diabetic neuropathy. *New England Journal of Medicine* **322**, 1031–7.

Robertson RP, Sutherland DER, Kendall DM, Teacher AU and **Gruessner RWG.** 1996: Metabolic characterization of long-term successful pancreas transplants in type 1 diabetes. *Journal of Investigative Medicine* **44**, 549–55.

Slover RH and Eisenbarth GS. 1997: Prevention of type I diabetes and recurrent ß-cell destruction of transplanted islets. *Endocrine Reviews* **18**, 241–58.

Stephanian E, Gruessner RG, Brayman KL *et al.* 1992: Conversion of exocrine secretions from bladder to enteric drainage in recipients of whole pancreaticoduodenal transplants. *Annals of Surgery* **216**, 663–72.

Stratta RJ, Cushing KA, Frisbie K and **Miller SA.** 1997: Analysis of hospital charges after simultaneous pancreas–kidney transplantation in the era of managed care. *Transplantation* **64**, 287–292.

Sutherland DER, Gores PF, Farney AC *et al.* 1993: Evolution of kidney, pancreas and islet transplantation for patients with diabetes at the University of Minnesota. *American Journal of Surgery* **166**, 456–91.

Taylor RJ, Bynon S and **Stratta RJ.** 1994: Kidney/pancreas transplantation: a review of the current status. *Urologic Clinics of North America* **21**, 343–54.

Troppmann C, Gruessner AC, Benedetti E *et al.* 1996: Vascular graft thrombosis after pancreatic transplantation: univariate and multivariate operative and non-operative risk factor analysis. *Journal of the American College of Surgeons* **182**, 285–316.

Troppmann C, Gruessner AC, Papalois BE *et al.* 1996: Delayed endocrine pancreas graft function after simultaneous pancreas–kidney transplantation. *Transplantation* **61**, 1323–30.

7 Heart transplantation

John V. Conte Jr and Ronald Freudenberger

Introduction

Human heart transplantation burst on to the clinical scene amidst great media attention in 1967 with the first successful human heart transplant in South Africa. This 'event', like so many surgical innovations, followed the traditional paradigm of surgical discovery. An idea is generated, followed by years of laboratory work in relative obscurity before it is introduced clinically. Once it has been introduced and clinical problems identified, additional years of research are needed to improve and refine the process before it becomes an accepted surgical procedure. This paradigm has never been so classically demonstrated as with the development of heart transplantation.

Frank Mann of the Mayo Clinic performed studies using a heterotopic canine heart transplant model. He postulated in 1933 that failure of the transplanted heart was due to biological incompatibility rather than to surgical technique. His description of a lymphocytic infiltrate of the failed allografts was the first description of cardiac rejection. This and similar models were used by Marcus and colleagues at the University of Chicago in 1953 in their experiments on organ preservation, which identified the deleterious effects of intracardiac air and the problems of tissue specificity. The advent of hypothermia and the cardiopulmonary bypass machine allowed experiments in orthotopic cardiac transplantation to develop. In 1953, Neptune performed heart–lung transplants after inducing profound hypothermia of both the donor and the recipients in 'an ordinary beverage cooler.' These experiments showed the return of cardiac activity after periods of up to 30 min. This and subsequent work by Webb and Howard in 1957 established hypothermia as one of the basic tenets of donor and recipient protection during transplantation. In 1958, Goldberg and colleagues at the University of Maryland reported the first series of orthotopic transplants using a left atrial cuff technique. This was followed subsequently by the development by Lower and Shumway of the process which would become the standard technique for cardiac transplantation for decades to come. They used separate left and right atrial cuff anastamoses together with aortic and pulmonary artery anastamoses to perform the first successful orthotopic canine cardiac transplants.

The Stanford group went on to develop a method of following serial electrocardiograms in order to monitor immunosuppression. With this guide to therapy, they achieved a 230-day survival in an orthotopic canine heart transplant. With ongoing studies of graft preservation and transplant physiology occurring in laboratories across the country, as well as other successful canine orthotopic transplants, the first human cardiac transplant was imminent.

With a laboratory experience encompassing over 100 canine heart transplants and additional experiments conducted on monkeys, calves and human cadavers, James Hardy at the University of Mississippi was ready to perform the first human heart transplant. This occurred in 1964 in a 68-year-old man with an ischemic cardiomyopathy. The concept of 'brain death' as we know it today was not accepted at that time, and therefore the policy was to await cardiac arrest of the donor prior to removing any organs. Since the timing of the death of the donor would be unlikely to coincide with terminal collapse of the recipient, it was elected to transplant this patient with a chimpanzee heart. The operation was completed but the patient only lived for a few hours.

The stage had been set for the first human heart transplant. Although several centers with strong experimental research programs were ready to go, they were upstaged by Christian Barnard of the Groote–Schuur Hospital in Cape Town, South Africa. Barnard learned the technique during a visit to the Medical College of Virginia in 1967. A few months later, with little animal experience, he performed the first transplant on 3 December 1967. The patient survived for 18 days before succumbing to pneumonia. Within the next month, Kantrowitz in Brooklyn and Shumway at Stanford performed heart transplants, and Barnard performed his second transplant. By the end of 1968, 102 cardiac transplants had been performed in 17 countries. The mean survival period was 29 days, and many centers became discouraged. By 1970, only a few dedicated institutions were continuing experimental and clinical work on heart transplants. It was during the next decade that the surgical paradigm was again invoked and laboratory and clinical investigations worked to improve the results of transplantation. At Stanford, the 1-year survival rate increased from 22% in 1968 to 65% by 1978. Shumway and his group at Stanford became the world leaders in cardiac transplantation when they reported on rehabilitation potential, early clinical results, infections, complications, hemodynamics, indications and contraindications, donor management, the technique of endomyocardial biopsy, a histological grading system for cardiac allograft rejection, rabbit antithymocyte globulin, graft arteriosclerosis and retransplantation.

It was also during this period that the acceptance of 'brain death' criteria and the development of national organ procurement networks greatly enhanced donor availability.

The promising results obtained with cyclosporine for immunosuppression at Stanford in 1980 led to an explosion of enthusiasm for cardiac transplantation. The post-cyclosporine era began and heart transplantation expanded worldwide. In 1980, only 17 centers worldwide were performing heart transplants. By 1995, 229 centers were reported to be active in heart transplantation by the Registry of the International Society for Heart Transplant. Currently, almost 3000 heart transplants are performed each year, with 1-year survival rates approaching 90% at experienced centers.

Recipient evaluation

Potential candidates

The etiologies of congestive heart failure that require cardiac transplantation are primary cardiomyopathy, and coronary artery disease with either resultant ischemic cardiomyopathy and symptoms of congestive heart failure or inoperable ischemic coronary disease with refractive chest discomfort. A small percentage of patients who undergo cardiac transplantation do so for valvular disease with severe left ventricular dysfunction and congenital heart disease. Other underlying etiologies in patients who have undergone cardiac transplantation include inoperable hypertrophic cardiomyopathy, sarcoidosis and amyloidosis. The latter two entities have been reported to recur post-transplantation and are considered to be contraindications by many centers.

In general, patients with advanced heart failure, NYHA class 3 or 4, on maximal medical therapy are candidates for transplantation. Maximal medical therapy includes vasodilators, particularly angiotensin-converting-enzyme inhibitors (ACEI), digoxin, diuretics and possibly beta-blockers. Those patients with increasing medication requirements, frequent hospitalizations or overall deterioration of clinical status should also be considered for evaluation for cardiac transplantation.

In addition to these clinical parameters, ejection fraction and hemodynamic parameters are generally obtained in order to risk-stratify patients further. Patients with low ejection fractions tend to have a poor prognosis. However, among patients with ejection fractions of less than 20% there is a limited ability to determine further prognostic information. The use of bicycle ergometry with gas exchange to determine the oxygen consumption at maximal exercise has proved to be a very useful tool. Data from Mancini and colleagues demonstrates that a maximal oxygen consumption of more than 14 mL/kg/min predicts a good prognosis. On the other hand, patients with a maximal oxygen consumption of less than 14 mL/kg/min have a poor prognosis and should be considered for cardiac transplantation.

Exclusion criteria

In 1992, a group of transplant surgeons, cardiologists, nurses and representatives from the United Network of Organ Sharing (UNOS) met to discuss various aspects of cardiac transplantation, including criteria for exclusion (see Box 7.1).

Irreversible pulmonary hypertension creates a high risk of postoperative right ventricular failure. A pulmonary vascular resistance index higher than 6–8 Woods units/m^2, a pulmonary artery systolic pressure greater than 50–60 mmHg, and a transpulmonic gradient greater than 15 mmHg, that does not decrease by 50% with the use of vasodilators, are all contraindications to cardiac transplantation. Various pharmacological agents, including dobutamine, nitroglycerine, prostacyclin and nitric oxide have been used to assess the reversibility of these pressures.

Coexisting medical illness with a poor prognosis remains a

Box 7.1 Contraindications to heart transplantation

Age > 65 years
Significant systemic or multisystem disease
Active or extrapulmonary infection
Significant hepatic disease (total bilirubin > 2.5 mg/dL)
Significant renal disease (creatinine concentration > 2.5 mg/dL, creatinine clearance < 35 mL/min)
Cachexia or obesity
Severe osteoporosis
Current cigarette smoking
Psychiatric illness
Recent (< 2 years previously) drug or alcohol abuse

contraindication to transplantation, as the patient is likely to have a poor short-term survival or a difficult postoperative course. Patients with irreversible pulmonary parenchymal disease are poor operative candidates. Irreversible pulmonary disease is defined as a forced expiratory volume in 1 s/forced vital capacity (FEV_1/FVC) ratio of less than 50% of the predicted value, or patients with restrictive lung disease with an FEV_1 of less than 50% of the predicted value. Patients with obstructive lung disease are at higher risk of perioperative lung infection, which adds to the risk of perioperative complications.

Irreversible renal dysfunction defined as a creatinine concentration greater than 2 mg/dL or a creatinine clearance rate of less than 50 mL/min is a contraindication to transplantation. An attempt is made to determine the degree of renal dysfunction that is reversible from that which is intrinsic and irreversible. Pre-existing renal dysfunction is likely to worsen with postoperative fluid shifts and the introduction of nephrotoxic immunosuppressants.

Primary hepatic dysfunction such as cirrhosis or any hepatic dysfunction with resultant coagulopathy increases the risk of perioperative complications, and is therefore considered to be a contraindication to cardiac transplantation.

Insulin-dependent diabetes mellitus with end-organ damage or high insulin requirements without end-organ damage are contraindications to cardiac transplantation. Patients with orally controlled diabetes without end-organ damage have successfully undergone cardiac transplantation with a similar outcome to those without diabetes. However, with steroid use, borderline diabetics may develop overt diabetes, and orally controlled diabetics tend to require insulin therapy.

Transplantation should be deferred in patients with active infection. Patients who have coexisting neoplasm should not undergo cardiac transplantation. Patients with a history of localized malignancy that was successfully treated, or those cured of their malignancy with a negative evaluation of metastatic disease, may be considered for cardiac transplantation.

Acute pulmonary embolism or infarction increases the perioperative risk of lung infection. It is generally recommended to defer cardiac transplantation until at least 6 weeks have passed.

Myocardial infiltrative or inflammatory diseases, such as sarcoidosis and amyloidosis, have been reported to recur in the transplanted organ. For this reason, the presence of these conditions is considered to be a contraindication to cardiac transplantation in most centers.

Psychosocial instability and substance abuse are risk factors for patient non-compliance. Graft loss secondary to non-compliance is well documented. Risk factors for non-compliance include previous substance abuse, mood and personality disorders, history of previous non-compliance and inadequate family support.

Donor evaluation

Preoperative donor assessment

Careful assessment of the donor heart is crucial to successful transplantation. The evaluation of all donors should begin with a detailed history and physical examination. The history should specifically look for the known cardiac risk factors (hypertension, cigarette smoking, hyperlipidemia, diabetes and family history) as well as other medical conditions which may affect the heart and a review of all medications taken. In addition, events surrounding the donor's demise need to be investigated, including a history of chest trauma and prolonged periods of hypotension. A history of drug or alcohol abuse also needs to be ascertained. Physical examination includes evaluation of the chest wall for evidence of blunt trauma, evaluation of pulses, and a thorough auscultation of the heart to look for murmurs or abnormal heart sounds.

Evaluation of the current status of the donor will include an assessment of the current hemodynamics based on arterial blood pressure, central venous catheterization, and the type and amount of inotropic agents. Chest radiographs can identify cardiomegaly, aortic contour, pulmonary artery size, abnormal calcifications and pulmonary processes.

Electrocardiograms are obtained in order to assess cardiac rhythm and rule out myocardial infarction (new or remote). A variety of non-specific ST-T wave changes are seen in brain-dead patients, which do not rule out the heart for transplantation. Echocardiography is imperative for all donors. It is used to assess cardiac anatomy, valve structure and function, wall motion, chamber size and ejection fraction.

When available, cardiac catheterization is used for high-risk patients. These include patients with risk factors for coronary artery disease, abnormal ECGs, older donors (including males over the age of 45 years), cigarette smokers and patients with other stigmata of atherosclerosis. The use of marginal donors has resulted in concomitant transplantation and coronary artery bypass grafting. The long-term results of these procedures are unknown.

Generally accepted donor criteria exist (see Box 7.2). Donors with structurally normal hearts, but with abnormal cardiac function, can sometimes benefit from invasive monitoring, aggressive

---

Box 7.2 General cardiac donor criteria

Negative history of cardiac disease
No history of severe thoracic trauma
No prolonged cardiopulmonary resuscitation, hypotension or hypoxia
Normal ECG and echocardiogram
Minimal inotropic support
Negative serology for HIV and hepatitis
Negative cardiac catheterization for donor
Age > 45 years or otherwise high risk

---

fluid and hemodynamic management and hormonal therapy. Several protocols utilizing thyroid hormones, steroids and vasopressin have converted marginal hearts into usable organs.

Intraoperative donor assessment

Visual and manual inspection of the donor heart is the final method of assessing suitability for transplantation. Abnormalities of the coronary arteries, venous return to the heart and wall motion should be sought. Unsuspected cardiac contusion is occasionally found. Palpation of the coronary arteries is performed in order to look for unsuspected atherosclerotic disease, particularly in patients at risk who do not undergo cardiac catheterization. Regurgitant or stenotic valvular lesions can sometimes be detected by gentle palpation of the roof of the left atrium, the aorta or the free wall of the right atrium.

Once the donor heart has been excised, the valves are inspected for vegetations, thrombus or structural abnormalities, and the septum is inspected for a patent foramen ovale.

Donor and recipient surgery

Once the preoperative evaluation has been completed, the procurement is performed as part of a multiorgan procurement. A midline sternotomy is performed, and the pericardium is opened widely and is suspended from the edges of the sternal retractor. A visual and manual inspection of the heart is made.

When cross-clamping is imminent, the patient is heparinized with 300 units/kg of heparin. When all of the teams are prepared to procure, the superior vena cava is ligated. The inferior vena cava is clamped at the level of the diaphragm and a venotomy is performed proximal to the clamp to allow the egress of coronary sinus return. The aorta is cross-clamped, and cold crystalloid cardioplegia is infused at a pressure of 150 mmHg, regulated by a pressure bag. An incision is made in the left atrial appendage or the superior pulmonary vein to allow drainage of pulmonary venous return and prevent distension of the heart. Several liters of cold saline and saline slush are poured over the surface of the heart to cool the heart topically. The heart is then taken out of the chest to a sterile back table. It is then placed in a sterile container filled with the preservation solution.

The recipient operative technique described by Shumway and Lower in 1960 is still the most commonly employed technique for cardiac transplantation. This technique of biatrial anastamosis has stood the test of time, and is the standard against which all techniques must be compared. A technique using bicaval anastamoses to replace the right atrial anastamosis has gained popularity in recent years, and may have some physiologic advantages. A technique of total cardiac replacement, in which separate pulmonary venous anastamoses and bicaval venous anastamoses are employed, also has its advantages. Evidence of the superiority of either of these techniques over the standard biatrial technique is inconclusive to date, and neither of them will replace the Lower and Shumway technique until such evidence is available. The timing of the recipient operation is important, and depends on whether the patient has had previous cardiac surgery, as well as the distance between the recipient hospital and the donor heart. Strategic planning is necessary to allow adequate time for line placement as well as sternotomy and insertion of the cardiopulmonary bypass cannulae.

Preservation solutions

There are as many preferences and philosophies with regard to preservation solutions and techniques of preservation of the donor heart as there are with regard to cardioplegia and protection of the heart for any cardiac surgical procedure. The simplest method employed by many centers uses crystalloid cardioplegia to arrest the heart and cold saline solution for storage. Others may use any combination of crystalloid cardioplegia, blood cardioplegia or a standard preservation solution such as the University of Wisconsin solution or modified Eurocollins solution to arrest the heart, and the same or another solution to store the heart. We have observed that arrest is faster when crystalloid cardioplegia is used than with any of the preservation solutions. This may be due to its lower viscosity. Modified Eurocollins or University of Wisconsin solution is then perfused prior to cardiectomy. Our opinion is that preservation will be better if the heart is preserved and stored in one of those solutions, rather than in normal saline solution.

Postoperative management

In the immediate postoperative period the management of the cardiac transplant recipient is analogous to that of most post-cardiotomy patients, with a few caveats. After surgery, arterial blood pressure, blood pH and urine output are closely monitored in order to confirm adequate cardiac output in the cardiac surgery intensive-care unit. An oximetric Swan–Ganz catheter is used to measure central venous pressure, pulmonary capillary wedge pressure and mixed venous oxygen saturations. Patients may have an intra-aortic balloon pump or ventricular assist device, require high doses of inotropic drugs or be pacemaker dependent. The maintenance of adequate filling pressures and optimum pH balance is essential. Monitoring of chest tube drainage is important, particularly in patients with previous cardiac surgery, in order to watch for early signs of cardiac tamponade. Patients are best cared for by experienced staff and a nurse caring for the recipient only.

Maintenance of a heart rate of 90–100 beats/min is one of the important aspects of early post-operative care. Most patients are in a sinus or junctional rhythm initially. Sinus-node dysfunction due to ischemia, the effects of hypothermic storage and vagal denervation usually improves within a few days post-transplantation. Isoproterenol (0.01–0.05 ng/kg/min), epinephrine (0.01–0.05 µg/kg/min) and dobutamine (5–10 µg/kg/min) are effective agents in the perioperative period because of their chronotropic effects. Oral theophylline preparations and beta-agonists are helpful at a later stage post-transplant. Permanent pacemaker insertion due to prolonged sinoatrial node dysfunction is seen in less than 6% of cases, and third-degree heart block is seen in less than 1% of cases.

Left ventricular function post-transplant is affected by a number of preoperative factors, including the hormonal effects of brain death, prolonged ischemic time, effects of hypothermic preservation, donor heart contusion, donor substance abuse (including cocaine), and the level of inotropic support prior to procurement. The net effect of these factors is that inotropic agents are routinely required post-transplant, but intra-aortic balloon pumps or ventricular assist devices are not usually required.

Right ventricular dysfunction post-transplantation is common. In addition to the factors that affect left heart function, the right ventricle is faced with the need to overcome the elevated pulmonary vascular resistance that is seen in the typical heart transplant recipient. Occasionally, kinking of the pulmonary artery caused by excessive length of the donor and recipient pulmonary arteries can cause right heart failure. This right ventricle dysfunction may range from mild dilation of the right ventricle to severe heart failure with tricuspid regurgitation, elevated central venous pressures, hepatic congestion and peripheral edema. Acute management is directed at decreasing the pulmonary vascular resistance and increasing the contractility of the right ventricle. The treatment can range from low doses of pulmonary vasodilators and inotropes to right ventricular assist devices.

Vasodilators that are commonly employed include nitroglycerine, isoproterenol, amrinone, dobutamine and prostaglandin E1. In severe cases, infusion of pulmonary vasodilators through the central venous pressure line and of epinephrine or norepinephrine through a left atrial line has been successful. Mechanical assist devices should be used as a last resort.

Ventilator management in patients following transplantation is largely determined by the overall condition of the transplanted heart. When transplantation is successful and there are no contraindications, patients can usually be wakened and weaned off the ventilator on the first postoperative day. Patients who require high doses of inotropes, an intra-aortic balloon pump or an assist device are best kept sedated and ventilated. Paralysis is avoided except in rare instances when cardiac output is so low that it is necessary to decrease oxygen consumption to the lowest level possible.

The basic immunosuppression strategy consists of a three-drug regimen based on cyclosporine and a 7-day period of antilymphocyte induction therapy using the monoclonal antibody OKT3 or the antithymocyte globulin ATGAM (see Box 7.3). Many cardiac transplant recipients have mild to severe renal insufficiency preoperatively, which may worsen in the perioperative period. This regimen of immunosuppression was selected to allow a gradual institution of cyclosporine to minimize the nephrotoxicity of high-dose cyclosporine induction, and to allow recovery of the pre-transplant renal insufficiency. Cyclosporine is started slowly intravenously (1–3 mg/h) until the patient is taking oral medications, when Neoral is started at a dose of 1–4 mg/kg/day. The goal is to increase the dose slowly to reach therapeutic levels on day 8, when the antilymphocyte therapy is completed. In patients with severe renal insufficiency, cyclosporine may be held for several days in order to allow maximum recovery of the kidneys.

Box 7.3 Model immunosuppression protocol

Preoperative
Immuran 4 mg/kg IV

Intraoperative
Solumedrol 500, 1 g IV

Postoperative
1. Solumedrol, 125 mg IV every 8 h for 24 h, then prednisone, 0.5 mg/kg PO every day, tapered as tolerated
2. Immuran, 2 mg/kg PO/IV every day
3. Cyclosporine, 1–4 mg/h IV, then Neoral, 0.5–2.0 mg/kg twice a day – aim for a whole blood level of about 350 after induction therapy

Antilymphocyte induction
ATGAM, 15–30 mg/kg IV – begin on postoperative day 1 per protocol

or

OKT3, 2.5–5.0 mg/kg IV – begin on postoperative day 1 per protocol

Dose is adjusted daily to keep CD_3 level below 5% or 50–100 cells/mm^3.

Most patients remain in the intensive-care unit (ICU) for 3–5 days. They are transferred to a monitored stepdown unit after they have been weaned off all inotropic agents, have had all lines and chest tubes removed and are taking oral medications. Sicker patients and those with a stormy postoperative course take longer. Physical therapy is started in the ICU as soon as the patient is extubated, and activity on the stepdown unit is increased quickly under the supervision of a physical therapist. The patient receives extensive nutritional counseling during this time, and they and their family must know the medication regimen thoroughly prior to discharge. Patients receive their first endocardial biopsy and an echocardiogram prior to discharge. Once they have been discharged, they are seen frequently in the clinic for the first few weeks and less frequently as time goes on.

Routine follow-up

The commonest causes of death in the first year post-transplantation are rejection and infection. Both of these complications occur most frequently in the first 2 months after transplantation. Therefore the most intensive follow-up post-transplantation is within this initial period, during which patients are instructed to remain in close proximity to the medical center. Patients are seen twice weekly as outpatients to examine them for evidence of infection, rejection or graft dysfunction. They undergo frequent EKG, chest X-ray and blood chemistry analysis in order to monitor renal and hepatic function as well as serum levels of the pharmacologic agents used. In addition, they undergo endomyocardial biopsy weekly during the first 6–8 weeks, and at gradually lower frequencies thereafter.

After the first 6 months, if there are no significant complications patients are usually followed up every month for the first 1–2 years. They undergo endomyocardial biopsy, serum chemistry, complete blood counts, EKG and other evaluations as necessary. Follow-up after this time period is adjusted according to the individual patient and the transplant center.

Routine immunosuppression

For most patients routine immunosuppression includes cyclosporine (a drug that inhibits lymphokine production by T-lymphocytes), azathioprine (which inhibits purine synthesis and cell proliferation) and corticosteroids (which inhibit gene transcription for the production of cytokines). Every attempt is made either to wean patients off or to wean them on to the lowest level of steroids possible. Several different steroid withdrawal regimens are used, with no consensus as to when to begin decreasing the dosage and how quickly this should be done. Success rates are in the range 40–70%. One strategy of steroid withdrawal is to start at 8 weeks, with the goal of being off steroids by 6 months post-transplant.

In addition to these agents, patients also receive oral nystatin or clotrimazole to prevent candidal infections. Oral acyclovir is often administered to prevent herpes zoster infection. Trimethoprim-sulfamethoxazole or pentamidine is administered to prevent infection with *Pneumocystis carinii*. Pyrimethamine and sulfadiazine are given to *Toxoplasma gondii*-seronegative patients who receive organs from seropositive donors.

Complications

Infection

One-third of all transplant patients develop an infection that requires intravenous antibiotics during the first year following transplantation. Infection is the commonest cause of death in the first year after transplantation. In the first year, 46% of infections are bacterial, with the peak incidence occurring during the first postoperative week. The majority of bacterial infections are lung infections, line infections and (rarely) sternal wound infections. Patients who were on mechanical ventilators prior to transplantation are at highest risk for developing a bacterial lung infection. Sternal wound infections account for 6% of serious wound infections, but result in a mortality rate of 22%. Opportunistic bacterial infections such as legionella and listeria also occur. However, these infections generally occur in the later postoperative period.

Viral infections occur with a peak incidence at 30–60 days post-transplantation. Cytomegalovirus (CMV) is the commonest pathogen responsible for serious infection in the post-transplant population. The majority of transplant recipients are seropositive for CMV and harbor dormant viral organisms. With the induction of immunosuppression, reactivation of this dormant virus or re-infection with another CMV strain may occur. If the recipient is seronegative for CMV and the donor is seropositive, there is a risk of transmission of this virus and appearance of a primary CMV infection.

Infection with CMV is most commonly localized to the lung, where it presents as pneumonia, with the appearance of fever, dyspnea, hypoxemia and a diffuse infiltrate. The next commonest area of localized CMV infection is the gastrointestinal tract. Gastrointestinal CMV infection can present as fever, diarrhea and massive gastrointestinal bleeding. Hepatic involvement manifested as hepatitis and eye involvement manifested as chorioretinitis and papillitis also occur. General or non-localized infection, manifested as malaise and lethargy with positive blood or urine cultures, may occur as well. Treatment is with 2–4 weeks of intravenous ganciclovir.

Fungal infections account for approximately 7% of infections post-transplantation. The peak incidence of these infections is during weeks 2 to 6. The commonest type is candidal infection, which is present in blood or as a sternal wound infection. Pulmonary aspergillosis, nocardia and cryptococcal infections also occur.

Protozoal infections peak at months 3 to 4. The commonest protozoal infection is *Pneumocystis carinii* pneumonia. Patients present with diffuse pulmonary infiltrate, dyspnea and hypoxemia. Prophylaxis with trimethoprim–sulfamethoxazole has resulted in a lower incidence of this infectious process. Dapsone is used for patients with a sulfa allergy. However, on discontinuation of the latter agent, infection with this pathogen may occur. Toxoplasmosis often occurs as a donor-transmitted disease.

Prophylaxis with pyrimethamine and sulfadiazine is effective in preventing active disease.

Rejection

Cell-mediated rejection is the commonest form of acute rejection, whereas antibody-mediated rejection is far less common. However, it is much more resistant to treatment. The Cardiac Transplant Research Database indicates that at the end of 1 year post-transplant, 37% of patients were free from rejection, 40% of patients had had one episode of rejection and 23% had had more than one rejection. The majority of all rejections occurred within the first 6 months after transplantation, and rejection accounted for 17% of all deaths within the first year.

Symptoms associated with rejection are non-specific and include malaise, lethargy, fatigue and low-grade fevers. If the rejection episode is severe and associated with graft dysfunction, dyspnea, an S3 gallop and lower blood pressure may be seen. However, most cases of rejection are associated with few specific symptoms or physical signs. Therefore, diagnosis of rejection is made on the basis of endomyocardial biopsy. In 1989, the International Society for Heart–Lung Transplantation standardized the grading system for endomyocardial biopsy allowing transplant physicians a uniform way to diagnose and treat rejection (see Table 7.1). Surveillance biopsies are performed frequently during the first 6 months. Since endomyocardial biopsy is an invasive procedure, there have been many attempts to develop a non-invasive method to determine rejection. Various forms of electrocardiography,

Table 7.1 Standardized cardiac biopsy grading

Grade	Formulation	Description
0	—	No rejection
1A	Focal, mild	Focal infiltrate without necrosis
1B	Diffuse, mild	Diffuse infiltrate without necrosis
2	Focal, moderate	One focus of aggressive infiltration and/or focal myocyte damage
3A	Multifocal, moderate	Multifocal aggressive infiltrates and/or myocyte damage
3B	Diffuse, borderline severe	Diffuse inflammatory process with borderline severe necrosis
4	Severe	Diffuse aggressive infiltrate, edema, hemorrhage, vasculitis, with necrosis

echocardiography and immunologic markers have been investigated with a view to developing a non-invasive means of detecting rejection. However, none of them have proved to be sensitive or specific enough to replace endomyocardial biopsy.

Treatment of rejection is generally reserved for higher grades of rejection. In general, patients with mild rejection are not actively treated but are followed closely for worsening rejection. Those with higher-grade rejection are treated with high-dose oral or intravenous steroids. Doses are in the range 1500–3000 mg of methylprednisolone, divided over 3 days, or 300–1000 mg of oral prednisone, tapered over 7–14 days. Rejection that is associated with hemodynamic compromise or graft dysfunction or rejection episodes that are resistant to the second course of steroid therapy are usually treated with monoclonal or polyclonal antibodies in addition to high-dose steroids.

Humoral rejection is diagnosed by immunofluorescent staining of the biopsy specimens.

Antibody and complement deposition is seen on the vascular endothelium. Humoral rejection is associated with a higher incidence of fatality and decreased long-term survival. In general, no treatment is recommended for humoral rejection unless there is concomitant graft dysfunction. In this case, high-dose steroids, antithymocyte globulin, cyclophosphamide and plasmapheresis have all been used with variable degrees of success.

Hyperacute rejection is a form of humoral rejection that causes immediate graft dysfunction at the time of implantation, and is due to preformed antibodies in the recipient. Patients who show hyperacute rejection have a poor prognosis.

Malignancy

Immunosuppressed transplant recipients have a 1–2% risk per year of developing a malignancy. This risk may increase as patients survive for longer after their transplant. It may also be higher in those with a history of previous malignancy. The overall risk is approximately 6%, about 100 times that in the general population. Solid organ transplant patients are not at higher risk of developing the common tumors such as cancer of the lung, prostate, breast and colon. Rather, they are at a higher risk of developing squamous-cell carcinoma of the skin, lymphoma, Kaposi's sarcoma, carcinoma of the vulva or perineum, carcinoma of the kidney and hepatobiliary tumors. Cutaneous malignancy is the commonest malignancy, and is associated with the use of azathioprine. The high incidence of skin carcinoma is believed to be due to the photosensitizing effects of the azathioprine metabolite, nitroimidazole.

A unique type of lymphoma, referred to as post-transplant lymphoproliferative disease, is non-Hodgkin's B-cell lymphoma. The mean time to presentation of these tumors is 12–18 months post-transplantation. The tumor appears to be induced by the Epstein–Barr virus. Data from the Cincinnati Transplant Tumor Registry suggest that up to 40% of patients with this disease may respond to a reduction in immunosuppressant therapy. Presentation of this type of lymphoma is similar to that of lymphomas in the non-transplant population, and may occur with lymphadenopathy, abdominal mass, gastrointestinal ulceration, seizures and fever of unknown origin. Chemotherapy, radiation therapy and surgical excision when possible should be considered. However, long-term survival rates are poor.

Cardiac allograft vasculopathy (CAV)

The leading cause of death after the first year post-transplantation is cardiac allograft vasculopathy (CAV). This is an unusual form of accelerated coronary artery disease. The phenomenon is detected angiographically in 30–50% of patients by 5 years after transplantation, and can be detected as early as 6 months after transplantation. This disease process differs from native coronary atherosclerotic disease in several important respects. It is diffuse, concentric and longitudinal, and develops rapid pruning and obliteration of distal branch vessels. Focal stenosis of these vessels may occur. However, this is less common than the diffuse types of stenoses that occur. Because of the diffuse narrowing that is found, coronary angiography (which relies on the adjacent 'normal' vessel caliber to diagnose stenotic lesions), is a relatively insensitive method for diagnosing CAV. More recently, intravascular ultrasound was shown to be a more sensitive way to diagnose this disease. Histologically, CAV reveals hyperplasia of the smooth-muscle cells and macrophages that migrate into the intima, which results in lumenal narrowing. These changes are almost identical to those which are seen in patients who develop restenosis after percutaneous transluminal coronary angioplasty.

Because of the denervation that occurs with the transplanted heart, patients do not usually present with angina. Presenting signs of this disease include graft failure, acute myocardial infarction and sudden death. Angiographic changes may occur as early as 1 year after transplantation. Therefore most transplant centers perform baseline coronary angiography at 1 month after transplantation and at yearly intervals thereafter.

CAV is thought to be multifactorial in origin, but is believed to be immune mediated, via injury to the vascular endothelium. Development of methods to prevent this from occurring has been difficult. The relationship between this disease and known risk factors for coronary artery disease such as hypertension, hyperlipidemia and smoking has not yet been firmly established. Links between CAV, and the number and severity of rejection episodes and the use of corticosteroids and cyclosporine, as well as infection with CMV, have been suggested but are not yet firmly established.

Treatment for CAV has included the use of calcium-channel blockers (which may increase lumenal diameter), percutaneous transluminal coronary angioplasty, atherectomy and coronary artery bypass grafting for focal lesions, with varying degrees of success. However, the only definitive treatment for this progressive disease is retransplantation. This remains a controversial area due to the shortage of donor organs and the relatively poor survival rate post-retransplantation.

Outcomes

Physiology of the transplanted heart

Soon after transplantation, the cardiac output is often depressed, and maintenance of a high central venous pressure and inotropic medication is important for maintaining the cardiac output. This is probably due to an early restrictive type of physiology caused by ischemia and the damaging effects of hypothermic preservation techniques, and abnormal atrial dynamics. Because of the mid-atrial anastomosis between the donor and recipient hearts, varying proportions of the donor and recipient are present. Furthermore, the recipient atria do not contract synchronously with the donor atria, because recipient sinus node electrical activity does not pass through anastomotic suture lines. This results in approximately 20% of the normal atrial contribution to the total stroke volume of the heart.

Many patients have normal resting intracardiac pressures after transplantation that can increase with exercise. This is due to an early restrictive hemodynamic pattern. When it is present early after transplantation it usually resolves. More recently it has been recognized that there is a subclinical, latent, restrictive component that is present and unmasked by volume challenge. This may be confounded by post-transplantation hypertension with resultant hypertrophy, and by bouts of rejection.

The transplanted heart displays a unique response to exercise. During early exercise the cardiac output increases by augmentation of end-diastolic volume and stroke volume. At more intense exercise levels, heart rate and contractility are increased by circulating catecholamines. The heart rate response is blunted in these individuals because of vagal denervation. The maximal cardiac output achieved is generally lower than that of normal individuals, because of a blunted heart rate response and a lower peak stroke volume.

Denervation of the heart leads to a resting tachycardia (95–115 beats/min) due to loss of vagal input. Moreover, the rate does not respond to carotid sinus massage or to drugs that are dependent on intact innervation of the heart, such as atropine. The blunted heart rate response to exercise that occurs relatively late is effected by high levels of circulating catecholamines. Administration of quinidine and disopyramide (agents that have vagolytic effects in the innervated heart), tend to increase atrioventricular conduction time due to their direct atrioventricular nodal effects.

Psychosocial aspects

Given 1-year survival rates of 80–90% and 5-year survival rates of 60–70%, patients who have undergone cardiac transplantation show an improvement in survival and a longer life expectancy. Several studies have addressed the quality of life in addition to the quantity of life. The National Transplantation Study examined quality of life in detail, and analyzed data from 85% of transplantation programs in the USA. This study found that 80–85% of the patients were physically active, and 90% of the patients who were analyzed described themselves as normal or stated that they had minimal signs or symptoms of disease. Only 7.2% rated their health status as poor, 9% of patients needed assistance in traveling around their community, and only 1% needed assistance with eating, dressing, bathing or using the toilet. Patients rated their life satisfaction, well-being and psychological affect as equal to that of the general population.

Despite these good ratings of physical activity and well-being, only 32–50% of patients are employed after transplantation. The reasons for this surprisingly low number are thought to be multifactorial. Employers may be reluctant to hire people who have undergone transplantation, due to fear of absenteeism and an increase in group health insurance rates. Patients may also be less motivated to work after a serious illness, due to fear of losing medical, disability or public assistance benefits.

Survival

Despite these potential complications, as indicated earlier, heart transplant patients experience a general improvement both in quality of life and survival. Data from the Cardiac Transplant Research Database indicate that the 1-year survival rate in major North American transplant centers is 85%. It is estimated that the 5-year survival rate in major North American transplant centers is 75%. Thus, despite its limitations, cardiac transplantation offers a viable option for improving both quality and quantity of life in selected patients.

Further reading

American Medical Association. 1968: Report of the ad hoc committee of the Harvard Medical School to examine the definition of brain death. A definition of irreversible coma. *Journal of the American Medical Association* **205**, 337–40.

Banner NR and **Yacoub MH**. 1990: Physiology of the orthotopic cardiac transplant recipient. *Seminars in Thoracic and Cardiovascular Surgery* **2**, 259–70.

Barnard CN. 1967: A human cardiac transplant: an interim report of a successful operation performed at Groote Schuur Hospital, Cape Town. *South African Medical Journal* **41**, 1271.

Baumgartner WA. 1990: Operative techniques utilized in heart transplantation. In Baumgartner WA, Reitz BA and Achuff SC (eds), *Heart and heart–lung transplantation*. Philadelphia, PA: WB Saunders, 113–33.

Carvel A and **Guthrie CC**. 1905: The transplantation of veins and organs. *American Journal of Medicine* **10**, 1101.

Emery RW, Eales F, Joyce LD *et al.* 1991: Mechanical circulatory assistance after heart transplantation. *Annals of Thoracic Surgery* **51**, 43–7.

Evans RW. 1993: Social, economic and insurance issues in heart transplantation. In Kaye MP and O'Connell JB (eds) *Heart and Lung Transplantation 2000*. Austin, TX: R.G. Landes Company, 1–14.

Griepp RB, Stinson EB, Clark DA, Dong E Jr and **Shumway NE**. 1971: The cardiac donor. *Surgical Gynecology and Obstetrics* **133**, 792–98.

Stinson EB, Griepp RB, Clark DA, Dong E Jr and **Shumway NE**. 1970: Cardiac transplantation in man. VIII. Survival and function. *Journal of Thoracic and Cardiovascular Surgery* **60**, 303–21.

Lung transplantation

8

John V. Conte Jr and Jonathan Orens

Introduction

The history of lung transplantation began in 1906, when Charles Guthrie and Alexis Carrel performed a heterotopic heart–lung transplant in which the heart and lungs of a kitten were transplanted into the neck of a cat. The recipient survived for 2 days. This procedure was reported to the Johns Hopkins Medical Society and was later published in the *Johns Hopkins Medical Bulletin*. Not surprisingly, given the stage of development of medical science at that time, interest was limited. It would be decades before knowledge of physiology and pharmacology, as well as surgical techniques, advanced far enough for physicians to comprehend transplantation as a viable clinical option.

More than 40 years after the first pioneering attempts at whole organ transplantation, a variety of surgeons were experimenting with the idea of lung transplantation. The Russian surgeon and physiologist Demikhov performed successful canine lobar homografts, although most of his work in the field of thoracic transplantation remained largely unknown until 1962, when it was published in the USA. Interestingly, Juvenelle was credited with performing the first canine autotransplant in 1950, although Henri Metras had already published his technique in Europe. Important and novel aspects of the technique described by Metras include reimplantation of bronchial arteries, and the use of an atrial cuff instead of reimplanting individual pulmonary veins. The atrial cuff technique has become standard, and bronchial artery reimplantation is now being intensely studied. In 1953, W.B. Neptune addressed some of the advantages of the atrial cuff technique, and attempted to delineate the role of immunosuppression, in this case by adrenocorticotropin hormone, in survival following transplantation. James Hardy, at the University of Mississippi, through his work on canine models furthered our understanding of the advantages of multidrug immunosuppression.

Hardy's extensive canine experience prepared him to perform the first human lung transplant in 1963. Although the recipient died on postoperative day 18 as a result of renal failure and malnutrition, Hardy proved that human lung transplantation was possible. However, for nearly two decades after his pioneering effort all attempts at human lung transplantation failed to achieve long-term survival. This included attempts at individual lobar transplantation by Shinoi and colleagues at the Tokyo Medical College in 1966, and combined heart–lung transplantation by Cooley and colleagues at the Texas Heart Institute in 1968. Despite their lack of success, investigators at several different institutions directed their efforts towards understanding the basic problems identified by the clinical failures, including operative techniques, organ preservation, immunosuppression and the physiology of the transplanted lung.

In 1981, Bruce Reitz and his colleagues at Stanford University performed the world's first successful lung transplant of any kind – a combined heart–lung transplant in a woman with primary pulmonary hypertension. In 1983, Joel Cooper performed the first successful isolated lung transplant in a patient with pulmonary fibrosis at the University of Toronto. Building on their experience with single lung transplantation, en-bloc double lung transplantation was attempted in 1986. Unfortunately, this technique was fraught with complications, and subsequently a technique of bilateral sequential lung transplantation, originally developed by Metras in 1950, became the procedure of choice for double lung transplantation. It was reintroduced by Pasque and his colleagues from Washington University in St Louis in 1990.

The next major clinical advance in lung transplantation occurred in 1992, when Vaughn Starnes and his colleagues at Stanford performed the first successful living related lobar transplantation in a pediatric patient. Although it was initially limited in scope, this technique has been expanded to bilateral lung transplants in adults for a variety of conditions, including primary pulmonary hypertension and cystic fibrosis.

Now that lung transplantation has become an accepted treatment option for patients with end-stage pulmonary disease, further research is in progress to improve outcome and survival among recipients. Lung transplantation as a clinical tool is limited by donor organ availability, acute and chronic rejection, infection and problems related to immunosuppression. Research is currently under way to improve organ preservation, develop xenotransplantation as a potential alternative or bridge to transplant, and ameliorate or prevent acute and chronic rejection.

Recipient evaluation

The ideal candidate for lung transplantation has end-stage lung disease without coexisting disease that would adversely affect survival following transplantation (see Box 8.1). Successful lung transplantation is performed for a number of major pulmonary disorders, including obstructive and restrictive diseases, pulmonary vascular disease and suppurative lung disease (see Box 8.2). Several issues must be considered with regard to the appropriate selection of candidates and the timing of transplantation. The

---

Box 8.1 Patient selection criteria

General principles
All patients who are selected for lung transplantation must meet the following criteria:
1. end-stage pulmonary parenchymal and/or vascular disease;
2. failed medical management;
3. life expectancy less than 2 years;
4. substantial limitations to activities of daily living;
5. New York Heart Association class III or IV functional level with rehabilitation potential;
6. no significant cardiac disease;
7. acceptable nutritional status;
8. satisfactory psychosocial profile and emotional support system.

Box 8.2 Diseases that are treatable by lung transplantation

Obstructive lung disease
Emphysema
α_1-Antitrypsin deficiency emphysema
Obliterative bronchiolitis

Suppurative lung disease
Cystic fibrosis
Bronchiectasis

Restrictive lung disease
Idiopathic pulmonary fibrosis
Sarcoidosis
Collagen vascular disease (without significant systemic manifestations)
Occupational lung disease
Eosinophilic granulomatosis
Lymphangioleiomyomatosis
Alveolar microlithiasis
Pulmonary alveolar proteinosis
Other pulmonary fibrotic disorders

Pulmonary vascular disease
Primary pulmonary hypertension
Eisenmenger's syndrome
Thrombo-embolic pulmonary hypertension
Veno-occlusive disease

natural history of the underlying disease as it relates to projected survival of the patient must be weighed against the morbidity and mortality of transplantation. The waiting period from the time of listing to the time of transplantation, as well as other factors such as concomitant illness, nutritional status and psychosocial stability, must also be considered (see Box 8.3).

Priority on the transplant waiting-list is determined by time on the waiting-list, with no consideration given to disease severity. However, patients with idiopathic pulmonary fibrosis receive a 3-month credit due to the rapidly progressive nature of this disorder and the large number of such patients who have died while awaiting transplant. In order to ensure consistency among transplant centers, three major societies have proposed disease-specific criteria for lung transplantation. However, although the United Network for Organ Sharing (UNOS), the International Society For Heart and Lung Transplantation (ISHLT) and the American Society of Transplant Physicians (ASTP) are each currently in the process

---

Box 8.3 Contraindications to lung transplantation

Relative contraindications
Obesity
Prednisone use > 20 mg/day or 40 mg every other day
Bilateral pleurodesis for cardiopulmonary bypass candidates
Physiologic age:
    > 65 years for single lung transplantation (SLT)
    > 60 years for bilateral single lung transplantation (BLT)
    > 55 years for heart and lung transplantation (HLT)
Psychosocial instability
Mechanical ventilation
Primary renal disease
Primary liver disease
Severe chest wall deformity
History of substance abuse

Absolute contraindications
HIV infection
Bone-marrow failure
Cirrhosis of the liver
Malignancy precluding long-term survival
Other life-limiting conditions
Active tobacco smoking or other substance abuse
Significant peripheral vascular disease
Impaired left heart function, unless considered for HLT
Severe symptomatic osteoporosis
Sputum with panresistant bacteria or *Aspergillus*
Active hepatitis B or C infection

Box 8.4 Disease-specific indications for lung transplantation

Chronic obstructive pulmonary disease
Postbronchodilator $FEV_1 \leqslant 25\%$ of predicted value
Resting hypoxia ($PO_2 < 55$ mmHg)
Hypercapnia
Significant secondary pulmonary hypertension
Clinical course
    Declining FEV_1
    Life-threatening exacerbations

Cystic fibrosis
Postbronchodilator $FEV_1 < 30\%$ of predicted value
Resting hypoxia ($PO_2 < 55$ mmHg)
Hypercapnia
Clinical course:
    Increasing frequency and severity of exacerbations
    Weight loss

Idiopathic pulmonary fibrosis
Vital capacity, total lung capacity $< 60\%$ of predicted value
Resting hypoxia
Significant secondary pulmonary hypertension

Primary pulmonary hypertension
New York Heart Association class III or IV functional level
Mean right atrial pressure $\geqslant 10$ mmHg
Mean pulmonary arterial pressure $\geqslant 50$ mmHg
Cardiac index ≤ 2.0 L/min/m^2
Failure of medical management

---

of developing such guidelines, individual programs continue to use their own unique selection criteria. Given the limited nature of the data on the natural history of processes for which transplants are performed, as well as the rapid rate of change in clinical practice, it is obvious that these guidelines should not be regarded as absolute (see Box 8.4).

Indications

Emphysema

For patients with severe end-stage emphysema, lung transplantation offers the possibility of improved survival and functional status. Although millions of people are affected by this disease worldwide, there are only limited data on the natural history of patients with severe emphysema. Traver and colleagues showed that the combination of a low 1-s forced expiratory volume (FEV_1), advanced age and chronic hypoxemia had a negative impact on survival. In this study population there was an overall 2-year survival rate of 44%. However, the 2-year survival rate in those patients with a post-bronchodilator FEV_1 of $\leqslant$ 30% of the predicted value and age $\leqslant$ 65 years was nearly 70%. In a similar group of patients with severe emphysema and hypoxemia, the Nocturnal Oxygen Treatment Trial (NOTT) documented an improvement in survival with the use of supplemental oxygen. Another large study of non-hypoxemic patients with a post-bronchodilator FEV_1 of $\leqslant$ 30% of the predicted value and age $\leqslant$ 65 years documented a 75% 2-year survival rate. Comparing the risks and benefits of transplantation with the natural history of emphysema, these patients should probably be listed for lung transplantation when the post-bronchodilator FEV_1 is $\leqslant$ 25% of the predicted value. In addition, problems such as the level of functional impairment, the severity of hypoxemia and hypercapnea, the presence of cor pulmonale, and the frequency of hospitalizations and recurrent infections may affect this threshold.

There is little consensus concerning which procedure is ideal for patients with end-stage emphysema. Single lung transplant is most commonly performed, although some centers offer sequential double lung transplantation for this disease. The functional and long-term survival data are reasonably good for single lung transplantation, and two patients may benefit from a single donor. However, native lung hyperinflation may occur in the immediate postoperative period, which may be very difficult to manage, particularly while the patient remains on mechanical ventilation. For this reason, patients with severe bullous disease are often offered double lung procedures. Lung volume reduction of the native lung may be useful in this setting.

Idiopathic pulmonary fibrosis

Idiopathic pulmonary fibrosis (IPF) is a progressive interstitial lung disease that is associated with very poor long-term outcome. Therapy consists of high-dose oral corticosteroids or cytotoxic drugs such as cyclophosphamide, but unfortunately only 10–30% of patients show a good clinical response. For those who fail medical therapy and have a low functional vital capacity (FVC) of $\leqslant$ 67% of the predicted value, the 2-year survival rate is less than 50%. Single lung transplantation is an effective treatment for this disease. The fibrotic process results in decreased lung compliance as well as loss of the vascular bed. Hence, following transplantation, ventilation and perfusion are both preferentially directed towards the allograft, resulting in good ventilation/perfusion matching. Although transplantation for IPF is the only life-sustaining option for those patients who fail medical therapy, the overall statistics after transplantation are sobering. The 2-year survival rate following single lung transplant for IPF is around 58% (for the period 1982–95). Patients with pulmonary hypertension are frequently offered bilateral lung transplantation. Patients with IPF should be referred early in the course of their disease, particularly if the FVC is ≤ 67% of the predicted value, because of the unpredictable rate of decline and the significant likelihood of death occurring while the patient is awaiting transplantation.

Primary pulmonary hypertension

Lung transplantation should be considered for patients with primary pulmonary hypertension (PPH) who have failed vasodilator therapy. Combined heart–lung and lung transplantation has been successfully performed for PPH since the early 1980s, and has resulted in an improved quality of life and prolonged survival. More recently, single or double lung transplantation has become more popular. This trend is based on the scarcity of donor organs, the ability of the recipient's right ventricle to recover its function following normalization of its afterload, and the high rate of chronic rejection in the transplanted lung in these recipients. However, a controversy exists between proponents of single and double lung procedures. Advocates of single lung transplantation argue that reasonable functional benefit and improved survival can be achieved while at the same time preserving a limited supply of donor organs as well as allowing a shorter operation with potentially lower morbidity. On the other hand, proponents of double lung transplantation argue that this procedure will allow maximum recovery of right ventricular function by maximally reducing the pulmonary vascular resistance and avoiding over-perfusion of the transplanted lung, as well as simplification of early postoperative management and improved toleration of acute allograft rejection. Sequential double lung transplantation may also provide a small functional benefit in the long term when compared to single lung transplantation. Further studies are needed to resolve this particular issue.

With the advent of new, more efficacious therapies such as continuous intravenous prostacyclin, there is no consensus on the timing of lung transplantation for patients with PPH. Many centers advocate listing patients for transplantation as soon as the diagnosis of

PPH is made, due to the long waiting period at most centers (12–18 months) and the unpredictable rate of progression, while others recommend that patients should only be listed on failure of medical therapy (i.e. vasodilators and anticoagulation). Accordingly, the overall clinical picture must be assessed for each individual patient in order to allow an ample waiting time for this potentially life-saving therapy.

Cystic fibrosis

Cystic fibrosis (CF) is a multisystem disease characterized by airflow obstruction and bronchiectasis with progressive tissue destruction due to recurrent suppuration. Patients with severe forms of the disease present in the first decade of life, and for some of them lung transplantation is a lifesaving measure. However, the multisystem nature of the disease poses clinical problems that frustrate a successful outcome after transplantation. Malnutrition and colonization of the lung with resistant bacteria and fungi are the main problems. CF patients who are colonized with bacteria resistant to even a single antibiotic should not undergo lung transplantation because of the high risk of death from these organisms during the postoperative period. In a series of 15 patients, the mortality rate due to antibiotic-resistant *Pseudomonas cepacia* (now *Burkholderia cepacia*) approached 46% when this organism was present in the sputum prior to transplantation. In contrast, there were no deaths in 8 patients who had been colonized with *Pseudomonas aeruginosa*. Several maneuvers have had variable rates of success in decreasing colonization with resistant bacteria, including holidays from systemic antibiotics, inhaled colystin, and sinus surgery. Double lung transplantation is the procedure of choice in these patients because of the underlying chronic suppuration and the risk of continued colonization and active infection.

The timing of transplantation in patients with CF must be individualized, but many centers use criteria based on mortality data from Karem and his colleagues. This group has documented a 2-year survival rate of nearly 50% when the pulmonary function studies revealed a significant reduction in the FEV_1 and FVC coupled with hypoxemia, hypercapnea and weight loss. Patients who have progressed to this stage will probably fare better with lung transplantation, for which the 2-year survival rate is around 64%. Cardiopulmonary exercise testing may be helpful for predicting survival and the timing of transplantation. Nixon and colleagues documented a correlation between maximal oxygen consumption and survival in CF patients.

Donor evaluation

Selection of donor organs is one of the keys to successful transplantation, regardless of the organ being transplanted. In few cases is this more important than in the selection of potential donor lungs. In the USA it is estimated that only 15–20% of potential multiorgan donors actually come to procurement. Failure to request donation at the time of declaration of brain death and failure to obtain consent from the next of kin are two of the commonest reasons for potential donors being lost. Of those donors who do come to procurement, it is estimated that only 10–15% are suitable as lung donors.

The lack of suitability of the majority of potential donor lungs is not surprising. Trauma patients often receive large volumes of crystalloid and blood products during resuscitation, a problem that is compounded by capillary leak syndromes which are commonly seen in this setting. The physiologic changes that accompany brain death compound the problem further. Trauma of almost any kind can cause pulmonary contusions and atelectasis, further impairing pulmonary function. Aspiration of blood, secretions or gastrointestinal contents frequently accompanies trauma, and commonly develops into pneumonia or other infectious complications. These patients are uniformly intubated and mechanically ventilated, thus disabling the natural defenses of the upper airways and further compromising pulmonary function. A study by Hsieh and colleagues found that among patients with closed head injuries who had ventilated for 24 h or more, 40% developed pneumonia, most often within 3 days of injury.

Hemodynamic instability is also common in brain-dead patients. Hormonal and metabolic derangements, low-grade infections, and multiple, less well-defined factors often combine to produce a low systemic vascular resistance, frequently compounded by diabetes insipidus. If this instability is treated primarily with volume infusions, pulmonary edema ensues, leading to disqualification as a potential lung donor. The large volume of fluid replacement preferred by abdominal transplant surgeons must be weighed against the lung transplant surgeon's desire to avoid pulmonary edema. Low-dose inotropic agents, antibiotics, vasopressin and central venous pressure monitoring can help to mediate this conflict of interest.

Neurogenic pulmonary edema is a less common but equally devastating cause of pulmonary edema in brain-dead patients. Its etiology is unclear, but may be due to catecholamine storm. Invasive monitoring is needed to permit aggressive diuresis, and hemodynamic and ventilator management.

All multiple organ donors should be evaluated as potential lung donors. The general criteria that have been in use since 1989 are accepted by most programs, although each program has its own specific method for evaluating candidates. The potential donor's medical history is reviewed, as are records of the current hospitalization. Brain death must be absolutely determined and documented. A history of significant pulmonary disease, including asthma, must be investigated. Seasonal wheezing is not a contraindication, but a history of long-term medical therapy or prior hospitalization is disqualifying, as is a history of recurrent bronchitis or concurrent pneumonia. Similarly, cigarette smoking itself is not a contraindication unless it has been prolonged (≥ 20 pack-years), chest radiography shows changes consistent with obstructive lung disease, or hypercarbia persists in the face of adequate alveolar ventilation. Prior thoracic surgery is not ideal, but is not an absolute contraindication to donation.

Information concerning the current clinical course and serologic data is crucially important. ABO mismatch or HIV antigenemia are absolute contraindications. Similarly, hepatitis B and C antibodies will exclude candidates in most centers. However, some programs are willing to accept donors who are positive for hepatitis B or C for recipients with matching serologies, and others will accept hepatitis B antibody-positive donors with a history of prior vaccination and a negative hepatitis B antigen. Sometimes serologies are ignored if the intended recipient is close to death and no other options are imminent.

Diagnostic evaluation of a potential lung donor is extensive. Chest X-rays are examined in order to rule out obvious injury, infection, intrinsic lung disease or pulmonary edema. Radiographic abnormalities that exclude donation include obvious pneumonia, parenchymal abnormalities (including masses or contusions) and significant pulmonary edema. Unilateral abnormalities will not necessarily exclude donation of the other lung, but will prompt increased scrutiny. A chest X-ray should be repeated every 4 h prior to procurement, as the clinical status may change abruptly. Some patients will have had computerized tomography (CT) scans during the current hospitalization, and these may contribute to the evaluation process. Small contusions in otherwise acceptable lungs may not exclude donation if the recipient does not have pulmonary hypertension, there is a good size match, and the transplant can be performed off bypass without systemic heparinization.

Acceptable gas exchange has traditionally been considered to be a PaO_2 of 300 mmHg on an FiO_2 of 1.0 and a positive end-expiratory pressure (PEEP) of 5 cmH$_2$O for 5 min, or a PaO_2 of 100 mmHg on an FiO_2 of 0.4. Even mild degrees of pulmonary edema, atelectasis or retained secretions can lead to ventilation/perfusion mismatching and impaired oxygenation. Although the threshold levels are clearly not normal, it has been shown that patients with at least this level of gas exchange can fare very well post-transplant. Patients who do not meet these criteria should have a trial of suctioning, diuresis and increased PEEP for a brief period before repeating an arterial blood gas analysis. If oxygenation does not improve and a chest X-ray excludes atelectasis, infiltrate, pulmonary edema and contusion, bronchoscopy should be performed in order to rule out mucous plugging of the airway. Arterial blood gases should be repeated frequently to allow ongoing assessment of gas exchange.

Culture results and sputum Gram stains should be reviewed. A positive Gram stain of the tracheal aspirate is found in at least 80% of donors, and should not be a contraindication to donation. It must be considered in the context of the whole clinical picture including chest X-ray, history, bronchoscopy and culture results.

As a rule, the ideal size for a particular recipient is their predicted total lung capacity rather than their current lung size. Unfortunately, the ideal lung is rarely encountered, and the severity of the recipient's disease must be taken into consideration. Simple height and weight matching is unworkable, due to pathologic changes in the size and shape of the recipient's thorax. For example, patients with emphysema have larger than expected chest cavities, while the chest cavities of patients with restrictive lung diseases tend to be smaller than expected. The chest will remodel itself to some degree post-transplant to accommodate the size of the transplanted lung. However, this cannot correct for a large size mismatch. An oversized lung will interfere with venous return and cause a mediastinal shift, resulting in homodynamic instability. It can also promote atelectasis, retention of secretions and the development of pneumonia. Alternatively, an undersized lung can cause pleural space problems or provide inadequate vascular capacity, resulting in postoperative pulmonary hypertension. Despite these real and theoretical concerns, it has been found that large lungs can sometimes adapt to a small recipient chest cavity. They may also be downsized by lobectomy or simple non-anatomic shaping. An additional factor to consider is that a larger lung can be used on the left side, given the potential for greater diaphragmatic excursion compared to the right side, where the liver limits pulmonary expansion. Similarly, patients with emphysema who are scheduled for single lung transplantation should have the right lung transplanted if possible, allowing the hyperexpanded native lung to expand downward and not compress the mediastinum and the allograft.

A variety of parameters have been used to match donors and recipients optimally. One method measures the vertical and horizontal dimensions of the lung on a chest X-ray at end expiration. Other approaches use height and weight measurements, or predicted total lung and vital capacities. Chest circumference measured below the nipple line has been used to match donors and recipients, but does not appear to offer any advantage over simple chest X-ray measurements.

The next step in the evaluation process is physical examination of the potential donor, most frequently in the intensive-care unit. Examination of the chest is performed, looking for evidence of trauma, chest wall abnormalities or asymmetry, while auscultation identifies cardiac murmurs as well as pleural or pericardial friction rubs. Bronchoscopy is then performed on all potential donors. This is sometimes done in the operating-room immediately prior to the procurement procedure. Anatomic abnormalities, particularly aberrant lobar orifices, must be ruled out. Evidence of aspiration of blood or gastrointestinal contents is sought. Mucosal surfaces are carefully examined, looking for evidence of acute or chronic infection. Frank purulence excludes the lungs from transplantation and is an ominous sign for utilization of the contralateral lung.

Visual and manual inspection of the lungs in the operating-room is the final step in the evaluation process. The entire surface of the lung must be examined, including opening and completely exploring both pleural cavities. Adhesions, apical bullae, contusions, pleural retraction and evidence of consolidation are sought. All but minor adhesions contraindicate donation, due to the inevitable injury to the pleural surfaces following dissection of dense adhesions. Mild apical bullous changes are acceptable, but large or multiple bullae indicate severe lung disease and exclude donation. Consolidation usually indicates infectious processes and excludes donation, particularly when the lung cannot be expanded by manual ventilation by the anesthesiologist. Manual palpation of the lung is gently performed in order to identify deep parenchymal lesions that would not otherwise be suspected. Once the lungs have been removed from the donor, one last inspection is performed.

Recipient operation

Cardiopulmonary pulmonary bypass is available on standby for all cases, and is planned in patients with pulmonary hypertension and preoperative right ventricular dysfunction.

Single lung transplantation

The patient is positioned in a thoracotomy position with the hips rotated towards the side of transplantation to facilitate groin cannulation for bypass, if necessary. A muscle-sparing thoraco-tomy is preferred. However, standard posterior lateral incisions are used as well. Immediately upon opening the chest the lung is collapsed and single lung ventilation is started. On arrival of the lung, vascular staplers are used to divide the vascular structures after 5–10 000 units of heparin have been administered. The bronchus is divided in a convenient location and the pneumonec-tomy is completed. The pericardium is opened to expose the left atrium and the proximal ends of the divided pulmonary veins. The new donor lung is placed in the chest and covered with iced lap sponges and saline slush. The bronchial anastamosis is constructed first because it is the deepest structure, the most technically chal-lenging and the most difficult to expose. Any size discrepancies are handled by intussuscepting the smaller bronchus into the larger bronchus. The left atrial and pulmonary artery anastomoses are then performed, and the clamps are subsequently released.

The EKG is monitored to watch for ST-segment elevations caused by washout of the hyperkalemic preservation solution. The lungs are ventilated with a PEEP of 10 cmH_2O initially to help to prevent reperfusion pulmonary edema by increasing the intra-alveolar pressure. If pulmonary edema develops, the PaO_2 is less than 300 mmHg on 100%, or there is a large compliance mismatch between the native and transplanted lung, independent lung venti-lation is used. The FiO_2 is weaned quickly, maintaining an oxygen saturation of 90%.

Bilateral lung transplantation

The approach to bilateral lung transplantation is somewhat differ-ent. Formerly, double lung transplantation with a tracheal anasta-mosis was used. This was later abandoned in favor of bilateral single lung transplantation, which was initially performed through separate thoracotomy incisions, but is now routinely performed through a sternal dividing bilateral subcostal or 'clamshell' inci-sion. Patients are positioned supine on the operating-table. The implantation technique is analagous to that of a single lung trans-plant. Cannulation for cardiopulmonary bypass can be done through the chest or the groin. This incision provides excellent exposure to the pleural surfaces, which is important because many of the patients undergoing bilateral lung transplantation will have dense, vascular pleural adhesions, and this exposure allows easier control of bleeding pleural surfaces.

Donor surgery

Lung procurement is performed through a midline sternotomy incision as part of a multiorgan procurement. Several methods of surgical procurement and preservation have been described which yield acceptable clinical results. These can be divided into three broad categories, namely a hypothermic flush perfusion technique, an autoperfusion technique and a systemic hypothermia technique using cardiopulmonary bypass. Of these, the most commonly employed method is a flush perfusion technique, which will be discussed in detail here. Hypothermia is achieved using a cold pulmonary artery flush through the main pulmonary artery, and an infusion of cold cardioplegia in the aortic root in conjunction with topical hypothermia. The solutions can be infused with the aid of a pressure bag, a roller pump, or by simple gravity drainage. The infusion of prostaglandin E1 or prostacyclin is used by most centers as a pulmonary dilator prior to the infusion of the pulmonary perfusate.

The technique begins with a sternotomy, and the pericardium and pleurae are opened widely to allow inspection of the heart and lungs. Once the heart and lungs have been found to be acceptable, the aorta and both cavae are dissected and encircled with vessel loops in the same way as they are for a standard cardiac donor retrieval. The innominate artery and vein and azygous vein are then ligated and divided. Immediately prior to clamping the aorta, the superior vena cava is ligated and the inferior vena cava is clamped. The cardioplegia and pulmoplegia infusions are started, and the lungs are ventilated continuously. Covering the surfaces of the heart and lungs with cold laparotomy sponges will help to maintain topical hypothermia during excision of the heart–lung block. The entire heart and lungs are removed en bloc and submerged in iced saline for division.

Postoperative management

Successful outcome after lung transplantation is highly dependent on a team-oriented approach to patient care, with input from surgeons, pulmonologists, cardiologists, anesthesiologists, infectious disease specialists, psychiatrists, nurses, respiratory therapists, transplant co-ordinators, social workers and nutritionists.

The co-ordination of care between these team members begins at the time of initial evaluation and continues throughout the postoperative period.

Management of lung transplant recipients must be tailored to the specific clinical setting. Those with primary lung disease and overall coexisting pathologic processes such as cardiac and renal dysfunction, poor nutritional status, and the presence of bacteriological infection or colonization, require individualized perioperative strategies. The type of procedure that is performed, as well as operative conditions including the use of CPB, transfusions, inotropic agents and single lung ventilation, may influence postoperative care. Finally, the quality of the allograft and cold ischemia time can change perioperative management based on the adequacy of initial lung function.

Patients are managed in the intensive-care unit for the first few days postoperatively. Universal precautions are of the utmost importance, although reverse isolation is not necessary. Patients are extubated and mobilized quickly, and invasive lines are removed as soon as possible in order to lower the risk of infectious complications. When appropriate, a thoracic epidural catheter can be used for pain control.

Respiratory

Early postoperative ventilator management is one of the most important aspects of the care of lung transplant recipients. General principles include maintaining adequate levels of oxygenation ($PaO_2 > 90$ mmHg), ventilation ($pCO_2 < 45$ mmHg) and a normal pH (7.35–7.45) with the lowest fraction of inspired oxygen and tidal volume possible in order to avoid oxygen toxicity and barotrauma. Standard extubation criteria are used, although a variety of ventilator strategies are frequently necessary (single-lumen vs. double-lumen endotracheal tube, one vs. two ventilators, extubation from double-lumen tube vs. changing to single-lumen tube, high vs. low positive end-expiratory pressure and early vs. delayed extubation).

One important factor that affects the initial ventilation strategy is the differential compliance between the native and implanted lungs. Patients with obstructive lung disease who receive a single lung transplant, particularly those with widespread destructive or cystic disease or those with a left-sided transplant, will initially be managed with a double-lumen tube. The native lung has significantly higher compliance than the allograft, and ventilation will preferentially go to the native lung, leading to air trapping and hyperinflation of the latter. This may compress the allograft, leading to atelectasis and impaired graft function. This is especially problematic with left-sided grafts, because the liver prevents the native right lung from expanding down into the abdomen. In this setting, the native right lung will expand medially and compress the mediastinum. Severe reperfusion injury of the allograft may exacerbate this shifting by causing a further reduction in allograft compliance. Two ventilators may be necessary, allowing ventilation of the native lung with a low inspiratory pressure, low tidal volume and prolonged expiratory time. Upon resolution of the reperfusion injury, the patient may be extubated or the double-lumen tube can be replaced with a single-lumen tube as indicated clinically. Patients with obstructive lung disease who receive a large donor lung may be successfully managed with a single-lumen tube initially because of the reduced risk of compression, atelectasis and mediastinal shift.

Perfusion differences between the two lungs may also influence early ventilator management in single lung transplant recipients. In patients with moderate pulmonary hypertension, blood flow will be preferentially shunted to the allograft, resulting in excessive perfusion of the allograft and reperfusion pulmonary edema (RPE). This can result in hypoxemia and severe early graft dysfunction. RPE is an idiosyncratic and poorly understood phenomenon that manifests as dense parenchymal infiltrates on chest X-ray, and significant hypoxia. It seems to be related to increased flow in the transplanted lung and long ischemic times, but it can occur in anyone. Immune-mediated injury may play a role in its pathogenesis. In addition, generalized pulmonary edema may develop in patients who require CPB, and large volumes of blood products and fluids compound the problem and further confuse management of the patient.

Patients who are undergoing single lung transplant with early evidence of RPE are ventilated via a double-lumen tube with two ventilators. A higher PEEP (7–12 cm H_2O) is used on the allograft side in an attempt to increase the intra-alveolar pressure, thereby reducing the pressure difference across the capillary bed and slowing the development of pulmonary edema. Early diuresis is also an effective adjunct. Vasodilators and inotropic agents are avoided if possible in an attempt to keep the overall amount of blood flow to the lungs, and to the allograft in particular, at normal-to-low levels during the first few days. In patients with restrictive lung diseases, the risk of developing hyperinflation of the native lung is small. Therefore a single-lumen endotracheal tube is placed once RPE resolves, and the patient is subsequently weaned and extubated. Patients with obstructive lung disease who develop RPE are managed with a double-lumen tube throughout, unless a need for bronchoscopy mandates exchanging to a single-lumen tube.

Patients who undergo double lung transplantation rarely have significant ventilation/perfusion mismatches. The pulmonary vascular resistance and compliance are similar between the two sides unless there has been a technical problem or the second side has suffered prolonged ischemic time. A single-lumen endotracheal tube is preferred in these patients due to ease of suctioning and bronchoscopy.

Respiratory therapists play an important role in the care of lung transplant recipients both during ventilation and after extubation. Aggressive bronchial hygiene is essential. Patients receive frequent suctioning and vibration while on the ventilator, and bronchodilators are routinely employed several times a day. Incentive spirometry, deep coughing exercises and percussion are performed frequently. Patients with large amounts of secretions also use vibrating types of spirometry devices. All patients receive fungal prophylaxis with inhaled amphotericin.

Fluid and nutrition

Close monitoring of the recipient's fluid status is imperative. Patients are deliberately kept relatively intravascularly hypovolemic during the initial stages. Judicious use of fluids, inotropic agents and blood products is guided by hemodynamic parameters and invasive monitoring. An excessive volume will result in interstitial edema, which is difficult to manage due to disruption of the pulmonary lymphatic system in the allograft. The use of colloid as opposed to crystalloid solutions is controversial. All drips are maximally concentrated in order to avoid excessive fluids. Diuretics are routinely employed postoperatively, limited by signs of inadequate perfusion such as prerenal azotemia.

Chest tube drainage is closely monitored. Previous thoracic surgery, extensive pleural scarring, CPB and liver dysfunction secondary to right heart failure all increase the risk of postoperative bleeding. Coagulation parameters are normalized with blood-product transfusions. Aprotinin has been shown to decrease postoperative bleeding, and antifibrinolytic adjuncts are routinely employed intraoperatively. Excessive bleeding mandates a return to the operating-room for exploration.

Many patients are nutritionally deficient prior to transplant. Enteral nutrition is started as soon as possible in these patients. Given the potentially catastrophic consequences of aspiration in this patient population, feeding is stopped well ahead of planned extubation, and swallowing studies are utilized liberally if there are any suspicions of dysfunction.

Laboratory and diagnostic studies

Laboratory studies initially include arterial blood gases, electrolytes, complete blood counts including hemoglobin, platelet counts, white blood cell counts and differentials, and coagulation studies as indicated. Daily cyclosporine or tacrolimus levels are required. Patients who are being given antilymphocyte induction therapy will receive daily lymphocyte subset determinations in order to guide therapy. Electrolyte testing is continued as long as diuretics are given, or until they are normalized and stable.

Chest X-rays are obtained daily in the intensive-care unit and as needed thereafter. Echocardiograms are obtained in the intensive-care unit as needed to rule out pericardial effusions or assess intravascular fluid status or cardiac performance in complex patients. Ventilation-perfusion scans and pulmonary arteriograms are sometimes required in the immediate postoperative period in order to define anastomotic patency.

Bronchoscopy is routinely performed in the operating-room at the end of the operation to check the bronchial anastamoses. In the intensive-care unit it is sometimes necessary to remove secretions when an endotracheal tube is changed, or if there is diagnostic confusion. Minimal fluid is used if a bronchoalveolar lavage is necessary.

Immunosuppression

The immunosuppression of lung transplant recipients varies significantly among transplant centers. Most programs utilize some form of cyclosporine- or tacrolimus-based triple therapy. Use of antilymphocyte induction therapy such as ATGAM, a polyclonal thymocyte preparation, or OKT3, a murine monoclonal antibody, is extremely variable and the subject of intense controversy. One approach is to use antilymphocyte induction therapy routinely in order to avoid early episodes of acute rejection and to allow the use of lower doses of cyclosporine in the early postoperative period. Early acute rejection has been associated with the development of obliterative bronchiolitis, a form of chronic rejection and a major cause of morbidity and mortality following transplantation.

All patients receive preoperative azathioprine in a dose of 4 mg/kg intravenously. This is continued postoperatively, 2–3 mg/kg/day, titrated to a white blood cell count of 6000 cells/mm^2. In the operating-room the patient receives 500 mg of methylprednisolone (Solumedrol) prior to reperfusion of the allograft, and this is continued for 24 h. Patients undergoing a bilateral lung transplant will receive a dose prior to reperfusion of each lung. In patients who are on steroids preoperatively, hydrocortisone, 1 mg/kg/day, is given until they are ready to begin oral prednisone, 0.4 mg/kg/day. Others begin steroid treatment after the cessation of antilymphocyte therapy. Cyclosporine is initiated at a dose of 1–4 mg/h IV immediately postoperatively in patients with normal renal function, and is switched to an oral dosage when it is tolerated to reach therapeutic levels of 350–400 ng/mL by whole blood radioimmunoassay. This protocol is maintained for 3–6 months, and is then slowly decreased to 250–300 ng/mL based on renal function and rejection profile.

Newer agents such as tacrolimus and mycophenolate mofetil are substituted for cyclosporine and azathioprine, respectively, in patients with recurrent or resistant rejection or with unacceptable toxicities.

Infectious disease prophylaxis

Infection is a major concern in any immunosuppressed patient. Prophylactic agents against bacteria, viruses and fungi are employed by most programs, but again protocols vary widely amongst programs.

Antibacterial prophylaxis is given perioperatively based on donor cultures and common institutional pathogens. These are discontinued 24 h post-transplant unless the donor has had positive cultures or the intraoperative bronchial cultures are positive. In this situation, a full course of treatment with sensitive antibiotics is warranted. *Pneumocystis carinii* prophylaxis is universal, although precise regimens vary, including trimethaprim–sulfamethoxazole, pentamidine and dapsone.

Antiviral prophylaxis is an important part of all lung transplant protocols. Of the potential pathogens, cytomegalovirus (CMV) is the most commonly encountered and potentially most lethal. CMV pneumonitis has been strongly correlated with the development of obliterative bronchiolitis. Severity of infection can range from asymptomatic shedding to lethal pneumonitis. Patients who are seronegative and receive lungs from seropositive donors are at highest risk for developing CMV disease despite aggressive prophylaxis. Some programs will not transplant CMV-positive donors into CMV-negative recipients because of this risk. Fungal infections are an infrequent occurrence in lung transplant patients, but carry high mortality. Most programs use some type of prophylactic regimen, but again these are extremely variable.

Complications

Although the long-term results of lung transplantation have improved as experience in all forms of lung transplantation has increased, complications remain life-threatening and difficult to treat. Complications in lung transplantation are of two general types, namely those that arise as a result of immunosuppression but which are similar to the complications suffered by recipients of other organ transplants, and those that are specific to lung transplant recipients. Only those specific to lung transplantation will be discussed in this section.

Airway

Airway healing has long been, and continues to be, one of the most technically challenging aspects of lung transplantation. Two classification systems have been proposed to grade airway anastomotic healing. Bronchial anastomotic complications can be generally grouped into full or partial thickness necrosis and dehiscence, ulceration and granulation, stricture and bronchomalacia. They are the most commonly encountered airway complications, and may all in fact be a complication of ischemia.

Bronchial arteries originate from the aorta or intercostal arteries. They branch at the carina and provide blood to the main and segmental bronchi via a peribronchial adventitial plexus. The normal bronchial arterial supply to the airways is interrupted in the course of procurement and is not re-established during implantation. Following lung transplantation, the blood supply to the anastamosis is primarily by retrograde flow through pulmonary arterial to bronchial collaterals. The distal main and segmental bronchi of the donor lung develop collaterals, while the more proximal main bronchi and carina do not. This fragile blood supply renders the anastomosis and the main bronchus just distal to the anastomosis particularly susceptible to ischemic injury, especially if there are several bronchial rings between the anastomosis and the take-off of the upper lobe bronchus. Devascularization of the recipient bronchus up to the carina compounds this problem by eliminating antegrade blood flow to the anastomosis via bronchial vessels.

Other factors which may influence the development of ischemic airway injury include hypotension, requirement for high-dose inotropic agents, prolonged ischemic time, poor preservation, rejection, infection, prolonged ventilation with high inspiratory pressures, devascularizing the main bronchus and use of steroids. Steroids have also been implicated as a factor in delayed or impaired healing of the airways. For many years, patients who had received steroids preoperatively were excluded from lung transplantation. However, improved surgical techniques, more effective immunosuppression with less reliance on high doses of steroids, and better understanding of the bronchial blood supply have allowed patients who required preoperative steroids to be transplanted with similar anastomotic complication rates to those who did not use preoperative steroids. In fact, some authors suggest that bronchial healing may be improved by the use of steroids during the induction phase of immunosuppression.

Necrosis and dehiscence occur during the first few weeks after transplantation. There is a wide spectrum of necrotic injuries, the most severe of which allow complete dehiscence – a complication which is difficult to treat and carries a high mortality rate. Strictures can occur from weeks to months after lung transplantation as a result of healing necrotic or ischemic tissue. Stenosis may occur later, and in airways that showed satisfactory initial healing. Such strictures are felt to develop in watershed areas between the donor's retrograde pulmonary artery–bronchial artery collaterals and the recipient's antegrade collateral circulation arising from the distal tracheobronchial tree. Granulation tissue is most probably an exuberant healing in response to ischemic injury such as a superficial ulcer. However, of all the commonly seen complications, the etiology of bronchomalacia is the most unclear. It is probably related to ischemic injury to the cartilaginous structures in the bronchus. It is easily diagnosed on bronchoscopy and is characterized by inspiratory dilation and expiratory collapse of the airway.

The incidence of anastomotic complications was as high as 80% in the early days of lung transplantation. These disastrous results were one of the main reasons why acceptance of lung transplantation lagged far behind that of other types of solid organ transplants. Two technical modifications which have improved the results and led to a resurgence of the procedure are shortening the donor bronchial stump to two or less cartilaginous rings proximal to the upper lobe take-off, and reinforcing the anastomosis with a vascularized tissue pedicle flap such as omentum, pericardium or an intercostal muscle pedicle flap. This reduced the airway complication rate to the range 15–23%. Later development of an intussuscepting anastomotic technique was credited with reducing the complication rates even further. Not all centers use this technique, and the benefits attributed to it are unclear. Many centers use an intussuscepting technique to accommodate size mismatches, and concentrate on avoiding devascularizing the bronchus, trimming the donor bronchus close to the upper lobe orifice and letting the anastomosis retract into the well-vascularized mediastinal tissue while performing end-to-end anastomoses. At present, airway complication rates are approximately 5–12% at experienced centers using a variety of techniques.

Treatment of dehiscence depends on its extent and timing. Circumferential and large dehiscences that present early are life-threatening and must be treated surgically with debridement of all necrotic tissue and re-anastomosis. Coverage with viable tissue is imperative, as is wide drainage to treat the pleural and mediastinal infections that almost universally ensue. If the necrosis extends to the lobar orifices, retransplantation is the only option. Areas of breakdown can be treated conservatively if there is a small, localized area of necrosis without pleural communication and they are discovered incidentally by surveillance bronchoscopy. Larger areas of necrosis and dehiscence are treated with silastic stenting. The strategy is to ensure airway patency while providing a scaffolding over which secondary healing can occur. These silastic stents can later be removed.

Strictures are treated by dilation performed with a rigid bronchoscope, olive-tipped bougies, balloon dilation or laser resection. Stenting may accompany dilation or it may be placed at a later date if airway obstruction recurs. The type of stent employed and the timing of implantation varies from one center to another, taking into account the advantages and disadvantages of both wire-mesh and silastic-tube types of stents. Airway obstruction due to granulation tissue is usually managed by laser ablation, while bronchomalacia is successfully managed by stenting alone.

Infection

Infection is the leading cause of morbidity and mortality following lung transplantation. Bacteria, viruses and fungi have all been implicated, with bacterial infections being the most common and usually the first to occur. Infectious complications may occur at any time postoperatively and are a leading cause of both early and late mortality. Transmission of pneumonia from the donor to the recipient commonly occurs. Initially antibiotic treatment should be directed against Gram stain and culture results from the donor. Recipients with infectious pulmonary disease prior to transplant are particularly prone to infectious complications, and offending organisms are frequently sequestered in the airways or sinuses of the recipient. In patients with cystic fibrosis, *Pseudomonas* species are often the culprits and are associated with severe pneumonias, higher risk of obliterative bronchiolitis, and higher mortality rates. Many programs consider colonization with *Cepacia* species to be a contraindication to lung transplantation.

CMV infections are the most worrisome of the viruses, and usually occur during the first 6 months after lung transplantation. The severity of CMV infections ranges from asymptomatic shedding through systemic CMV syndromes to fulminant CMV pneumonitis. CMV may be reactivated in the recipient with the initiation of immunosuppression, or it may be transmitted from the donor to the recipient. Seronegative patients receiving organs from seropositive donors are at highest risk of developing CMV disease, although the disease is common in seropositive recipients receiving organs from seropositive donors. In addition, CMV infection has been strongly correlated with the development of obliterative bronchiolitis. Some programs use CMV matching when selecting donors. However, the scarcity of donors frequently makes this impractical. Some form of CMV prophylaxis is standard practice. Regimens vary widely between LT centers, but many have been shown to decrease the incidence, severity, morbidity and mortality of infection.

Fungal infections are less common, but can be lethal. Airway colonization of both donors and recipients with *Candida* species is common, but invasive candidiasis is uncommon. *Aspergillus* species also commonly colonize recipient airways. Any invasive fungal infection must be treated aggressively with the appropriate intravenous antifungal agents, and in cases of invasive aspergillosis, surgical resection is required. Inhaled amphotericin is frequently used as prophylactic treatment.

Pneumocystis carinii was formerly a common perioperative pathogen. Before the institution of routine prophylaxis, its incidence approached 85% in some series. Trimethoprim–sulfamethoxazole prophylaxis has almost eliminated this problem. In sulfa-allergic patients, dapsone or inhaled pentamidine has been used effectively. Most programs continue some type of prophylactic regimen indefinitely.

Reperfusion pulmonary edema

Reperfusion pulmonary edema (RPE), defined as edema in the allograft immediately following transplantation, is also known as reperfusion injury or the pulmonary reimplantation response. It is characterized radiographically by diffuse pulmonary edema, and histologically by the presence of neutrophil infiltrates within the alveolar interstitium and perivascular tissue spaces, as well as increased vascular permeability. It may develop immediately upon reperfusion, as frothy pulmonary edema, or as late as several days after lung transplantation, as mild radiographic infiltrates. Difficulties occur with both oxygenation and ventilation in the most severe cases. Airway pressures may be elevated and pulmonary hypertension often follows. It was first described by Veith and colleagues in canine lung transplantation and has been a major problem in human LT, although the etiology remains unclear. Potential causes include ischemic cellular injury, oxygen-derived free-radical-induced lipid peroxidation injury mediated by white blood cells, complement-cascade-mediated injury, disruption of pulmonary lymphatics and rejection. Factors that may influence development include poor lung preservation with inadequate flushing and pulmonary vasoconstriction, long ischemic times, and the use of cardiopulmonary bypass.

The RPE syndrome may be short-lived and resolve within days, or it may lead to early allograft failure and death. There is currently no effective method of prevention and no way to predict which patients will develop RPE. Standard ventilator management using high inspired oxygen concentrations and increased end-expiratory pressures may in fact exacerbate the injury. However, patients who survive the early postoperative period with supportive care can anticipate adequate pulmonary function upon recovery. Supportive care in this setting includes minimizing oxygen demand and maintaining low pulmonary capillary wedge pressures with sedation and diuresis. Clinically, nitric oxide has been reported to be beneficial in patients with severe reperfusion injury, and some patients have even been maintained on extracorporeal membrane oxygenation (ECMO) until reperfusion injury resolved.

Experimentally, a variety of strategies have been shown to reduce the degree of injury but have not been demonstrated to be reliably and significantly effective. They include nitroprusside, a neutrophil endopeptidase inhibitor (ulinastatin), anti-intracellular adhesion molecules, lidocaine, neutrophil elastase inhibitors (ONO-5046 Na), L-arginine, pentoxifylline and others.

Bleeding

Bleeding is not often a major problem in lung transplant cases. However, when it occurs it is often severe. There are two large vascular anastomoses performed for each lung transplanted, and suture-line bleeding must be suspected whenever significant bleeding is encountered. Posterior mediastinal bleeding from lymphatic tissue or bronchial vessels was a common problem in heart–lung and double lung transplantation, and use of a cardiopulmonary bypass further increases the risk. A bilateral thoracosternotomy incision ('clamshell') improves exposure to the posterior mediastinum, and has reduced the frequency of this as a source of troublesome bleeding. Pleural bleeding is a common source of ongoing slow blood loss, particularly in patients with inflammatory lung diseases such as cystic fibrosis, or in patients who have previously undergone cardiothoracic procedures. The improvement in pleural exposure afforded by the clamshell incision, as well as use of the argon-beam coagulator and routine antifibrinolytic use, have greatly diminished the pleura as a source of significant bleeding. Patients with pulmonary hypertension are particularly susceptible to bleeding due to secondary liver dysfunction and associated coagulation abnormalities, in addition to the routine use of anticoagulation in some of these patients. Surgical exploration should be considered early on due to the increase in pulmonary edema and worsening of coagulation abnormalities that result from massive transfusion.

Pulmonary

Phrenic nerve injury is not uncommon after lung transplantation, most often being temporary if due to stretching, or permanent if it results from division, crush or thermal injury. Unilateral paresis occurs in up to 30% of patients, with recovery sometimes requiring several months. The incidence is even higher after bilateral lung transplant, or if the recipient had previous thoracic surgery or significant pleural adhesions. The clinical outcome following this complication may be severely compromised, often causing difficulties in separating from assisted ventilation.

Retention of secretions and atelectasis may also cause significant problems in the immediate postoperative period. Vagal denervation and decreased mucociliary clearance seem to be responsible. Aggressive chest physiotherapy and suctioning or bronchoscopy are necessary, and the incidence of pneumonia in this setting is very high.

As mentioned above, over-distension of the native lung with concomitant crowding and atelectasis of a single allograft is relatively unique to patients with obstructive lung disease. Reperfusion injury and decreased compliance in the allograft, requiring increased peak pressures for adequate ventilation, may exacerbate gas trapping in a native emphysematous lung. This process is more common in patients with extensive destruction of their remaining lung, and in those who have received left-sided allografts. Cephalad pressure exerted by the liver prevents the remaining right lung from expanding downward, and forces it to expand medially, compressing the mediastinum. Severe respiratory and hemodynamic compromise can result. Positioning the patient with the allograft side up, independent lung ventilation with low volumes to the native lung, bronchodilators and aggressive pulmonary toilet have been shown to be beneficial. The severity of this condition can be so extreme that many centers now perform lung volume reduction on the native lung at the same time as the transplant, as prophylaxis.

Rejection

As with all organ transplantation, allograft rejection is a significant problem in lung transplantation. Early studies of heart–lung transplant recipients identified a much higher incidence of rejection in the lungs than in the heart. The reasons for this finding are unknown, but there are many possible theories. Lungs are unique among organ transplants in that they are constantly exposed to inhaled antigens that cause inflammation and may cause up-regulation of the immune response. Environmental exposure also increases exposure to a variety of infectious agents that may enhance alloimmunity. In addition, lungs are transplanted with significant quantities of lymphatic tissue. This is populated by a large number of immunocompetent cells that may play a role in up-regulating the native immune system against any foreign antigen.

Allograft rejection is classified as hyperacute, acute or chronic. Hyperacute rejection occurs immediately upon reperfusion, and is caused by pre-existing antibodies to donor blood group, HLA or other antigens expressed by the allograft. Fortunately, this is rare, due to ABO matching and routine screening for preformed antibodies. In patients with high levels of preformed antibodies (> 20% panel-reactive antibodies) against a panel of commonly encountered antigens, a cross-match against the donor's serum is required to prevent this lethal complication.

Acute rejection is a cell-mediated process directed against specific cell-surface antigens that are encoded by the major histocompatibility complex (MHC). T-cell lymphocytes are the primary effector cells of acute rejection. Acute rejection is diagnosed by both clinical and histological criteria, and is reported to occur in 60–90% of lung transplant recipients. In fact, the vast majority of recipients have at least one episode of acute rejection. At Papworth Hospital 75% of recipients developed rejection during the first 30 days, and 60% of all cases of rejection occurred within the first year. Presenting symptoms include dyspnea, fatigue, dry cough, low-grade fever, malaise, new or changing infiltrates, and a change in spirometric parameters, all in the absence of active pulmonary infection. A recent radiologic study found that the presence of septal lines and new or increasing pleural effusions without vascular redistribution or increased cardiac size are useful markers of acute rejection. Pulmonary function is impaired during episodes of acute rejection, as manifested by decreased FEV_1, FVC and lung diffusion of carbon dioxide (D_LCO). Home hand-held spirometry seems to be an effective method of monitoring for acute rejection, despite the fact that these devices are non-specific, they cannot differentiate between rejection and infection, and simple spirometry can be skewed by function of the residual native lung.

Clinical presentation is commonly viewed as diagnostic in the early post-transplant period, when it is difficult to differentiate between infection, rejection and reperfusion injury histologically. However, further reliance on the clinical picture alone beyond the immediate postoperative period is not indicated. Typically, subjective symptoms develop relatively late in the rejection process, and diagnosis is frequently dependent on the clinical response to empiric therapy. A recent review of transbronchial biopsies concluded that over 50% of patients with histological evidence of mild rejection and 75% of patients with moderate acute rejection were asymptomatic at the time of diagnosis. Histologic examination of transbronchial biopsy specimens is considered to be the gold standard for diagnosis of acute rejection after the immediate postoperative period. Unfortunately, there is no consensus as to the optimal schedule for surveillance biopsies. Most programs follow a specific protocol that includes frequent biopsies during the first year and tapers off thereafter, as well as biopsies whenever clinical suspicion is aroused. Acute rejection becomes significantly less common after the first year.

On histologic examination, acute cellular rejection is characterized by mononuclear infiltrates in the perivascular tissue spaces. Immunologic studies have shown a variety of cell types, including cytologic and helper T-cells, macrophages, dendritic cells, plasma cells and eosinophils. In early or mild rejection, the infiltrates are sparse, with the density and cellularity of the infiltrates increasing and extending into the interstitium with increasing severity. Subendothelial infiltration of lymphocytes can be observed, and is designated as vasculitis or endotheleitis. Alveolar damage in the form of hemorrhage, hyaline membrane formation, alveolar exudates with necrosis and accumulation of mononuclear cells in the air spaces constitutes the final phase of the rejection process. The Lung Transplant Study Group of the International Society of Heart–Lung Transplantation has developed a standardized classification system to grade acute lung rejection on the basis of histological findings.

Treatment of acute rejection varies among institutions, and is based on both clinical and histological findings. Acute rejection of a histological grade of A3 or higher, or grade A2 rejection accompanied by clinical symptoms or functional deterioration is considered by most programs to be an indication for intervention. The potential side-effects of treating low grades of rejection, especially the risk of infection, must be balanced against the potential benefit. One study of clinically silent A2 rejection showed that 37% of untreated patients showed improvement or resolution on follow-up biopsy and 63% showed worsening. Those who failed to improve had more frequent episodes of acute rejection, and a greater percentage subsequently developed obliterative bronchiolitis.

Standard treatment for an initial episode of acute rejection includes pulsed intravenous methylprednisolone, often with modification of the maintenance immunosuppressive regimen. The standard dose is 500–1000 mg/day for 3 days, followed by an increase in oral prednisone to 0.5 mg/kg/day and a subsequent taper. Treatment of patients with persistent or recurrent rejection is controversial. Potential therapies include a second steroid challenge, antilymphocyte therapy, adding immunosuppressive agents such as FK506 (Tacrolimus) or mycophenolate (Cellcept), methotrexate, total lymphocyte irradiation, photopheresis and aerosolized cyclosporine.

Obliterative bronchiolitis

Obliterative bronchiolitis is the pulmonary manifestation of chronic rejection. It is analogous to tissue responses that occur in other types of solid organ transplantation, and is characterized by a fibroproliferative process leading to the obliteration of tubular structures in the transplanted organ. In the heart, it is manifested by the development of graft coronary artery disease, in the liver by a syndrome of vanishing bile ducts, and in the kidney by chronic vascular and tubular fibrosis.

The incidence of obliterative bronchiolitis is reported to be as high as 60% in long-term survivors of lung transplant, with very high mortality within 1 year of the diagnosis. Risk factors associated with the development of the disease have some form of acute or chronic lung injury in common. Well-documented risk factors include rejection and infection, particularly CMV infections. Obliterative bronchiolitis presents with a progressive loss of lung function caused by airflow obstruction.

Pulmonary function testing shows a decreased FEV_1, FVC, TLC, and D_LCO, with a disproportionately greater decrease in FEV_1 and a decrease in the FEV_1/FVC ratio consistent with an obstructive pattern. Radiographic changes include a loss of peripheral vascular markings, lung distension with hyperlucency of the peripheral lung fields, and pleural thickening. CT scans reveal irregularly distributed areas of hyperlucency, fibrosis, bronchiectasis and occasionally focal calcification.

The histopathologic process consists of inflammation and fibrosis of the lamina propria and obstruction of the bronchiolar lumen, with inflammation and bronchiectasis of larger airways. Obliterative bronchiolitis is heterogeneous, with normal bronchioles often juxtaposed with obliterated remnants. Interestingly, patients can display histologic changes without clinical symptoms, and vice versa. A clinical staging system has been developed to describe the syndrome based on pulmonary function and histologic findings. Patients inevitably proceed along a course marked by a progressive decline in pulmonary function, often accompanied by recurrent infections. No effective treatment has been found, although most centers will augment the patient's immunosuppressive regimen. This approach is controversial, and may actually be detrimental due to the increased risk of infection with greater immunosupression, but it is considered to be a desperate measure in the face of dismal outcomes.

Outcomes

Since the first lung transplant was performed by Hardy over 35 years ago there has been a significant improvement in survival and functional outcome. Lung transplantation, as well as other solid organ transplants, only really became practical for patients with end-stage lung disease with the introduction of cyclosporin A in the early 1980s. Since that time, and in addition due to improvements in surgical technique, lung transplantation has been routinely considered to be a lifesaving measure, and is expected to improve the functional capabilities of patients with end-stage lung disorders. However, obliterative bronchiolitis continues to be the major long-term limitation of lung transplantation.

Survival

Data from the St Louis International Lung Transplant Registry indicate a 71% 1-year and 45% 5-year survival rate for recipients of all types of lung transplantation. These figures are relatively similar to those reported by the International Society for Heart and Lung Transplantation (ISHLT). Short- and long-term survival remains dependent on the original underlying disease. Patients with emphysema have the best survival statistics, while those undergoing retransplantation fare the worst. A number of factors are responsible for early mortality ($\leq$90 days), including infection (35% of cases), primary graft failure/reperfusion injury (13%), heart failure (9%), acute rejection (5%), bleeding (6%) and anastomotic dehiscence (5%). Factors responsible for late mortality differ, although infection remains the commonest cause of death (30% of cases) in patients who survive beyond 90 days. A higher incidence in patients who develop obliterative bronchiolitis may be related to a higher rate of pneumonia and bacterial colonization in these patients. Chronic rejection (obliterative bronchiolitis) occurs in up to 40% of patients by 2 years, and is the cause of death in 50% of those affected. Other causes of late mortality include malignancy (6% of cases), respiratory failure (5%) and bleeding (4%).

Functional outcome

Functional outcome was recently reviewed in the 1997 ISHLT report, which included data from April 1994 to December 1996. At 2 years post-transplant, 85.7% of recipients reported no activity limitations, 13.4% were able to perform activity with some assistance, and 0.8% required total assistance. Despite functional improvements achieved by transplantation, only a minority of patients (30.2%) were working full-time by 2 years post-transplant. During this same time period, the majority of patients (54.1%) required repeated hospitalizations through 1 year of follow-up, falling to 42.2% during the second postoperative year. The commonest reason for repeat hospitalization was allograft rejection and infection.

Pulmonary function and exercise tolerance

Although the data are limited, investigators have reviewed specific measurements of lung function and exercise tolerance following lung transplantation. Functional improvements may be frustrated by complications such as pleural scarring, chest wall changes and phrenic nerve injury. In addition, with single lung transplantation the functional outcome depends on the underlying disease, as the native lung contributes to the overall lung function and can develop further complications. Following single lung transplantation, FEV_1 is expected to rise to only 50–57% of the predicted value for patients with chronic obstructive pulmonary disease, and the FVC to about 69% of the predicted value for pulmonary fibrosis patients. Double-lung transplant recipients enjoy a greater improvement in overall lung function, an FEV_1 of 78–85% and an FVC of 66–92% of the predicted value. Interestingly, during cardiopulmonary exercise testing neither work rate nor maximal oxygen consumption (VO_{2max}) achieved differ significantly between recipients of single lung transplant and double lung transplant. In patients without significant complications, there is no evidence of ventilatory limitation during exercise (defined by the ratio of expired volume to maximal voluntary ventilation, or V_E/MVV) assessed at 3 months and through the first postoperative year, regardless of whether a single or double lung transplant was performed. Other studies confirm a significant rise in VO_{2max} and 6-min walking distance and an improvement in New York Heart Association functional class following all forms of lung transplantation.

Quality of life

Despite widespread use of lung transplantation as a therapeutic modality, there have been few published studies assessing quality of life in recipients. Gross and colleagues documented the overall improvement in quality of life following lung transplantation as assessed by the Medical Outcomes Health Survey (MOS)-20 health profile. Over the long term, improvements persist except in those patients who develop chronic rejection. However, although there are significant benefits with regard to exercise tolerance, pulmonary function and quality of life following lung transplantation, only a minority of patients return to work on a full-time basis.

Financial considerations

There is little published data on the overall cost of lung transplantation. However, the procedure and postoperative care appear to be the most expensive of all solid organ transplants. A pilot study by Ramsey and colleagues from the University of Washington

Medical Center that was published in 1995 delineated the costs of the transplant procedure and postoperative care. The mean patient charge per transplant procedure was $164 989 (median $152 071), including surgical fees and immediate postoperative care. Other published cost analyses include one from Canada and one from the USA. Initial costs were $114 953 (Canadian dollars, 1992–93) and $137 234 (1989–92), respectively. Longer-term postoperative care is also costly, averaging $106 588 for the first year, compared to that of other solid organ transplants such as heart, liver and kidney ($45 262, $93 267 and $23 316, respectively, for the first postoperative year).

Further reading

Egan TM, Boychuk JE, Rosato K *et al.* 1992: Whence the lungs? A study to assess suitability of donor lungs for transplantation. *Transplantation* **53**, 420.

Griffith BP and **Zenati M**. 1990: The pulmonary donor. *Clinics in Chest Medicine* **11**, 217–26.

Hardy JD, Webb WR, Dalton ML *et al.* 1963: Lung homotransplantation in man. *Journal of the American Medical Association* **186**, 1065–74.

Khettry VR, Kroshus TJ, Hertz MI *et al.* 1997: Early and late airway complications after lung transplantation: incidence and management. *Annals of Thoracic Surgery* **63**, 1576–83.

Marshall SE, Lewiston NJ, Kramer MR *et al.* 1991: Prospective analysis of serial pulmonary function studies and transbronchial biopsies in single lung transplant recipients. *Transplantation Proceedings* **23**, 1217–19.

Reitz BA, Wallwork JL, Hunt SA *et al.* 1982: Heart–lung transplantation: successful therapy for patients with pulmonary vascular disease. *New England Journal of Medicine* **306**, 557–64.

Shinoi K, Hayata Y, Aoki H *et al.* 1966: Pulmonary lobe homotransplantation in human subjects. *American Journal of Surgery* **111**, 617–28.

Sibley RK, Berry GL, Tazelaar HD *et al.* 1993: The role of transbronchial biopsies in the management of lung transplant recipients. *Journal of Heart and Lung Transplantation* **12**, 308–24.

Starnes VA, Barr ML and **Cohen RG**. 1994: Lobar transplantation: indications, techniques and outcome. *Journal of Thoracic and Cardiovascular Surgery* **108**, 403–10.

Williams T, Grossman R and **Maurer J**. 1990: Long-term functional follow-up of lung transplant recipients. *Clinics in Chest Medicine* **11**, 347–58.

Organ allocation and donor management

9

Rebecca A. Schroeder and Paul C. Kuo

Introduction

Care of the potential organ donor begins as soon as a patient is identified as brain dead. Too often in a busy intensive-care unit such patients are pushed off to the side to await the arrival of the transplant co-ordinators or even the procuring surgical teams. Little attention is given to the dramatic physiologic changes that accompany brain death, as well as the progression of pathologic processes that may render potential grafts totally unusable. It is important to remember the final purpose of these organs and their role in preserving and improving life in the recipient population. Continuation of meticulous critical care practice is essential, although with somewhat different goals in mind.

Most organ donors have sustained massive neurologic injury as a result of head trauma or a severe cerebrovascular accident. Almost all patients who have these injuries should be regarded as potential donors. Exceptions to this generalization include untreated septicemia, acquired immunodeficiency syndrome (AIDS), viral hepatitis, viral encephalitis, Guillain–Barré syndrome, current intravenous drug use, active tuberculosis and malignancy, with the exception of primary brain tumors. Acute poisoning is considered by some to be an exclusion criterion, although 12 cases have been reported from Belgium in which death was the result of poisoning with methaqualone, benzodiazepines, tricyclic antidepressants, barbiturates, insulin, carbon monoxide, cyanide, methanol, acetaminophen or a combination of the above. The 1-year survival rate for all organs taken together in this series was reported to be 75%, with a 'favorable' outcome reported for 87%. In no case could a death in the recipient be related to toxic exposure in the donor. Advanced age has been a reason to turn down potential donors. However, this situation has been changing, with some centers now accepting kidneys and livers from donors over the age of 65 years.

Definition of brain death

The definition of brain death has undergone significant evolution within the last three decades, and its impact on organ transplantation has been profound. Until 1968, those few organ transplants that were performed involved organs from living or non-heart-beating donors. Prior to that time, the concept of brain death without physiologic death of the entire organism had been advanced by Mollaret and Goulon, who described a state of 'coma depasse' which was characterized by loss of all reflex and neurologic electrical activity. With the passing of the Uniform Anatomical Gift Act in 1968, as well as the establishment of the Harvard criteria published in the same year, organ donation from brain-dead but heart-beating patients was legally established. The major criteria were defined as unreceptivity and unresponsiveness, no movements or respiratory efforts, no reflexes, and a flat electroencephalogram (EEG). This concept was further refined by the Uniform Determination of Death Act issued as a joint effort by the American Bar Association and the American Medical Association at the National Conference of Commissioners on Uniform State Laws in 1981. According to this document, 'an individual is dead if there is irreversible cessation of circulatory and respiratory functions, or if there is irreversible cessation of all functions of the entire brain, including the brainstem.'

Also in 1981, the President's Commission on Ethical Problems in Medicine published further guidelines governing the declaration and definition of brain death. According to this panel, cerebral and brainstem functions must be absent, the cause of death must be known and exclude recovery, and cessation of all brain function must persist during a period of observation and treatment. These guidelines defined the concept of 'whole brain death'. A significant difference between these and the Harvard criteria is the allowance for persistent spinal cord function in the presence of brain death. Furthermore, the commission delineated other issues that must be addressed when dealing with a declaration of brain death. That is, specific criteria defining brain death must be explicit, accessible to verification and adaptable to differing clinical situations. In addition, they must minimize errors in misclassifying patients as alive, avoid unreasonable delay and, most importantly, completely eliminate the error of declaring a living person as dead.

Brain death, as both a legal and a medical concept, is defined differently in different countries around the world. For example, in Australia brain death is legally defined as 'irreversible cessation of all function of the brain', which is similar to the definition in use in the USA. This implies permanent destruction of the functional abilities of all portions of the brain – that is, both the brainstem and higher cortical functions. Thus, the presence of any neurological function, including primitive reflexes, would disallow the diagnosis of brain death. Alternatively, in the UK, the presence of irremediable brainstem injury sufficient to cause cessation of all brainstem reflexes is presumed to imply permanent loss of the abilities to regain consciousness and ventilation.

Theoretically, these criteria could be met by severe but isolated brainstem injury or stroke, although this clinical scenario would be extremely rare. The commonest cause of severe brainstem injury is herniation of the brainstem through the foramen magnum secondary to massive increases in intracranial pressure (ICP), a condition that would also cause irreversible injury to but not cessation of function of the cerebral cortex. Technically, this describes 'brainstem death' as opposed to 'whole brain death' as is required in the USA. The criteria published by the Conference of Medical Royal Colleges otherwise resemble those for whole brain death accepted in the USA. No country has yet accepted the concept of 'cerebral death', an idea that would equate cessation of cognition and awareness or a persistent vegetative state with death, and it is unlikely that current legal systems will deem this acceptable in the foreseeable future.

Unfortunately, a subset of patients who would seem to be ideal organ donors but who fall into this category of cerebral death are infants born with anencephaly (the complete absence of any cerebral cortex). Although these infants may breathe spontaneously at birth and have stable cardiovascular systems for short periods of time due to the presence of a primitive brainstem, they uniformly die within weeks. Whereas in Germany there have been reports of these infants being resuscitated at birth and their organs immediately procured, there is very little likelihood that this will be possible in the USA in the foreseeable future.

Explicit clinical criteria for the declaration of brain death have changed over the years since the publication of the President's Commission guidelines, most often due to changing medical technology and management practices. However, common to all protocols is a careful and detailed neurological examination that must document the absence of movement, including decerebrate and decorticate posturing, and shivering. There must be no seizures and no response to verbal stimuli or deep pain, and no respiratory efforts in the face of hypercarbia. Cranial nerve reflexes, including pupillary light reflexes, corneal reflexes, gag and cough reflexes, and the oculocephalic and oculovestibular reflexes must also be absent. Most importantly, the cause of the current condition must be known and sufficient to account for brain death, and there must be no improvement over a period of observation, most commonly 2–24 h. Finally, the patient must not be hypothermic and the condition must not be due to acute drug intoxication or poisoning.

Clinical and radiographic or electrical confirmatory testing is necessary to document brain death. An atropine challenge must result in no response in heart rate. Apnea testing is well known, but must be performed under strict conditions. The patient is pre-oxygenated for at least 5–10 min, and is then disconnected from the ventilator while continuing apneic oxygenation in order to avoid arterial oxygen desaturation, which may cause hemodynamic instability and cardiac arrest. Reaching an arterial pCO_2 of 60 mmHg is generally considered to be an adequate challenge. EEG is frequently performed although, as noted above, it is not adequate in isolation to satisfy the criteria for brain death. In fact, even in the face of established brain death and an isoelectric EEG, some evidence of isolated nerve activity may be present in the form of spontaneous depolarizations detected by deeply placed electrodes. This technique is also plagued by inconsistencies in inter-operator variability and other technical problems, and only provides information about the supratentorial structures. Somatosensory, visual and brainstem auditory evoked potentials have been of limited or no practical value, in addition to being complex and costly. Blood flow studies of various types, including xenon-enhanced computed tomography, transcranial Doppler studies and other nuclear medicine scanning techniques have been used. Specifically, a technetium-tagged tracer, ^{99m}Tc-HMPAO, has shown a 100% correlation with four-vessel angiography in demonstrating no cranial blood flow in at least one clinical trial. However, four-vessel angiography remains the gold-standard test for diagnosing brain death. In fact, Nau and colleagues have concluded after studying multiple modalities that it is the only reliable test for documenting brain death by whole brain criteria, especially in the case of confounding factors.

Organ allocation

Guidelines for the sharing and distribution of donated organs have been developed and published by the United Network for Organ Sharing (UNOS). This governing body was established as a non-profit corporation with the purpose of establishing a national organ procurement and transplantation network under the Public Health Service Act with the mission of improving the effectiveness of the nation's renal and extrarenal organ distribution and transplantation systems. The goals of the corporation include 'increasing availability of and access to donor organs for patients with end-stage organ failure; to develop, implement, and maintain quality assurance activities; and to systematically gather and analyze data and regularly publish the results of the national experience in organ procurement and preservation, tissue typing, and clinical organ transplantation'. It is managed by a Board of Directors elected from among the membership, as well as a slate of principal officers, also elected by the members. In addition, there are permanent standing committees to deal with issues of communications, ethics, finance, histocompatibility laboratories, kidney and pancreas transplantation, liver and intestinal organ transplantation, thoracic organ transplantation, membership and professional standards, minority affairs, organ procurement organization, patient affairs, pediatric transplantation and scientific advisory issues.

Transplant programs and locally based organ procurement organizations (OPO), as well as histocompatability laboratories, may apply for admission as institutional members, and are reviewed for minimum qualifications prior to approval. The criteria for admission include specific education and training requirements for transplant surgeons as well as mandatory minimum capabilities for laboratories. For new programs, UNOS has defined specific criteria that are necessary prior to granting certification. For example, a potential kidney transplant program must have a UNOS-approved histocompatability laboratory, a UNOS-certified surgeon, a UNOS-certified transplant nephrologist, and perform a minimum of 15 kidney transplants per year, or 45 transplants in 3 years. Programs may be reviewed for possible probationary action if survival rates fall below a defined threshold. OPOs may be based at a specific transplant center, or be situated independently, and serve multiple programs. For certification, they must demonstrate an ability to interact with national organ sharing networks, have access to particular technology in organ preservation, handle a minimum of 50 organ procurements per year, and serve an exclusive geographic area. There are also particular requirements with regard to the necessary organizational and financial structure.

The country is divided into 11 geographic regions, each containing various numbers of OPOs within its borders. The allocation of organs is co-ordinated by the 'host OPO', and proceeds uniformly from a local to a regional and finally a national basis. The allocation of specific organs varies widely among different organ types. A basic outline is presented below that is intended to describe the general guiding principles which govern the distribution of procured organs. However, these guidelines are subject to constant review and revisions as new issues and problems are identified.

In general, kidneys are first allocated locally, then within the UNOS region and finally nationally. One exception to this practice is kidneys that would provide a 'zero antigen mismatch' between donor and recipient. Donors are evaluated in order to define the characteristics of the major histocompatibility complex (also known as HLA antigens). Patients with high plasma-reactive antigen (PRA) levels have a better chance of a negative cross-match if their HLA status can be matched as closely as possible. If any procured kidney qualifies as a zero antigen mismatch for any potential recipient on the UNOS waiting-list, it is offered to that patient within the time limitations for organ preservation. Otherwise the organ is offered to the patient who ranks highest according to a complex formula which involves time on the waiting-list, degree of antigen compatibility and degree of PRA, again in the order of local, then regional and finally national allocation. Other factors that complicate kidney allocation even further are the potential for kidney–pancreas, double kidney or liver–kidney transplantation, as well as a system of organ 'paybacks' intended to compensate OPOs who provide many organs to transplant centers outside their local region. Medical urgency is only taken into account when a kidney transplant is needed in conjunction with another abdominal or thoracic organ.

Livers are also distributed according to a complex point system, again with preference being given to local areas followed by UNOS regions. Livers are only offered nationally if no suitable candidate is identified locally. However, medical urgency plays a crucial role in deciding to whom a liver should be offered. These rules are constantly being developed in order to ensure fairness of organ allocation and optimize the rational use of scarce organs. As recently as August 1997, UNOS published updated guidelines, under which patients who would have been classified as status 1 prior to that time have been separated into two categories. Those who qualify for the new status 1 category must now be suffering from acute fulminant liver failure with a life expectancy of less than 7 days without a transplant, and must be over the age of 18 years. For the purposes of definition, acute fulminant liver failure involves the onset of stage II hepatic encephalopathy within 8 weeks of the onset of liver disease without pre-existing liver disease, as well as laboratory evidence of severe liver dysfunction. Primary non-function or hepatic artery thrombosis of a recently

Table 9.1. Child–Turcotte–Pugh (CTP) scoring system

	Number of points		
	1	**2**	**3**
Encephalopathy	None	1–2	3–4
Ascites	None (or controlled by diuretics)	Slight	Moderate
Bilirubin (mg/dL)	< 2.0	2–3	> 3.0
Albumin (g/dL)	> 3.5	2.8–3.5	< 2.8
Prothrombin time* (s prolonged over baseline)	< 4.0	4–6	> 6.0
Bilirubin (mg/dL) (for primary biliary cirrhosis, primary sclerosing cholangitis or other cholestatic liver disease, substitute for the above values)	< 4.0	4–10	> 10.0

* INR (International Normalized Ratio) is alternative to prothrombin time (< 4.7/1.7–2.3/ > 2.3).

transplanted liver and acute decompensated Wilson's disease also qualify a patient for status 1 classification. All status 1 patients within a UNOS region receive priority with regard to consideration for a potential organ over local and regional status 2A or 2B candidates.

All other patients who are awaiting liver transplantation are now classified according to a scoring system known as the Child–Turcotte–Pugh (CTP) scoring system (see Table 9.1). The remaining patients who had been classified as status 1 are now grouped under the heading status 2A. These patients must require a critical-care setting for treatment of chronic liver disease, have a life expectancy of less than 7 days without a liver transplant, and have a CTP score of >10. In addition, these patients must meet at least one of the following criteria: active variceal bleeding or portal hypertensive gastropathy requiring in excess of two units of blood and unresponsive to treatment, including transjugular intrahepatic portosystemic shunt placement (TIPS); hepatorenal syndrome; refractory ascites that is unresponsive to treatment; stage III or IV encephalopathy that is unresponsive to medical therapy; severe coagulopathy with ongoing bleeding, again refractory to replacement therapy. Extrahepatic sepsis that is unresponsive to therapy, severe irreversible multi-organ system failure or a requirement for high-dose or two or more pressors to maintain adequate blood pressure disqualify a patient from the status 2A category. Patients who would formerly have been in the status 2 group now fall into the status 2B group. These are patients who have a CTP score of $\geqslant 7$ and one or more of the following criteria: documented variceal bleeding or portal hypertensive gastropathy requiring two or more units of blood and unresponsive to treatment; hepatorenal syndrome; spontaneous bacterial peritonitis; refractory ascites. All of the remaining patients who are on the active waiting-list are classified as status 3. These patients require continuous medical care, although not necessarily as hospital inpatients, and have a CTP score of $\geqslant 7$. Pediatric patients may be classified as status 1 if they are located in the intensive-care unit due to acute or chronic liver disease with a life expectancy of less than 7 days without a transplant. Children who are awaiting transplant may be classified as status 2B if they suffer from an inborn error of metabolism that causes the accumulation of substances that are toxic to the central nervous system regardless of their location, and as status 1 if they are hospitalized for an acute exacerbation of their disease.

Generally speaking, livers are offered first to local status 1 patients, then to local status 2A followed by 2B and 3 patients, before being offered to status 1 patients in the UNOS region and finally to patients on the national list. Donor organ size plays an important role, as placing an organ that is too large for a particular recipient, or 'cutting down' the liver to an acceptable size, are both hazardous options. Moreover, livers are offered on the basis of ABO blood group rather than by HLA-matching criteria. Blood-type compatibility, time on the waiting-list and medical status classification are calculated into the point system, which determines the order on the waiting-list within each status group.

Thoracic organs as a group are first allocated locally, but thereafter according to a zonal system. Unlike renal and liver allografts, much stricter geographic limitations are mandatory due to the limited cold ischemic times tolerated by these organs. Three zones are delineated by concentric circles of 500 and 1000 nautical mile radii, with the donor hospital at the center. These are designated zones A (within 500 miles), B (within 1000 miles) and C (greater than 1000 miles). In addition, the medical status of waiting candidates is taken into account. As with the rules that govern liver allocation and patient classification, the guidelines concerning thoracic organ allocation have recently been rewritten. A status 1A patient is one who is in an intensive-care unit and requiring continuous infusions of inotropic agents to maintain adequate cardiac output, or who requires cardiac or pulmonary assistance in the form of left or right ventricular assist devices or an intra-aortic balloon pump. Dependence on a total artificial heart device has been eliminated as a qualifying criterion, as these patients are assumed to be too unstable to tolerate transplantation. Qualification by ventilator dependence has been limited to those weighing ≤ 45 kg, as these patients are excluded from receiving a mechanical assist device because of their size. Status 1A patients must also be hospitalized at the listing transplant center. Status 1B patients require either a circulatory assist device or admission to an acute care hospital for continuous infusions of IV inotropic agents, although that hospital need not be the listing transplant center. This group also includes those patients who may be on assist devices but not in an acute hospital setting. Status 2A patients are dependent on continuous IV intropic agents, but may be managed outside the hospital, while the group status 2B encompasses all other patients who are awaiting heart or heart–lung transplants.

Hearts and heart–lung combinations are generally allocated as a group, with priority being given to status 1A patients, ABO compatibility and patients who have accumulated time on the waiting-list within the local region. This is followed by local heart–lung candidates according to the same criteria, and finally by status 2A and 2B patients. If no suitable candidate is located within the local area, the organs are then offered within Zones A, B and C (in that order) to status 1A and 1B candidates for hearts alone, followed by heart–lung candidates and finally status 2A and 2B heart candidates.

Only after the heart has been allocated are the lungs offered to patients who are awaiting single or double lungs alone. A similar zonal geographic system is utilized when offering lung allografts, and priority is given to waiting candidates with ABO compatibility, and to those with the longest waiting times. Interestingly, there is no status system to give priority to sicker patients who are awaiting lung transplants.

Pancreas transplants are offered in the greatest variety of combinations, as candidates may be awaiting an isolated pancreas, a kidney–pancreas combination or a combined solid organ–islet cell transplant from the same donor. Absolute priority nationwide is given to zero-antigen-mismatch organs. After this, length of time on the waiting-list is considered. Whole pancreas transplants are offered first locally for isolated pancreas and kidney–pancreas combinations, then regionally, and finally on a nationwide basis. In addition, certain antigen combinations are given priority. If a UNOS Organ Center has been unable to place a pancreas for 5 h or if procurement is imminent, it may be offered on the basis of a facilitated protocol according to which programs agree to accept organs procured by institutions outside their own OPO, and to accept organs for zero-antigen-mismatch candidates. Only if suitable recipients cannot be identified according to the above criteria will the host OPO offer the pancreas locally, regionally and then nationally for clinical islet transplantation. If the organ remains unused, it may be offered for research.

Patients who are awaiting stomach or small or large bowel transplants are becoming somewhat more common, and are also included in the UNOS candidate waiting-lists. Status 1 patients are those with existing liver function abnormalities and/or those for whom potential sites for intravenous feeding have become severely limited. Those for whom intestinal transplantation has been deemed urgent are also classified as status 1. All other patients are classified as status 2. Organs are offered with medical status taking second priority to geographic location. Many of these patients are also awaiting liver transplants and are governed by the rules that cover multi-organ candidates. They accrue time on the liver waiting-list, and when an offer of a liver is made for them, local arrangements are often made as to whether the intestinal component may accompany the liver.

Other isolated issues that govern the allocation and potential offers of organs are numerous. For example, HIV-antibody-positive donors are excluded from donation, although UNOS policy does not categorically exclude HIV-antibody-positive candidates from receiving a donated organ. Those who test positive for HTLV-I-Ab are also considered to be unacceptable as donors. Individuals who have received human pituitary-derived growth hormone are also deferred as organ donors. Foreign nationals are not considered differently to American or resident aliens on UNOS waiting-lists, although the number of such patients who are transplanted may not exceed 5% of the total transplants performed at a particular center without incurring an outside audit by UNOS. Formal contractual arrangements with foreign governments violate UNOS policy.

Physiology of brain death

Brain death, whether it results from catastrophic neurologic injury or severe anoxic or metabolic insult, occurs over a variable length of time and is associated with a host of physiologic, histologic, endocrine and metabolic processes which affect the function of many organ systems. Most frequently, the declaration of brain death is not made until well after this cascade of events has been initiated, and significant injury to the potentially transplantable organs may have already occurred. A thorough understanding of the nature of these events is therefore necessary if organs are not to be 'lost'. Proactive management of potential donors, including aggressive invasive monitoring, hemodynamic management and meticulous attention to detail, becomes important, especially in the multi-organ donor.

Observations of physiologic and clinical changes immediately preceding brain death secondary to enormous increases in ICP were documented many years ago, and the Cushing triad of hypertension, bradycardia and alterations in breathing patterns is well known. This elevation in mean arterial pressure represents a last-ditch effort on the part of the cerebral vasculature to maintain cerebral perfusion in the face of drastically elevated ICP. Bradycardia develops as a result of both parasympathetic nervous system activation and reflex slowing of the heart rate secondary to baroreceptor function. However, during the past few decades a number of models of brain death under very carefully controlled conditions have been developed which have provided a much more detailed picture of what is happening as this process occurs.

Research by Shivalkar and his colleagues has contributed enormously to the current understanding of events that accompany brain death. In a canine model, they compared brain death caused by a gradual increase in ICP to that caused by an explosive rise in ICP. Interestingly, the rate of ICP increase affected the degree of physiologic derangement, but the general sequence of events was the same. In general, brain herniation or 'coning' following severe cerebral injury represents a progressive central nervous system ischemic injury that begins supratentorially and proceeds caudally to involve the crucial brainstem regions of the pons and medulla and finally the spinal cord. Initially, parasympathetic activation is seen after failure of the Cushing reflex to maintain cerebral perfusion and the ischemic threshold of the brain has been exceeded. Progressive bradycardia and hypotension develop, as does centrally altered breathing as the ischemic zone reaches the midbrain respiratory control centers. As the area of injury reaches the most distal midbrain regions, the vagal cardiomotor centers become ischemic, which destroys the source of vagal outflow, and parasympathetic activity is terminated.

Following the actual occurrence of brain death as defined by current conventional criteria, a situation of unopposed sympathetic stimulation occurs, which lasts for a period of minutes to hours. This so-called 'autonomic storm' is characterized by tachycardia, hypertension, hyperthermia and dramatically increased cardiac output. The degree of metabolic derangement appears to be related to the speed of development of brain death and the rate of increase of the ICP. In Shivalkar's canine model, a slow rate of increase in ICP (group 2) yielded a 200-fold increase in plasma epinephrine levels, while 23% of the myocardium was considered to show mild ischemic damage. On the other hand, an 'explosive' increase in ICP (group 1) leading to brain death was associated with a 1000-fold increase in circulating epinephrine levels and a severe hyperdynamic response. On microscopy, 93% of the myocardium was shown to be severely ischemic, with 100 times more focal infarctions than in group 2, and severe myocytolysis, swollen mitochondria and necrotic nuclei were common. This sequence of events has been confirmed in baboon hearts, which showed that the greatest degree of myocardial damage occurs in the left ventricle, while necrotic changes were seen in the conduction systems of almost half of the subjects. Furthermore, clinical corroboration using quantitative birefringence microscopy has been documented in humans, with 43% of hearts from brain-dead donors showing impaired function prior to procurement, despite similar age, sex, level of inotropic support and incidence of cardiac arrest.

During this autonomic storm, a variety of electrocardiographic changes are seen. In a baboon model, five distinct stages have been described. First there is a sinus bradycardia followed by a sinus tachycardia without ischemic changes, with each phase having a duration of the order of minutes. Subsequently, for a period of about 15 min, multifocal ventricular ectopic beats are frequent. In the fourth stage, sinus tachycardia with marked ischemic changes develops, and this can last for up to several hours. The final stage is characterized by sinus rhythm with a reduction in R-wave amplitude and persistent ischemic changes in 50% of subjects. This last pattern of ischemia can last for more than 12–15 h. Of interest, the first and second stages of this sequence are abolished by vagotomy, while many of the histological changes described above fail to develop after sympathectomy. It should be noted that the transient bradyarrhythmias that are seen during the early and acute phase of brain herniation are unresponsive to atropine sulfate, and treatment often requires epinephrine or isoproterenol.

Peripherally, the autonomic storm is accompanied by severe vasoconstriction, and a subsequent shift of the circulating blood volume to the capacitance vessels. This results in a significant increase in venous return to the right side of the heart, and the development of short-lived but dramatic increases in pulmonary arterial pressures. At the same time, left ventricular dysfunction secondary to catecholamine-induced cardiomyopathy leads to increased left atrial pressures, further contributing to increases in pulmonary pressures. Capillary wall disruption and leakage of protein-rich fluid into the interstitium may develop during this period of pulmonary hypertension. In fact, some investigators feel that this may at least partly account for the development of neurogenic pulmonary edema that frequently follows severe neurologic injury.

Immediately after this period of autonomic hyperactivity, a situation of multifactorial hypotension ensues. The myriad causes of this hypotension include loss of autonomic regulation of the peripheral vasculature, and resultant unopposed vasodilation and decreased myocardial inotropic performance. This seems in part to be a result of severe catecholamine depletion as well as intrinsic myocardial injury sustained during the period of the autonomic storm. Direct myocardial injury was first proposed when investigators in South Africa noted that hearts taken from healthy, anesthetized baboons and stored in a hypothermic perfusion system for 48 h functioned much better than those taken from brain-dead baboons. The only difference between the two groups was the induction of brain death, and for the first time it was proposed that brain death itself was responsible for organ dysfunction in transplanted organs. More recently, it has been shown that whether inotropic support is provided or not, depletion of high-energy phosphates and glycogen reserves in the myocardium is seen after brain death. In addition, histologic studies have shown that within 4–7 h of brain death, irreversible focal ischemic injury and myocytolysis of varying degrees have occurred in 5% and 12% of the left and right ventricular myocardium, respectively. It has been proposed that one important factor in direct injury to myocardial cells involves increased calcium uptake and subsequent myocyte necrosis. Although autopsy studies in human patients who died at various times following sudden increases in ICP indicate that it takes 6–12 h for myocardial damage to become evident histologically, they have also shown that 8–12% of patients who die from acute cerebral lesions prior to this temporal window show such cardiac injury. The significance of this period of extreme catecholamine depletion, hypotension and myocardial failure is not limited to the potential heart or lung donor. This period of autonomic chaos has been documented in 50% of patients during the development of brain death, and inadequate peripheral perfusion is probably much more common. Hypoperfusion to all organs of the body occurs during this period, at first due to intense vasoconstriction, and subsequently due to inadequate cardiac output combined with systemic vasodilation. All organs that are being considered for transplantation are therefore at risk during this period.

Hormonal changes resulting from brain death have been the subject of intense study within the transplant community. A general shift from aerobic to anaerobic metabolism is evidenced by a measured reduction in pyruvate, glucose and palmitate utilization.

By administering ^{14}C-labelled glucose to groups of sedated or brain-dead Chacma baboons, investigators have been able to show markedly reduced substrate uptake, as well as pathologic accumulation of lactate and free fatty acids in the plasma, all of which are indicators of anaerobic metabolism. In addition, brainstem ischemia secondary to herniation is followed by a sudden decrease in the levels of several free circulating anterior and posterior pituitary hormones. The development of diabetes insipidus due to a deficiency of antidiuretic hormone (ADH) has been estimated to occur in up to 87% of patients with brain death resulting from trauma or global ischemia, and it certainly causes or exacerbates the hypotension that is almost universally observed in potential donors. In addition, a recent study from Russia documented a marked fall in the levels of ADH, follicle-stimulating hormone, prolactin, thyroid-stimulating hormone, T_3 and T_4, although the levels of adrenocorticotrophic hormone (ACTH), growth hormone and luteinizing hormone remained unchanged. The significance of these other pituitary hormone changes has not been well studied.

Decreased ADH levels have been consistently noted in patients with severe neurologic injury, and they seem to have far-reaching consequences. Patients who have developed diabetes insipidus prior to declaration of brain death are frequently managed with desmopressin (DDAVP), an ADH analog that exhibits minimal pressor activity. However, several investigators have demonstrated an improved hemodynamic status in response to infusions of arginine vasopressin. Kinoshita noted that the addition of vasopressin to epinephrine infusions (0.3 µg/kg/min) lowered the dose of epinephrine necessary to maintain peripheral perfusion. In another study, Yoshioka was able to maintain brain-dead patients with continuous vasopressin and low-dose epinephrine infusions for an average of 23 days, a feat which could not be achieved with epinephrine alone. These studies suggest that there is some intrinsic and crucial contribution made by ADH to maintenance of the hemodynamic integrity of the cardiovascular system, and that its absence may be a predominant factor responsible for the eventual cardiac arrest or collapse that is observed in almost all brain-dead patients.

The other hormonal issue that has generated a significant amount of interest with regard to the management of brain-dead patients is control of thyroid hormone function. Novitsky and colleagues have been most active in this arena. They have consistently documented decreased levels of circulating T_3 and T_4, although the levels of thyroid-stimulating hormone (TSH) did not change. In one trial, T_3 at a dose of 2 µg/h was given to brain-dead baboons who showed increased rates of metabolic utilization of glucose, pyruvate and palmitate as well as a reduction in the concentration of lactate and free fatty acids. This indicates a correction of the metabolic defect in oxidative metabolism noted in brain-dead patients. These findings have been challenged by research by Howlett and colleagues. However, in their studies they did not measure circulating T_3, so it is difficult to compare the results of these studies. Yet in a prospective, randomized, placebo-controlled study of 37 human organ donors receiving T_3 (2 μg/h), no improvement in hemodynamic stability or myocardial function as measured by transesophageal echocardiogram was noted. It remains controversial whether a deficiency of T_3 is responsible for the decrease in oxidative metabolism and a degree of the myocardial dysfunction that is seen in brain-dead patients. It is likely that a situation similar to sick euthyroid syndrome occurs, in which only predisposed patients actually benefit from treatment. Several medical centers, including Papworth Hospital in the UK, have developed a 'Hormone Package' consisting of T_3, ADH and insulin or T_3, cortisol and insulin, that is provided to potential organ donors. They have demonstrated marked improvements in cardiac function in treated subjects compared to untreated controls. However, this has not yet led to wide acceptance of this practice.

Regardless of the cause of death in the organ donor, some pathologic processes occur almost universally. For a variety of reasons, including the original injury and appropriate treatment of the latter, electrolyte disturbances are routine in potential organ donors. Not surprisingly, hypernatremia is most commonly a result of diabetes insipidus and diuretics given to lower the ICP. Hypokalemia, hypomagnesemia, hypocalcemia and even hypophosphatemia are also common and require prompt replacement therapy. Hyperglycemia is frequently a result of inappropriate administration of large amounts of dextrose-containing solutions, either for treatment of diabetes insipidus or in fluid resuscitation, but it may also be due to peripheral insulin resistance or, more rarely, intrinsic pancreatic traumatic or ischemic injury, or even unrecognized diabetes mellitus. Hypothermia is almost universal, again for a variety of reasons. Loss of thermal regulation by the central nervous system rendering the patient poikilothermic is responsible in some cases, but radiant and convective heat loss in the critically ill patient is also important. However, once a patient becomes cool, their ability to rewarm themselves is non-existent, and active rewarming measures are mandatory. Hypothermia decreases renal concentrating abilities and leads to a cold diuresis. It shifts the oxyhemoglobin dissociation curve to the left, causing decreased oxygen delivery at the tissue level, and leading to local tissue ischemia. At the same time, it also causes myocardial depression, pulmonary hypertension, cardiovascular instability, arrhythmias and eventually cardiac arrest. Coagulation disturbances are also commonly seen. As many as 88% of patients develop disseminated intravascular coagulation after coagulation-cascade activation and factor consumption secondary to massive tissue thromboplastin release, which accompanies severe neurologic injury. Alternatively, factor and platelet dilution may occur after massive blood loss and fluid resuscitation. Furthermore, significant hypothermia alone is a well-recognized cause of coagulopathy, and readily exacerbates any derangement of coagulation of another cause.

Box 9.1 Physiologic changes associated with brain death

Neurologic changes
Increased intracranial pressure, herniation

Cardiopulmonary changes
Hypertension followed by hypotension
Tachycardia
Bradycardia
Arrhythmia (premature ventricular beats, asystole)
Myocardial dysfunction
Myocardial ischemia
Increased pulmonary artery pressures
Pulmonary edema
Cardiac arrest

Endocrine/metabolic changes
Decreased aerobic metabolism
Increased anaerobic metabolism
Decreased circulating pituitary hormones*
    Diabetes insipidus
Electrolyte disturbances
    Hypernatremia
    Hypokalemia
    Hypomagnesemia
    Hypocalcemia
    Hypophosphatemia
    Hyperglycemia

Hematologic changes
Coagulopathy
    Disseminated intravascular coagulation
    Factor and platelet dilution

Other changes
Hyperthermia followed by hypothermia

* Other than ADH, exactly which hormones become deficient is controversial.

Management of the potential organ donor

At the time of declaration of brain death, the management goals for the patient are changed dramatically from preserving life and neurological function to preserving and optimizing the function of specific organs at the expense of other systems. At a general level, the basic critical-care principles remain the same, but a different balance must be struck which takes into account which organs are being considered for procurement and transplantation.

Optimizing cardiovascular system function can be a challenging task, and it is frequently made more complicated if the thoracic organs are being considered for transplantation. Stresses of enormous proportion accompany the evolution of brain death itself, not to mention the negative consequences that treatment of severe neurological injury may involve. Significant volume depletion by mannitol and other diuretic therapy aimed at minimizing ICP, in addition to the consequences of the catecholamine surge and subsequent deficit, often leave the potential donor hypotensive and inotropic-dependent. Myocardial dysfunction results from excessive inotrope usage, brain death physiology or severe hypovolemia. Fluid resuscitation guided by central venous monitoring or even pulmonary artery catheter placement is mandatory, hopefully reducing the dependence of the patient on inotropes for the maintenance of systolic arterial blood pressure greater than 90–100 mmHg. Colloids or crystalloids may be used for volume repletion to achieve a central venous pressure of 9–12 mmHg. Glucose-containing solutions should not be used, in order to avoid hyperglycemia and consequent osmotic diuresis. A pulmonary artery catheter may be indicated secondary to evaluation for thoracic organ donation, or due to coexisting medical conditions in the donor such as valvular disease, cardiomyopathy, severe lung disease or persistent hypotension.

Hypotension that is resistant to fluid repletion is common among organ donors, and is most frequently treated with peripheral vasoconstrictors. Dopamine has been the pressor of choice, presumably due to its mesenteric vasodilating capabilities, although this has not been well documented in humans. The use of inotropes is discouraged by many centers due to concerns about catecholamine-induced cardiomyopathy in the donor, and catecholamine depletion of the myocardium due to endogenous catecholamine release, with attenuation of responses to subsequent catecholamine administration. In addition, high doses of vasopressor agents decrease the blood flow to vital organs, possibly resulting in ischemic injury to the very organs that are intended for transplant. In general, low doses of dopamine (< 7.5 µg/kg/min) are considered to be acceptable. Further vasopressor therapy must be guided by invasive monitoring assistance. The addition of arginine vasopressin may also be considered at this point. However, the unrestrained use of fluid to maintain acceptable organ perfusion must be balanced against the risk of inducing volume overload and pulmonary edema. This would disqualify the lungs from potential donation, in addition to potentially impairing gas exchange and causing arterial hypoxemia and end-organ ischemia.

Additional cardiovascular issues that require attention often include arrhythmias and sudden cardiac arrest. In fact, in a review of brain-dead patients who were maintained on ventilators, 62% suffered cardiac arrest within 24 h, and 87% did so within 72 h. It must be remembered that atropine in the brain-dead patient is ineffective, and direct beta-agonists such as isoproterenol or epinephrine are necessary. In addition, other injuries such as myocardial contusions incurred at the same time as the neurologic trauma may manifest themselves and complicate the clinical picture.

The goals for respiratory management of the patient include ensuring adequate oxygen delivery to other organs and maintaining an acid–base equilibrium, in addition to achieving optimal lung function and preventing further injury to the lungs if they are being considered for transplantation. Mechanical ventilation is always necessary. In general, the inspired fraction of oxygen should be kept at less than 50%, peak inspiratory pressures (PIP) at less than 30 cmH_2O with tidal volumes of 15 mL/kg, and less than 5 cmH_2O peak end-expiratory pressure (PEEP). Oxygen saturations of at least 95% and a pH of 7.4 are also considered to be standard. In addition, meticulous respiratory care is necessary in order to minimize colonization of the trachea with pathogenic organisms, as well as to minimize the incidence of pneumonia and atelectasis. Excessive PEEP levels must be avoided in order to decrease the incidence of barotrauma and compromise of venous return to the heart.

A variety of other issues that are more specific to brain-dead organ donors are also important. As discussed earlier, hypothermia frequently develops for a variety of reasons, and active measures must be taken to prevent further heat loss and to rewarm the patient if hypothermia has already developed. This includes the use of forced warm air devices, warming intravenous fluids and ventilating the lungs with warmed, humidified air. Central temperature monitoring is necessary, and the temperature should be kept at or above 35°C. The issue of prophylactic antibiotic use is controversial and center-specific. Coagulopathy, again of multifactorial origin, is also common. Although the risk of microvascular thrombosis is high, therapies such as ε-aminocaproic acid are not recommended. Defects in coagulation should be treated with replacement therapy guided by deficits of specific factors or platelets. Similarly, endocrine and metabolic disorders should be treated according to frequent laboratory measurements of electrolytes and glucose levels.

The provision of nutrition to the potential organ donor is another topic of interest. Significant increases in safe cold ischemia times for livers and other abdominal organs have been achieved with the development of University of Wisconsin (UW) solution, which provides (among other things) products for continued cellular metabolism. Most organ donors spend a minimum of 2 to 3 days, and sometimes in excess of 1 week, on mechanical ventilation and without nutrition during the process of identification, confirmation of brain death and preparation for organ procurement. Interestingly, in studies in rats, livers from fasted donors appeared to tolerate long-term preservation better than livers from fed donors, but improved survival was seen in rats that had been fed glucose (a 40% solution in drinking water) for 4 days prior to transplant. The investigators proposed that this was due to elevation of liver glycogen levels in the allograft. This would result in improved capacity for anaerobically derived ATP during the ischemic period, and better maintained hepatocyte viability. With shorter periods of glucose intake, smaller degrees of benefit were seen, but intake was still felt to be helpful. If this observation is confirmed in further laboratory investigations, it is possible that once a patient has been declared brain dead and further neurological injury is no longer an issue, the provision of glucose infusions (but avoiding hyperglycemia) may become common practice.

Specific organ considerations

Apart from the general issues of critical care of the potential organ donor discussed above, there are multiple issues specific to each of the solid organs which profoundly affect the current performance of organ transplantation, or the ways in which it may be performed in the future. Many of these are related to efforts to meet the ever increasing need for donated organs, and to enlarge the donor pool.

Heart

Thoracic organs that are being considered for transplantation are subjected to the most stringent selection criteria of all solid organs. For example, in the UK, a potential heart donor must be under the age of 50 years, with a normal 12-lead EKG, no family history of cardiac disease, no history of prolonged asystole and no need for high-dose inotropic support. Requirements in the USA are even more restrictive. However, these criteria seem to be well justified. The early mortality rate for adult patients has remained unchanged for the past 5 years at 9–10%. However, the mortality rate in recipients who have received hearts with impaired function was found in one retrospective review to be 44%, compared to 6% for those with undamaged hearts. Likewise, another review of survival indicated that donors over the age of 40 years yielded a higher 1-year mortality rate in the recipient, while those over 50 years of age were associated with a more than twofold increase in early postoperative recipient mortality. Older age in the donor was found to be second only to retransplantation as a predictor of early mortality. However, the issue of age is becoming somewhat controversial. In a more recent review of 77 donors over the age of 40 years, no difference was found in 1-year recipient survival rates, although there was a greater need for pacemaker insertion in the older donor group. At the Mayo Clinic, a heart from a donor over the age of 40 years is considered to be acceptable if it has a normal ejection fraction, normal coronary arteries on angiography, and is expected to have a cold ischemic time of less than 240 min.

These limitations have resulted in increasing efforts on the part of transplant surgeons to identify those organs that have not sustained significant injury or do not suffer from intrinsic disease and would function well post-transplant. It is well recognized that non-cardiac causes of myocardial dysfunction or inotropic requirement often accompany severe neurologic injury and brain death. Hemodynamic management is obviously important. Although invasive monitoring is required, attempts to optimize preload and afterload, decrease the need for inotropes and improve myocardial function will sometimes reveal a heart which has the capacity for normal performance. In addition, hormonal replacement has received a significant amount of attention. It has been noted that thyroid hormone and vasopressin given to brain-dead organ donors have been beneficial to cardiovascular function and improved long-term graft survival. In a retrospective review, unstable donors who were treated according to a T_4 replacement protocol showed 95.2% graft survival, compared to 83.3% in those donors who were already considered to be suitable for transplantation and were not treated with any hormones ($p < 0.01$). Similarly, one group of investigators claimed to be able to increase their donor pool by 30% by using a hormonal replacement protocol involving steroids, insulin, T_3 and arginine vasopressin. In a trial of 52 donors who were originally deemed to be unacceptable,

44 donors (92%) were 'rescued' with this regimen. Of a total of 150 procurements, only four were finally excluded due to left ventricular hypertrophy or palpable coronary disease, although the investigators do not specify how patients were selected for procurement. The overall survival rate was 76% in the 'rescued' group, compared with 84% in the control group at 13–48 months. Unfortunately, no level of significance was reported.

Ischemic preconditioning of the myocardium, a topic of interest in organ preservation during cardiopulmonary bypass, has also received some attention. In isolated working rat hearts, one cycle of 5 min of normothermic ischemia was followed by 5 min of reperfusion prior to induction of global hypothermic ischemia for 10 h at 4°C. This protocol resulted in decreased creatine phosphokinase leakage, and better functional recovery as measured by maximum developed left ventricular pressure, although the high-energy phosphate content did not differ between the experimental and control groups. In other studies, ischemic preconditioning has been shown to decrease the extent of necrosis and the incidence of arrhythmias and contractile dysfunction caused by prolonged regional and global ischemia.

Lung

Clinical goals for acceptable lung donation include peak airway pressures of less than 30 cmH$_2$O, with tidal volumes of 15 mL/kg and a positive end-expiratory pressure of 5 cmH$_2$O. Physiologic pH and minimum oxygen saturations of 95% should also be maintained, while avoiding hyperoxia. Major pulmonary contusion, atelectasis resistant to lung inflation techniques and/or pneumonia are grounds for exclusion, as are chronic lung disease, heavy smoking and pulmonary aspiration. Not surprisingly, an elevated alveolar–arterial gradient and tracheal colonization with fungus or sputum samples with many polymorphonuclear leukocytes have been associated with increased morbidity and operative mortality. There has been some controversy over the propriety of procurement of lungs from trauma patients in whom pulmonary injury may not yet have manifested itself. However, in a retrospective review of 125 isolated lung or heart–lung transplants comparing a trauma group to a non-trauma group, no difference was found at 30 days post-transplant.

As with potential donor hearts, ischemic preconditioning has been investigated as a potential method for minimizing preservation injury in lungs. In one study using rats, the left main bronchus and pulmonary artery were occluded for 5 min, followed by 10 min of reperfusion and ventilation. This was in turn followed by procurement and cold ischemic storage for 6 or 12 h, and then transplantation. Although lung water was no different from that of controls, the levels of thiobarbituric acid-reactive substances, which provide an indirect measure of oxidative stress, were reduced in both the 6- and 12-h groups. Interestingly, oxygen exchange was only improved in the 12-h group. It remains to be seen whether ischemic preconditioning will actually yield a clinically significant improvement.

Liver

The issue of organ allocation with respect to liver transplantation has recently been influenced by a small collection of studies concerning outcome in different patient populations. A small retrospective review of status 1 patients found that 1-year patient and graft survival rates were better for those with acute disease processes than for those with acute exacerbations of chronic disease (61% and 46% vs. 45% and 46%, respectively). If this is replicated in further studies, it could have profound implications for organ allocation policies. However, another expanded review from the same group in combination with other centers in the region revealed no strong survival-based difference in transplants performed for critically ill patients of acute or chronic etiologies. Yet the newest available UNOS guidelines do take into account the etiology and chronicity of patients with fulminant liver failure, allocating highest priority to those with acute disease only. Whether this will lead to more efficient utilization of this scarce resource has yet to be determined.

Kidney

Management goals for potential kidney donors include maintaining urine output above 100 mL/h, and if possible avoiding the use of catecholamines. Size-matching was thought to be important when deciding what types of patients would be appropriate for particular organs. However, recent research has shown that this has no effect on graft survival.

Pancreas

Recently, human islet isolation and transplantation have generated increasing interest. However, the overall success rate is quite low.

A retrospective review of 153 human islet isolations performed at the University of Alberta, Canada, over a period of 3 years indicates that multiple donors are necessary in order to provide a transplantable islet-cell mass. In addition, of 55 reported adult transplants in type 1 diabetics, only 11% showed 1-year insulin independence. Interestingly, success is often defined as islet-cell function of any type. Hence by measuring C-peptide in recipients the success rate is increased to 33%.

Non-heart-beating donation

Each year there is an ever increasing discrepancy between the number of patients awaiting solid organ transplants and the number of organs available. Several strategies have been tried in an attempt to increase the size of the donor pool, including public education and the utilization of organs formerly considered to be unsuitable for transplantation. A further strategy involves the use of organs from patients who technically do not meet the criteria for the definition of brain death. In general, these are patients who have sustained massive neurologic trauma from a variety of causes, but who continue to demonstrate certain brainstem reflexes or an intact drive to breathe. These donors are known as non-heart-beating (NHB) donors, and a tremendous amount of research has been done by many investigators looking at the feasibility of using these organs after a conventional declaration of death been made – that is, after the heart has ceased to beat and the patient has ceased breathing. It has been estimated that the donor pool could be enlarged by 20–25% if non-heart-beating donations were routinely used.

Multiple animal models of non-heart-beating donation have been developed to evaluate cardiac function after transplantation. In a pig model, ultrastructural damage and an inability to beat for more than 15 min after reperfusion occurred after only 30 min of in-situ ischemia. After only 10 min of ischemia, significant decreases in energetic compound content, coronary flow and left ventricular developed peak pressure were seen. However, these hearts received no pharmacologic intervention or cold ischemia. On the other hand, canine hearts have been successfully transplanted after up to 1 h of hypoxic arrest using cardioprotective agents including verapamil, prostacyclin and a hydroxy-radical scavenger. Other research in lambs and rabbits has also shown that hearts can be transplanted after ischemic arrest for periods of 10–30 min and successfully weaned from cardiopulmonary bypass.

The physiology of the lung seems to make it uniquely suited to non-heart-beating procurement. Cellular respiration appears to occur directly at the gas–cellular interface, rather than via vascular perfusion, and seems to be predominantly passive – that is, not an energy-requiring process. Thus the provision of oxygen to the lung either by ventilation or by apneic insufflation may prevent ischemic injury at the cellular level during the period of cardiac arrest required in order to declare death. In fact, pulmonary cells have been shown to be functionally and histologically viable for up to several hours after death. Trials in dogs have shown successful transplantation after 1–2 h of warm ischemia. In some of these trials the lungs continue to be ventilated and in others they are not, but most show adequate gas exchange post-transplant. Moreover, in lungs from rats that had been subjected to 2–3 h of ischemia *in situ*, no difference was seen in gas exchange or lung function compared with controls who experienced no warm ischemia. Interestingly, lungs that had been subjected to episodes of hypotension prior to the *in-situ* ischemia developed elevated airway and pulmonary artery pressures and gross pulmonary edema within 10 min of reperfusion.

Experience with human NHB donors is limited to abdominal organs, and is becoming more controversial. However, several centers have had protocols in place and have been performing such transplants for several years. The University of Wisconsin has been using organs from NHB donors since 1974, has had a specific protocol since 1993, and has reported their experience. Over a 17-month period, 16 non-heart-beating donors were identified from a total of 130 organ donors. Only 10 donors finally came to procurement, due to advanced age or sudden cardiac arrest. Five liver transplants and six kidney–pancreas transplants were performed. The preservation times for these and conventionally procured organs were similar. One liver recipient developed primary nonfunction that was thought to be secondary to a technical error. Organ function post-transplant was similar to that of conventionally procured organs, and all of the patients were alive after a mean follow-up period of 12.7 months. Of the 27 kidneys procured from these same donors, 19 of 21 patients had functioning grafts after a mean follow-up period of 8.3 months. However, the postoperative need for dialysis was 14.3%, compared with 8.6% for kidneys from heart-beating donors. Of additional interest is a lung which was transplanted from one of the NHB donors to a patient supported on extracorporeal membrane oxygenation (ECMO) while awaiting transplantation. The patient was weaned and extubated after 4 days, but no further follow-up was given. Surgeons at that institution currently accept liver and pancreas grafts from NHB donors with warm ischemic times of up to 1 h and kidneys with warm ischemic times of up to 2 h.

A group in Sweden has also reported on 17 livers procured from NHB donors between 1984 and 1987. One organ developed primary non-function, while 77% demonstrated good function after 1 month. Peak aspartate aminotransferase levels were no different to those of organs procured from conventional donors. The University of Pittsburgh has also reported on seven livers procured from NHB donors, five of whom were undergoing cardiopulmonary resuscitation at the time of procurement and were managed with a rapid flush technique via the femoral vessels. One recipient died as a result of technical failure in the operating-room, and one recipient developed hepatic artery thrombosis. All of the others were discharged with grafts showing good function.

The technical details of organ procurement from these patients have been a source of controversy. The University of Wisconsin has published its protocol for the procedure, according to which patients with severe neurological injury without hope of meaningful recovery, but who do not meet the criteria for brain death, are considered for donation. Support is withdrawn in the operating-room after femoral cannulas have been placed. Phentolamine, 10–20 mg, is administered to prevent agonal vasoconstriction. A total of 10 000–20 000 units of heparin and 12.5–25 g of mannitol are also infused. All patients become hypotensive in response to phentolamine. The patients are then extubated. After declaration of

---

Box 9.2 Establishing the diagnosis of brain death

Clinical signs
Cerebral unresponsiveness
Absent pupillary, corneal, oculovestibular and oculocephalic reflexes
Lack of spontaneous motor activity
Lack of response to verbal stimuli or deep pain
Lack of gag reflex
Negative atropine challenge (2 mg)
Negative apneic challenge in response to hypercarbia ($PaCO_2 \geqslant 60$ mmHg)

Confirmatory tests
Electroencephalogram
Visual evoked potentials
Auditory evoked potentials
Somatosensory evoked potentials
Transcranial Doppler
Technetium–HMPAO scintigraphy
Xenon-enhanced computed tomography
Four-vessel angiography

death signified by cessation of breathing and heartbeat, the cannulas are flushed with University of Wisconsin solution, an incision is made, the thoracic aorta is clamped and organs are removed en bloc. The usual operating time is 15 min. An exact definition of the lack of heartbeat is left to the discretion of the anesthesiologist. It is possible that agonal respiratory efforts or heartbeat may continue for several hours, disqualifying the patient from organ donation. More recently, attempts by another academic program to institute such a protocol have been met with objections by the public media concerning the administration of a drug that may be construed as hastening the onset of death by causing hypotension, namely phentolamine. At the present time it is unclear what the outcome of this controversy will be.

Conclusion

Traditionally, the vast amount of attention given to organ donation recipients has not been granted to care of the organ donor. With the current shortage of organs and the increasing numbers of patients who die while awaiting a suitable organ transplant, vigorous attempts to increase the size of the donor pool are warranted. These include basic strategies such as public education to increase awareness of transplantation and hopefully to address specific concerns in local communities. More controversial and exotic tactics, such as xenograft use, are unlikely to enter common practice in the near future, although utilization of the non-heart-beating donor may be of significant benefit if the ethical and legal concerns can be overcome. However, the basics of critical care, especially hemodynamic manipulation and respiratory care, remain the bedrock of ensuring that organs procured from any donor are in optimum condition for function in the recipient.

Further reading

American Medical Association. 1968: A definition of irreversible coma: ad hoc committee of the Harvard Medical School to examine the definition of brain death. *Journal of the American Medical Association* **205**, 337–40.

American Medical Association. 1981: Guidelines for the determination of death: report of the medical consultants on the diagnosis of death to the President's Commission for the Study of Ethical Problems in Medicine and Biomedical and Behavioral Research. *Journal of the American Medical Association* **246**, 2184–6.

Bittner H, Kendall S, Chen E and **Van Trigt P**. 1996: The combined effects of brain death and cardiac graft preservation on cardiopulmonary hemodynamics and function before and after subsequent heart transplantation. *Journal of Heart and Lung Transplantation* 15, 764–77.

Cooper DKC, Novitsky D and **Wicomb WN**. 1989: The pathophysiological effects of brain death on potential donor organs, with particular reference to the heart. *Annals of the Royal College of Surgeons of England* **71**, 261–6.

D'Alessandro A, Hoffman R, Knechtle S *et al.* 1995: Successful extrarenal transplantation from non-heart-beating donors. *Transplantation* **59**, 977–82.

Darby J, Stein K, Grenvik A and **Stuart S**. 1989: Approach to management of the heartbeating 'brain dead' organ donor. *Journal of the American Medical Association* **261**, 2222–8.

Goarin J, Cohen S, Riou B *et al.* 1996: The effects of triiodothyronine on hemodynamic status and cardiac function in potential heart donors. *Anesthesia and Analgesia* **83**, 41–7.

Howlett TA, Keogh AM, Perry L, Tovzel R and **Rees LH**. 1989: Anterior and posterior pituitary function in brainstem-dead donors. *Transplantation* **47**, 828–34.

Muto P, Freeman R, Haug C, Lu A and **Rohrer R**. 1994: Liver transplant candidate stratification systems: implications for third-party payers and organ allocation. *Transplantation* **57**, 306–8.

Novitzky D, Cooper D and **Reichart B**. 1987: Hemodynamic and metabolic responses to hormonal therapy in brain-dead potential organ donors. *Transplantation* **43**, 852–4.

Novitsky D, Cooper DKC, Muchmore JS and **Zuhdi N**. 1989: Pituitary function in brain-dead patients. *Transplantation* **48**, 1078.

Wheeldon D, Potter C, Oduro A, Wallwork J and **Large S**. 1995: Transforming the 'unacceptable' donor: outcomes from the adoption of a standardized donor management technique. *Journal of Heart and Lung Transplantation* **14**, 734–42.

Yoshioka T, Sugimoto H, Uenishi M *et al.* 1986: Prolonged haemodynamic maintenance by the combined administration of vasopressin and epinephrine in brain death: a clinical study. *Neurosurgery* **18**, 565–7.

10 The future of transplantation

Eric A. Elster, E. Darrin Cox and Allan D. Kirk

Introduction

Transplantation has rapidly gained acceptance as the treatment of choice for most non-malignant end-stage organ diseases. In the past 50 years, this field has evolved from an experimental curiosity to the preferred option for most patients with kidney, liver, lung, islet and heart failure. However, unlike many established therapies, transplantation remains a rapidly changing discipline. Progress is being driven in large part by the continued shortcomings of the field, namely chronic allograft rejection, long-term side effects of the immunosuppressive agents used to prevent rejection, and a limited donor supply.

The current experimental literature is ripe with novel approaches to circumvent transplantation's woes, and as such there is an enormous unrealized potential for improvement. Paradigm shifts in our understanding of the etiology of rejection are occurring and giving rise to novel treatments to stave off immune-mediated rejection. Lasting graft acceptance without the need for chronic immunosuppressive therapy appears to be nearing clinical reality. New methods of transplantation, such as split-liver transplants or islet-cell transplantation, and new sources of transplantable organs, such as living donors and xenotransplants, are being developed that may potentially alleviate the profound shortage of suitable organs. This chapter will outline several advances in transplantation that are likely to have a clinical impact within the next 10 to 15 years.

New approaches to preventing allograft rejection

Allografts are invariably rejected unless the recipient's immune system is significantly modified. At present, this modification occurs in the form of chronic immunosuppression. Although modern immunosuppressive regimens are very effective in preventing acute T-cell-mediated rejection, they remain suboptimal for two primary reasons. First, immunosuppressive medications have no lasting effect – patients must take them for life. The result is an expensive therapy with progressive, chronic toxicity. Prolonged drug exposure over a period of years leads to opportunistic infections, osteoporosis, hypertension and an increased cancer risk, among other things. Second, no immunosuppressive drug or drug regimen completely prevents a detrimental immune response towards a graft at doses that are chronically tolerable. Thus, with time, most grafts undergo a gradual immune-mediated injury that is termed chronic rejection. Chronic rejection is also compounded by the direct renal toxicity of some clinically used immunosuppressants. Thus transplant patients currently trade an acute illness for a more tolerable chronic condition.

Goals for improvements in immune modification following transplantation have been shaped by the above problems. Investigators are now actively looking for a method of short-term immune manipulation that induces a long-term change in the way in which the immune system views a foreign organ. This goal, known as allograft tolerance, has been clinically elusive but has been realized experimentally with increasing success. If tolerance could be achieved, the benefits would be obvious – no chronic drug toxicity, no chronic medication expense or compliance problems, fewer organs lost to chronic rejection and, as a result, less burden on already strained organ supplies and financially strapped health systems.

What is tolerance?

Much confusion exists in the current literature with regard to what is meant by the seemingly simple word 'tolerance'. Tolerance is the durable persistence of a tissue in the absence of a *detrimental* immune response, without ongoing therapeutic intervention. This does not mean that there is no immune response towards the graft, only that the response is one that does not lead to an immune-mediated attack. This definition does not involve the origin of the tissue – there is no distinction between self and non-self. The same mechanisms that the body employs to establish and maintain tolerance to self are also required to establish and maintain tolerance to transplanted tissues. Because tolerance is a dynamic process involving active immune mechanisms, it can in some instances be reversed. Thus experimental data frequently use the word 'tolerance' to describe a transient rejection-free state. For clarity, others have proposed the term 'rejection-free survival' as an alternative way to describe experimental and clinical results.

The bedrock principle for the past 50 years has been that the immune system mediates allograft rejection. Therefore immunosuppression must be the key to graft acceptance. The theory that the immune system's primary function is to distinguish self from non-self gained wide acceptance as a result of the classic experiments by Medawar. Furthermore, it was proposed that the process of self-tolerance was a unique function of the neonatal immune system, and that the adult was not able to alter their immune specificity in any reliable way. It is clear that individuals acquire the ability to determine self from non-self at an early developmental stage. However, the main point to be derived from this fact is that tolerance is a learned phenomenon, not an innate characteristic of the individual. It is now becoming increasingly clear that this ability to distinguish self from non-self is fine-tuned throughout life as one continually encounters new antigens and as physiologic states change (e.g. during puberty and pregnancy). Thus the individual is continually encountering antigens, both new and old, and determining its response to those antigens. Transplantation is just another event during which a new antigen is encountered. As the immune system plays a key role in determining the response to these new antigens, it may be possible to redirect it rather than simply suppress it. It is also clear that the context in which an antigen is encountered is every bit as important as the foreignness of the antigen. A foreign antigen encountered without any evidence of disease or cell damage is likely to be regarded as a benign part of self. Unfortunately, transplants are performed by largely traumatic methods, and are associated with many disease-related processes, including ischemia, reperfusion injury, cell death and vascular injury. Thus, when thinking about the immune processes that govern the difference between rejection and tolerance, it is necessary to consider the context of the antigen as well as its source.

Recently, it has become apparent that tolerance to one's own tissues is not absolute and is closely regulated. Research is focusing on using the body's natural ability to acquire and maintain tolerance to transplanted tissues, rather than relying on chronic immunosuppression for graft survival. Since tolerance requires active immune function, there is in fact growing evidence that immunosuppression may actually prevent tolerance as well as rejection. In other words, *appropriate* immune system function rather than a *lack* of function is the key to rejection-free graft survival.

Consideration of the transient nature of immunity further supports this conceptual framework. A persistent immune response would quickly become burdensome and detrimental to the individual. Natural active mechanisms down-regulate the immune response at appropriate times in the response cycle. Accordingly, mechanisms exist to turn off the immune system and return it to an inactive state. Thus even when rejection has been initiated, it is likely that it can be reversed by exploitation of an existing physiological ability to down-regulate counter-adaptive immune activity. This understanding necessitates a major shift in clinical focus away from current pharmacotherapeutics of transplant surgery.

The signals that govern tolerance

It was once thought that lymphocytes were activated whenever they bound to their intended antigen. However, it has become clear that although this event is necessary, it is not sufficient for lymphocyte activation. Additional signals are required to reinforce the appropriateness of a response and to direct the response towards activation or specific inactivation. Work by multiple investigators has further refined a two-signal model of immune responses that has now been validated. The antigen signal, known as signal 1, must be directed by a second signal, known as signal 2, that denotes the context of the antigen recognition. Signal 1 is delivered by the antigen receptors, antibodies and T-cell receptors (TCR), and is responsible for the specificity of the response. Currently, most pharmacotherapeutics, including OKT3, ATG, cyclosporine, tacrolimus and to some extent steroids, block this signal, either by preventing TCR signal transduction or by preventing TCR expression. Signal 1 blockade does not induce tolerance, and subsequent withdrawal of the blockade results in graft rejection. Tolerance is a *specific* immune response and, as such, the signal of specificity (signal 1) must be intact.

Signal 2 determines the appropriateness and direction, be it activation or inactivation, of the response by determining the context in which the foreign antigen is encountered. Tissue injury and infection represent appropriate contexts in which to mount a protective immune response. Antigen-presenting cells (APC) receive and translate a variety of signals that connote illness or injury, including cell death, stress molecule expression and complement deposition, into co-stimulatory signals that are delivered to lymphocytes along with signal 1.

Although previous conventional strategies concentrated on manipulating signal 1, it is becoming apparent that signal 2 is more important. APCs recognize injury or infection and convey this information to immune effector and regulatory cells in the regional lymphoid tissue. These cells then become primed for a finite, antigen-specific, co-ordinated immune attack. Alternatively, native parenchymal cells – that is, non-immune cells – tend to present antigen without signal 2. The response would be development of autoimmunity, resulting in an antigen-specific, co-ordinated immune down-regulation. Finally, certain molecules provide negative signal 2s that are delivered by APCs when an antigen has been eliminated and an immune response is no longer needed. Thus an encounter with antigen on an APC can either induce or suppress activation, and an encounter with antigen on a parenchymal cell in its native state generally leads to a down-regulatory or immuno-suppressive response.

Two co-stimulatory molecules that are found on T-cells are CD28 and CD152 (CTLA4). Co-ligation of CD28 with the TCR leads to T-cell activation. CD152 binding induces anergy (a state of inactivation) or apoptosis (programmed cell death). The ligands for both CD28 and CD152 are CD80 (B7-1) and CD86 (B7-2). These ligands are not found on resting parenchymal cells, but are expressed on APCs and activated endothelium. Another ligand receptor, CD154 (CD40L), which is found on T-cells and activated platelets, binds CD40, which is found on APCs and epithelium, and provides further contextual information for the interaction.

Co-stimulatory molecules are important in many aspects of specific immune responses. In the presence of trauma (e.g. an organ transplant), platelets become activated after exposure to the subendothelium. CD154 on activated platelets binds to CD40 on endothelial cells and APCs and leads to an up-regulation of molecules required for efficient antigen presentation. These include major histocompatibility complex (MHC) class I and II to deliver signal 1, and CD80 and CD86 to deliver signal 2. Chemotactic factors are secreted, as are cytokines, sometimes referred to as signal 3. The APC then migrates to the secondary lymphoid tissue where it interacts with T-cells. MHC binds to the TCR and CD80/86 binds to CD28. The net result is the activated immune response that drives rejection.

Interruption of this series of binding events can dramatically alter the resulting response. CD40 appears to be the starting point for a co-ordinated defensive immune response. Thus blocking the interaction of CD40 with CD154 prevents the APCs from communicating the context of injury. Blocking CD80 and CD86 conveys the antigen signal, but in a way that looks like a parenchymal cell rather than an APC, a context in which the immune system should not respond. Thus when co-stimulation occurs, the system interprets the antigen as a pathogen, but when co-stimulation is blocked, it interprets it as self.

A final issue concerning the balance between immunity and tolerance is that of multiplicity. Immune responses possess tremendous potential to induce collateral damage and autoimmunity. Therefore there must be confirmation of a significant antigen presence prior to initiation of the immune response. Many T-cells acting in concert must recognize an antigen prior to a response being deemed appropriate. The APC serves as a place where many T-cells can recognize an antigen and reinforce each other's response through intracellular interaction. If only a few cells with a given specificity are present, the default response is to prevent reactivity. This is another means by which autoreactive T-cells that occur infrequently as a result of thymic selection rarely induce autoreactive immune responses. As will be discussed below, one method of inducing tolerance involves T-cell depletion with gradual reconstitution, so that at no time is a 'quorum' of antigen-specific T-cells available for response.

Methods for inducing tolerance

Co-stimulation blockade

As discussed above, current immunosuppressive regimens block signal 1. With growing awareness that T-cells are important regulators of tolerance, there has been increasing interest in allowing normal TCR function but blockade of signal 2, or co-stimulation, to foster rejection-free survival and persistent T-cell tolerance to the grafted organ. TCRs still become engaged by binding to cells on the allograft, but by concurrently blocking CD28 or CD40 pathways these cells become anergic or undergo apoptosis. Other non-allospecific T-cells are unaffected and pre-existing immunity is unaffected. Theoretically, a chronic state of immunosuppression would not be necessary, and there would not be an increased risk of opportunistic infection or cancer. A number of recent reports verify this approach. Larsen showed that blocking both CD28 and CD40 pathways in mice aborts T-cell clonal expansion *in vitro* and *in vivo*, promoting long-term survival of allogeneic skin grafts and inhibiting chronic rejection in cardiac allografts. Anti-CD154 given to rhesus monkeys as monotherapy at the time of transplantation has resulted in long-term rejection-free survival, and clinical trials in humans are anticipated with this approach. Additional preclinical investigation is proceeding using agents that interrupt CD40, CD80 and CD86. It is likely that a combination of several of these agents will be required to induce tolerance reproducibly without immunosuppression.

Transient T-cell depletion

Recently, several investigators have shown that tolerance can be achieved in non-human primates by complete ablation, both in the periphery and in the central lymphoid tissues, of all mature T-cells at the time of or just prior to transplantation. When the T-cell population is reconstituted over the next few months, cells that are reactive to the graft are not found in the circulation. This approach has induced a durable state in which subsequent donor-specific grafts are not rejected but third-party grafts are maintained. The effect lends itself to explanation by the multiplicity theories discussed above, and has been shown to be independent of the thymus.

This 'depletion' approach has recently been transferred to the clinical setting by Calne and colleagues with the antibody Campath-1H, a humanized anti-CD52 antibody. Campath-1H is a powerful lytic agent for both T- and B-lymphocytes that leaves bone-marrow stem cells unaffected. A total of 31 patients have been transplanted using this agent in concert with half-dose cyclosporine as the sole maintenance therapy, with very acceptable results. This area is still the subject of intense clinical investigation.

Gene therapy

Gene transfer techniques have improved in efficiency and efficacy during the past decade, and *in-vivo* gene transfer techniques are now utilized clinically in other fields of medicine. As these techniques have improved, their applicability to laboratory transplantation has become feasible, and they appear clinically promising. Gene therapy strategies currently under study in transplantation focus on the cytokines that regulate the immune response or the major histocompatibility complex genes that mediate rejection.

Gene transfer protocols can be broadly classified as indirect and direct mechanisms. Indirect methods involve the transfer of genetic information into a target cell *in vitro*, and then subsequent transfer into a recipient. Indirect methods include retroviral-mediated transduction, liposome-mediated cell fusion, and stable transfection. Direct methods do not require the intermediate *in-vitro* step, and thus involve the transfer of genetic information directly into target tissues or organs. Direct methods include direct injection of DNA into target organs, intravenous injection of DNA–liposome mixtures into recipients, and infection by adenovirus constructs carrying specific genes. Specific examples are discussed below.

As was mentioned previously, the immune response that develops in response to a graft is influenced by regulatory cytokines. Cytokines are potent immunoregulatory molecules that work locally. Systemic cytokine release is poorly tolerated and results in a syndrome of septic-type shock commonly known as the systemic inflammatory response syndrome (SIRS). Thus systemic administration of regulatory cytokines is not a viable means of influencing an immune response. However, local delivery of these agents should be well tolerated, and would potentially be effective in altering the direction of an immune response at the time of antigen encounter. Gene therapy is well suited to achieving local cytokine delivery. Examples of experimental immune-modulating transcripts delivered to allografts include transforming growth factor-β (TGF-β) and IL-10. This approach can also be used to alter the nature of the antigen, MHC class I. Each has been shown to delay the onset of allograft rejection, but lasting rejection-free survival has not been achieved.

Qin and colleagues transferred the gene for TGF-β into cardiac muscle using a mouse ear–heart model, and transferred the gene using a plasmid directly injected into cardiac grafts during the transplant procedure. Gene expression persisted for 2 weeks and, more importantly, the allograft survival rate was doubled. They then directly transferred viral IL-10 into the same model. IL-10 is another down-regulatory immunomodulator. Viral IL-10 is structurally homologous to human IL-10, but does not induce T-cell co-stimulation. Allograft survival increased almost threefold in treated mice.

These studies and others have shown that it is possible to produce persistent, biologically controlled long-term expression of gene products from genes transferred *in vivo*. In fact, the immune system may play a key role in the regulation of gene expression. Local immunomodulation, confined to the transplanted tissue or organ, is thus possible. It remains to be seen whether this fairly cumbersome process can be adapted to a clinically applicable approach.

Immunologic unresponsiveness has also been demonstrated using recipient cells transfected with donor MHC class I or II genes. This work was first performed in the rat cardiac allograft model. Liver allograft survival was prolonged in a similar model after direct intrathymic DNA injection and subsequent expression of allo-MHC I antigen in the thymus. It has long been established that tolerance to self-MHC antigens develops via the presence of this antigen on thymic epithelium. It is hypothesized that the introduction of donor-type MHC antigen directly into the thymus just prior to or at the time of transplant may obviate the need for cellular intermediates.

Currently, gene therapy as applied to organ transplantation is limited by many factors, including low-level or transient gene expression, by available methods of gene transfer, undesirable immune responses to vectors employed in gene transfer, limited understanding of the complexities of the major histocompatibility complex and its role, and incomplete understanding of the optimum cytokine milieu. As gene transfer technology improves and our understanding of these complex issues increases, gene therapy may allow the safe and effective manipulation of the immune response.

Chimerism and central tolerance

As discussed previously, the thymus is the central organ for T-cell development, and is a critical site for the deletion of autoreactive T-cells. For this reason, the ability to induce tolerance in the thymus is known as *central* tolerance. This is in contrast to *peripheral* tolerance, which may be induced by mature T-cells that encounter antigen in the peripheral tissues in the absence of co-stimulation. Peripheral tolerance has been discussed above, and includes co-stimulation blockade and the multiplicity-based approaches.

Many investigators have clearly shown that prolonged states of rejection-free survival can be induced and maintained indefinitely by central methods. In general, these methods involve the transfer of hematopoietic cells from the donor under conditions that allow for the development of hematopoietic chimerism, such as chemical or radiation-induced immunodeficiency. It is hypothesized that physical space must be created in the hematopoietic compartment to allow donor stem cells to engraft. Whole body irradiation or high doses of syngeneic marrow in concert with lymphocyte depletion are thus required.

Donor antigen is clearly required for any specific immune event to occur, be it rejection or tolerance. It has become increasingly clear that the character of that antigen and the means by which it is administered are important factors in determining the response of the immune system. Several investigators have had success in achieving tolerance by supplementing the transplanted organ antigen with additional antigen in the form of bone marrow.

Using a variety of conditioning regimens, donor bone marrow is transplanted and engrafts throughout the body. This situation is known as mixed chimerism, since donor and recipient hematopoietic elements coexist. The mechanism by which this promotes graft acceptance remains unclear. Thymic re-education in the face of new 'self' antigen has been proposed. Other investigators have improved their experimental success by directly injecting donor antigen into the recipient thymus. There is also evidence that the marrow cells establish a self-regulating network that maintains a state of unresponsiveness to the graft.

Given the success of preclinical tolerance induction regimens using mixed chimerism, several human trials have been approved and are now in progress. It is likely that this strategy will form part of the anti-rejection armamentarium in the near future. The primary drawback of this approach is still the requirement for recipient preconditioning (preventing broad applicability in cadaveric situations) and the need for ionizing radiation, although recent studies have shown that these requirements may be unnecessary if donor cells are introduced under the cover of co-stimulation blockade. Thus a combined approach that uses both peripheral and central tolerance induction strategies may be the ultimate solution.

New approaches to eliminating the shortage of donor organs

The critical shortage of organs has led to a search for other sources of functional grafts. Certainly improved anti-rejection strategies such as those listed above will help by reducing the number of individuals who return to the waiting-list. However, even with perfect graft survival, there are not enough organs available annually to serve the current waiting population. This lack of usable organs is highlighted by a 1992 study from Seattle, which identified a maximum of only 7000 brain-dead donors in the USA. Even assuming 100% utilization, these donors would only provide 14 000 kidneys, a figure that falls far short of the total number of patients in need of renal transplantation. In addition, the list of those waiting for organs greatly underestimates the number of individuals who would benefit from transplantation. Several strategies are being developed to address this problem, ranging from optimization of existing systems to the creation of other alternatives, including allotransplantation.

Optimal utilization of the current allogeneic donor pool

Living donation

Living kidney donation has the potential to eliminate the waiting-list for kidney recipients completely. It has the best results for renal transplantation independent of MHC matching. This is undoubtedly due to the excellent condition of both the donor and the recipient for these elective procedures. The extremely short periods of ischemia and the controlled conditions surrounding a living donation minimize the extent of lymphocyte activation, especially co-stimulation and adhesion.

The overriding principle in all living donor procedures is the safety of the donor. This must take precedence over any concerns for the recipient. It is well documented that renal donation in appropriately screened donors is safe. Although the procedure was originally limited to genetically related individuals, its safety has allowed a liberal expansion of the donor pool to include unrelated friends and even random altruistic individuals. A significant increase in living donation has also been spurred on by the development of laparoscopically assisted donor nephrectomy, and this trend is expected to continue as that procedure becomes standard at more transplant centers.

This idea is now being expanded to liver transplantation, and it is likely that improvements in islet-cell transplantation will see a resurgence in living pancreas donation as well. Living donor liver transplantation was initially developed for children, and required a left lateral hepatectomy in the donor. The procedure has now been performed for adults in selected centers. Both extended left and formal right hepatectomies have been performed. These procedures are significantly more complex and dangerous for the donor, and deaths have occurred. Consequently, this alternative is limited to highly skilled and experienced liver transplant centers.

Living donor pancreas transplantation has been generally unsuccessful, largely due to the complications associated with the exocrine drainage of a distal pancreatectomy graft. There is clearly adequate islet mass in a pancreas to support insulin independence for two individuals. With the recent improvements that have been achieved in islet-cell procurement and transplantation, this approach will certainly be re-evaluated in the near future. It is likely that islets procured from a distal pancreatectomy specimen and used for living islet donation may prove the most successful.

Split liver transplantation

The technique for transplantation of an adult left lateral segment into a child was initially developed to address the size mismatch problems caused by the relative lack of pediatric donor livers and attempts to use adult liver grafts in children. An expansion of this technique was used to begin transplanting living donor grafts from adults to children. First reported in 1984, this technique focuses on using segments two and three (left lateral segment) and/or segment four to provide size-matched organs for children. This early experience in children has given rise to the technique of split liver transplantation (SLT), in which a cadaveric organ is divided into two parts, which effectively doubles the transplantation population and provides size-matched organs for pediatric patients.

Worldwide experience over the past 10 years has shown an increased patient survival rate and graft survival rate due to improved patient selection and refinement of the technical details of the procedure. Currently, there are two methods for SLT – the *ex-vivo* and *in-situ* techniques, each of which is appropriate in certain settings.

In the *ex-vivo* approach, the organ is procured in the standard manner and the liver is preserved with standard solutions. The graft is then divided into two parts on a back table (*ex vivo*) based on segmental anatomy. The common bile duct is retained with the right graft, which can either contain the main portal vein and celiac trunk, or else extension grafts can be used on the right hepatic artery and right portal veins. These extension grafts, made of allogenic iliac, splenic or superior mesenteric arteries or iliac vein, allow tension-free anastomoses. The left hepatic vein orifice is oversewn and the graft is implanted in the recipient using standard techniques and a choledocholedocostomy with a T-tube for biliary drainage.

The left graft, which is smaller, is used for either a child or a small adult. The left hepatic artery is preferably procured with the left graft, as well as the left portal vein and the left bile duct. Alternatively, the left graft can retain the celiac trunk and the main portal vein. In order to transplant these left grafts, surgical techniques such as venoplasty must be employed to complete the suprahepatic venous anastomosis. Biliary drainage is constructed with a Roux-en-Y left hepaticojejunostomy. The absence of a portal vein bifurcation is a contraindication to the use of a procured liver with a split technique.

The disadvantages of this procedure have limited its usefulness to elective cases where organ procurement can be well orchestrated. The extra time it takes to split a liver *ex vivo* can cause prolonged ischemic injury, which exacerbates reperfusion injury and increases the incidence of rejection. In order to combat such problems, several groups have taken the next logical step in liver splitting by using the *in-situ* technique, which limits the period of cold ischemia. This procedure, which adds 1 to 2 h to organ procurement, begins with control of the supraceliac and infrarenal aorta, as well as control of the inferior mesenteric vein, in order to permit cooling in case of donor instability. As with a standard procurement, liver segments two and three are mobilized with the left hepatic artery. The left hepatic artery is then dissected, its branches to segments one (caudate lobe) and four are divided, and the left hepatic vein is carefully isolated. The liver parenchyma is split with the middle hepatic vein retained on the right graft. The grafts are then taken, leaving the celiac trunk, main portal vein and common bile duct with the right graft. Finally, the grafts are transplanted as with the *ex-vivo* technique.

Early results obtained with the *in-situ* technique have been encouraging, with similar patient survival rates and decreased incidence of biliary complications compared to the *ex-vivo* technique. The primary drawback of this method is the additional time spent in the operating-room preparing and procuring the graft, which may delay the procurement of other vital organs. However, the widespread implementation of these techniques (*in situ* being preferable) would effectively double the number of livers available for transplantation. Co-operation between liver transplant centers with regard to sharing of split organs would also improve the utilization of this technique.

Creation of a new donor pool: xenotransplantation

Many researchers have looked towards xenotransplantation – organ transplantation from one species to another – as a solution to the problem of shortage of organs. Many obstacles have blocked the implementation of such a strategy, including immune, non-immune and ethical concerns. This is highlighted by the fact that since the first attempts at xenotransplantation in 1963, all attempts to cross the species barrier have failed, including more than 25 attempts from non-human primates and occasional attempts to use even more distant species. Despite these hurdles, many advances have been made both in our understanding of the immune processes that prevent successful xenotransplantation and in the implementation of this knowledge in providing a renewable and sustained source of donor organs and tissue.

The advantages of xenotransplantation, other than the

inexhaustible supply of organs, include the opportunity for genetic manipulation of the donor organ to increase disease resistance and minimize the need for recipient immunosuppression. In addition, these organs would permit elective operations without the delay and expense of organ procurement as well as risk for donors. The inevitable decline in recipient health that accompanies a prolonged waiting period for available organs would also be avoided. These benefits need to be balanced against disadvantages such as the risk of zoonosis (the transfer of diseases from animals to humans) and physiological incompatibility with the host.

When considering xenotransplantation, it is not known which species might meet the criteria for immune and physiological acceptance. Xenografts have been divided into two groups based on the immune relationship of the donor species to humans. Concordant grafts are derived from closely related species such as the Old World monkeys and apes. Discordant grafts are derived from distantly related species, including New World monkeys and non-primates such as pigs.

The controversy between concordant and discordant grafts has focused primarily on the use of non-human primates and pigs. Concordant non-human primates offer fewer immune and physiological barriers to transplantation. They are immunologically closely related to human beings and therefore require less immunomodulation, and their physiological function is quite similar to that of humans. However, there are several disadvantages associated with these animals which make their use unlikely to be successful. Certain primates, such as chimpanzees, are endangered and breed slowly. Even if they could be used, their numbers would be exhausted within less than a year. Furthermore, as primates are highly intelligent and social animals, ethical concerns about their use are a key and appropriate obstacle.

Pigs, on the other hand, are easy to breed, exist in abundant supply and as a staple in the diet of many cultures, and are likely to raise fewer ethical objections to xenotransplantation. However, many immunologic and non-immunologic disadvantages associated with the use of pigs need to be overcome in order to make xenotransplantation a clinical reality. Immunologic barriers to discordant transplantation can be divided into three groups, namely hyperacute rejection, acute vascular rejection (also called delayed xenograft rejection) and cell-mediated xenograft rejection.

Hyperacute rejection

Hyperacute rejection (HAR) is the immunological divider between concordant and discordant species. It develops rapidly, even within minutes of reperfusion, and is not reversible. Histologically, interstitial hemorrhage, platelet thrombi, neutrophil infiltration and fibrin deposition are seen. This reaction is limited to both discordant grafts and non-ABO-mismatched concordant grafts. Immunocompetent hosts that possess natural xenoreactive anti-bodies initiate HAR by binding to xenoantigen on the endothelium of the graft. These antibodies are primarily directed against one carbohydrate antigen, the saccharide Galα1–3Gal, which is produced by the enzyme galactosyl transferase. Concordant species lack this enzyme and therefore do not express the antigen. Consequently they are protected from HAR with standard ABO typing.

Upon binding of these xenoreactive natural antibodies (XNA) to Galα1–3Gal on graft endothelium, complement is activated and the process of HAR begins. Initially IgM XNA activates the classi-cal complement pathway, with later production of IgG. These IgM antibodies are expressed by all concordant species and probably develop in response to bacterial exposure. Injury caused by reper-fusion contributes to further complement activation, exacerbating the response. In discordant species, complement regulatory mole-cules such as decay-accelerating factor (DAF), membrane cofactor protein (MCP) and CD59 do not function effectively against human complement. Since porcine DAF and MCP (which inhibit C3 convertase) and CD59 (which inhibits the membrane attack complex) are ineffective in regulating the human complement cascade, xenografts are subjected to unregulated complement-mediated injury.

Strategies to overcome HAR have centered on down-regulating the expression of Galα1–3Gal and increasing the expression of complement regulatory proteins in porcine xenografts. One of the first groups to address this problem attempted transfection of African green monkey fibroblasts with Gal cDNA to express Galα1–3Gal. These cells were then transfected with human α-galactosidase, which cleaves α-linked galactosyl residues and exposes subterminal saccharides. Antibodies to these saccharides also develop, but to a lesser extent then Galα1–3Gal. In order to circumvent HAR fully, these cells were also transfected with α(1,2)fucosyl transferase, which substitutes Galα1–3Gal with H substance (O blood-group antigen). This strategy eliminated HAR in this model.

A similar approach has been used by others in a porcine model to increase the expression of H-transferase and therefore amelio-rate complement-mediated lysis. The other arm of HAR inhibition concerns the development of animals that are transgenic for expression of the complement regulatory proteins DAF, MCP and

CD59. Recent studies have shown that combining these two approaches prevents HAR in primates. Thus the approach that would seem mostly likely to prevent HAR would involve the creation of transgenic animals that had been specifically bred to be resistant to this immediate immune attack.

Acute vascular rejection

Another obstacle to successful transplantation using xenografts is acute vascular rejection. This process develops several days after transplantation and is mediated by a number of factors, including induced xenoreactive IgG, complement, neutrophils, platelets and macrophages. The binding of xenoreactive antibodies to the graft appears to serve as a trigger for activation of the other pathways. This theory is further supported by the fact that antidonor antibodies are present in the host's circulation. Depletion of these antibodies either prevents or delays acute vascular rejection, and treatment with antidonor antibodies leads to acute vascular rejection. Recent work suggests that antibodies directed against Galα1–3Gal play a significant role. In order to overcome this response, a reduction in the expression of Galα1–3Gal to a level lower than that needed for HAR is thought to be required.

Cell-mediated rejection

Even if the graft survives the immediate threats to its survival, the recipient's cellular immune system will still respond to the xenograft. Previous experience with xenotransplantation has indicated that cell-mediated rejection is even more vigorous than that noted in allografts, and involves a broader array of cell types, including macrophages, natural killer (NK) cells and T-cells. One explanation for this response may lie in the link between the innate immune system, composed of the complement system among others, and cellular immunity. It is now clear that elements of innate immune responses are potent inducers of acquired immunity. Vigorous platelet and complement activation creates a milieu that is likely to be interpreted by both donor and host antigen-presenting cells as worthy of response, and as such is likely to lead to co-stimulation. T-cells are thus directly activated by graft APCs and indirectly activated via recipient MHC-restricted APCs. After co-stimulation, activated T-cells then up-regulate cellular effectors, leading to graft failure. One arm of this response, namely natural killer (NK) cells, has been shown to express cell-surface receptors for Galα1–3Gal, leading to activation against grafts. Moreover, NK cells are generally down-regulated by killer-inhibitor receptors that recognize homologous MHC class I. Xenografts, being devoid of human class I, may thus not regulate NK responsiveness appropriately. Methods for thwarting cell-mediated rejection include conventional immunosuppression, co-stimulation blockade and transgenic techniques to minimize innate immune responsiveness and NK activation.

Non-immune factors

Physiological discrepancies and the possibility of zoonosis are still the two main non-immune barriers to xenotransplantation. It is unlikely that organs from discordant species would adequately replace the function of complex organs such as the liver. Many key enzymes and hormones produced by these organs are species-specific, and therefore do not function appropriately in humans. In addition, discordant proteins are immunogenic to humans. Whether this problem can be overcome by exogenous protein supplementation or genetic engineering of the graft to produce compatible products remains to be seen. The ability to transfect these organs with such genes does raise the possibility that this technology can be used as an adjunct to deliver substances to treat the primary pathology in certain conditions.

The risk of zoonosis – that is, transfer of infectious disease to the host or the population at large – remains an area of intense study. With regard to the porcine model, many microbial agents have been detected and eliminated. However, there is still the risk of activation of endogenous porcine retroviruses that have yet to be characterized. The foreseeable future for xenotransplantation lies with development of additional animal models followed by extra-corporeal organ use. Only when these methods are efficacious can attempts be made to use xenotransplantation as a bridge to allo-transplantation or, alternatively, primary xenotransplantation.

New types of transplants: cellular grafts

Embryonic stem cells

The next step in transplantation technology will involve progressing from whole organ grafts to free tissue grafts. One possibility is the transfer of cells that are capable of differentiation into various cell lines. Embryonic stem (ES) cells and their functional equivalent, embryonic germ (EG) cells, may provide such a vehicle for free tissue transfer. ES cells are derived from blastocysts and have maintained their pluripotency despite having the ability to divide and self-renew. EG cells have the same characteristic, but are derived from fetuses. These cells can be maintained in culture in an undifferentiated state indefinitely, or until they are injected into host tissue. Once they are inside a host, these pluripotent cells can form embryoid bodies (EBs) which contain all the elements of the germ line – mesoderm, endoderm and ectoderm. From these germ-line precursors all cell types, including endothelial, hematopoietic, muscle and neuronal cells, can be expressed as tumors.

Before this ability to differentiate into embryoid bodies can be used to replace diseased or damaged tissue, several obstacles must be overcome. At present these pluripotent stem cells can be differentiated into EBs containing two cell lines, such as heart tissue and blood islets. Although culture conditions can favor one cell type over another, no one has been able to produce EBs that are specific for one cell type. The hope is that with genetic manipulation, specific EBs will be developed that can be used to treat a variety of diseases, ranging from Parkinson's disease and multiple sclerosis to type 1 diabetes mellitus. Neuronal transplants may be the first to become a clinical reality because of the central nervous system's 'immunologically privileged' status. Transplants placed in other sites must overcome rejection, although standard immunosuppression or newer paradigms such as co-stimulation blockade may control such responses. Alternatively, these cells may be genetically engineered to avoid immune detection. Finally, the ethical problem of using human fetal tissue as a source of ES and EG cells remains an area of public concern.

Islet-cell transplantation

The primary defect in type 1 diabetes mellitus is an insufficient number of insulin-producing β-cells in the pancreatic islets. The resulting hyperglycemia causes end-organ damage through a number of pathways, resulting in the clinical signs of diabetes. The ultimate goal of islet-cell transplantation is to establish an insulin-independent, normoglycemic state in the recipient. However, even improved metabolic control with decreased insulin requirements is a worthy goal if this can be achieved safely.

Currently, islet-cell transplantation is still limited by the same obstacles that face solid organ transplants – that is, donor supply and rejection. These problems are more acute in islet transplantation, as it is now clear that islets outside their natural organ architecture are significantly more susceptible to rejection and to toxicity from immunosuppressive drugs. In addition, the procurement methods for islet transplantation have remained problematic in that the yield of islets from a single pancreas often falls far below the number that is needed to achieve insulin independence.

Islet-cell isolation and purification

Islet cells represent only 1–2% of the mass of the entire pancreas, but must be reliably isolated and purified in order to achieve successful transplantation. Collagenase, an enzyme derived from *Clostridium histolytica*, is used to disrupt pancreatic tissue and liberate cellular fractions. The enzyme is administered via the pancreatic ductal system in order to distend the entire organ and ensure thorough distribution. Once they have been enzymatically liberated, the islet cells must be isolated and purified. The whole pancreas is placed in an automated digestion chamber and the released fractions are passed through cold media in order to suspend collagenase activity and prevent the digestion of islet cells. Purification is achieved with a computerized cell separator. Current methods allow the retrieval of increasingly large quantities of islet cells in small volumes. Pancreatic preservation times of less than 8 h have been shown to yield increased graft survival rates, highlighting the need for efficiency.

Islet-cell delivery

In contrast to whole organ transplantation, free tissue transfer allows non-surgical methods of graft placement, decreasing the cost and morbidity, and even the mortality, associated with invasive procedures. The preferred site for islet-cell transplantation is the portal vein, which is easily accessed by percutaneous transhepatic catheterization. Placement in the portal system eliminates the potential for systemic hyperinsulinemia, which can have dangerous side-effects such as changes in lipid metabolism and subsequent atheroma formation. Therefore, portal venous placement allows for easy access and physiologic control of diabetes.

Immunosuppression strategies

Current immunosuppressive drugs are diabetogenic and are therefore not optimal for the treatment of islet-cell rejection. Tacrolimus, cyclosporine and prednisone suppress insulin secretion or induce insulin resistance. These effects, when combined with a reduction in β-cell mass related to the immune response, can render a transplant ineffective. Several other strategies are now being implemented in order to minimize such complications and broaden the indications for transplantation. The first to be employed is the use of newer immunosuppressive agents, such as rapamycin and mycophenolate mofetil. In addition, the use of anti-lymphocyte globulin (ALG) has been shown to be associated with minor graft success. OKT3 has not been successful, since the cytokine release associated with its use induces β-cell death. Co-stimulation blockade with anti-CD40 ligand may decrease dependence on such drugs or render their use unnecessary.

Islet-cell survival has been improved by use of the chimerism methods described previously. Initially this approach was thought to be limited by the need to cytoablate the host's bone marrow. However, subsequent investigators have shown that multiple infusions may achieve the same goal. Ongoing studies are examining the use of such strategies in islet-cell transplants.

Immunoisolation is the term used to describe attempts to isolate islet cells from the immune system using synthetic barriers to cellular movement. Microencapsulation of islets within semipermeable membranes made of alginate polylysine has been successful in animal models. The idea is to allow glucose inflow and insulin outflow, while preventing access to the islet-cell population by antibodies, macrophages, T-cells and other immune modulators. Because a large mass of islet cells must be used for this technique, the limited organ supply currently restricts its usefulness. If the technology can be perfected, other cell sources such as xenotransplants may be considered to meet the needs of the diabetic population.

Islet-cell transplant success to date has been measured by the presence of c-peptide, the portion of the molecule that is cleaved when insulin is produced, or insulin independence. Success has been strongly associated with preservation times of less than 8 h, transplantation of > 6000 islet equivalents/kg, implantation into the portal vein as opposed to other anatomical sites, and the use of ALG as an anti-T-cell agent. Of 240 islet-cell allografts performed by 1993, only 20 patients were insulin independent for at least 1 week during their post-transplant course. The goal of islet-cell transplantation is to provide superior metabolic control and insulin independence prior to the development of the various complications of diabetes. Interestingly, research concerning ways to overcome rejection may even provide a therapy for the underlying autoimmune disease that creates the need for transplantation in this disease.

Summary: what will the future bring?

As outlined above, a multitude of novel approaches to transplantation are entering clinical trials or will do so during the next decade. These ideas address most of the limitations in the field that are recognized today. Although it may seem ambitious to state that this century will see elimination of the problems of rejection and organ supply, hopefully this will be the case. It is also probable that evolving vaccination strategies will eliminate most of the viral illnesses that lead to terminal hepatic disease, immune strategies will be applied to prevent autoimmune organ disease, and artificial organ development will progress to the point where many diseases that currently require tissue transfer will be treated with a mechanical interface. As such, the distant future of transplantation is likely to see a gradual reduction in the need for the discipline.

As the new century dawns, it is amazing to consider that at the beginning of the last century it was not possible to approximate blood vessels surgically, preserve tissue, culture cells or even enter the thoracic cavity – all procedures which are taken for granted today. In fact, a mere 50 years ago there had not been a single successful transplant of any type, and success in non-renal transplants has really been a product of the past 20 years. Thus if the coming years are, at the very minimum, as productive as the preceding ones, patients may experience a vastly improved future in which transplantation can be applied electively to all of those who need it.

Further reading

Billingham RE, Brent L and **Medawar PB**. 1953: Actively acquired tolerance of foreign cells. *Nature* **172**, 603–6.

Kirk AD, Harlan DM, Armstrong NN *et al*. 1997: CTLA4-Ig and anti-CD40 ligand prevent renal allograft rejection in primates. *Proceedings of the National Academy of Sciences of the USA* **94**, 8789–94.

Kirk AD, Burkly LC, Batty DS *et al*. 1999: Human anti-CD154 monoclonal antibody treatment prevents renal allograft rejection in non-human primates. *Nature Medicine* **5**, 686–93.

Knechtle SJ. 1996: Gene therapy and transplantation – a brief review. *Transplantation Proceedings* **28** (**Supplement 1**), 19–23.

Larsen CP and **Pearson TC**. 1997: The CD40 pathway in allograft rejection, acceptance and tolerance. *Current Opinion in Immunology* **9**, 641–7.

Larsen CP, Elwood ET, Alexander DZ *et al*. 1996: Long-term acceptance of skin and cardiac allografts after blocking CD40 and CD28 pathways. *Nature* **381**, 434–8.

Lee LA, Gritsch HA, Sergio JJ *et al.* 1994: Specific tolerance across a discordant xenogeneic transplantation barrier. *Proceedings of the National Academy of Sciences of the USA* **91**, 10864–67.

Madsen JC, Superina RA, Wood KJ and **Morris PJ**. 1988: Immunological unresponsiveness induced by recipient cells transfected with donor MHC genes. *Nature* **332**, 161–4.

Owen RD. 1945: Immunogenetic consequences of vascular anastamoses between bovine twins. *Science* **102**, 400–1.

Qin L, Chavin KD, Ding Y *et al.* 1994: Gene transfer for transplantation. Prolongation of allograft survival with transforming growth factor-beta 1. *Annals of Surgery* **220**, 508–19.

Sykes M and **Sachs DH**. 1988: Mixed allogeneic chimerism as an approach to transplant tolerance. *Immunology Today* **9**, 23–7.

Thomson JA *et al.* 1998: Embryonic stem cells derived from human blastocysts. *Science* **282**, 1145–47.

Index

Page numbers printed in *italic* refer to tables or boxed material

ENGLISH-SPEAKING JUSTICE

REVISIONS

A Series of Books on Ethics

General Editors:
Stanley Hauerwas and Alasdair MacIntyre

English-Speaking
Justice

GEORGE PARKIN GRANT

UNIVERSITY OF NOTRE DAME PRESS

Notre Dame, Indiana 46556

United States Edition 1985 by
University of Notre Dame Press
Notre Dame, Indiana 46556
Printed in the United States of America

Library of Congress Cataloging in Publication Data

Grant, George Parkin, 1918-
  English-speaking justice.

  Reprint. Originally published: Sackville, N.B.,
Canada : Mount Allison University, 1974.
  Includes bibliographical references.
  1. Justice—Addresses, essays, lectures. 2. Liberalism
—Addresses, essays, lectures. I. Title.
JC578.G7 1985   320.5'1   84-40293
ISBN 0-268-00914-7
ISBN 0-268-00915-5 (pbk.)

To ALEX COLVILLE and DENNIS LEE
two artists who have taught me about justice

Editorial Introduction

About George Parkin Grant's writings on moral
and political theory two things need to be said at
the outset. They are among the most interesting
North American work in that area to be produced
since 1945; and they are almost entirely unknown
in the United States. Partly this is because of our
philistine parochialism which steadfastly refuses to
acknowledge either the diversity or the interdependence of the various North American cultures, so
that Mexican as well as Canadian voices go unheard.
And partly it is because Grant himself has consistently directed what he has to say to the contemporary concerns of his own political and cultural
milieu, that of English-speaking Canadians.

It is no accident that an unusually high proportion of his writings originated as speech: most notably his Massey Lectures for the Canadian Broadcast-
ing Corporation, published in 1969 as *Time as
History*, but also in lectures to audiences at con-
ferences, at universities and at the Royal Society of
Canada. Grant exhibits, as few recent writers on
moral and political theory do, a consistent attempt

to speak immediately to the peculiar needs of time and place. This gives to his work a flavor that is very different from that of most academic writing, one that links his style to the content of his preoccupations.

Two of those preoccupations are important for readers of *English-Speaking Justice*. In his most widely read book *Lament for a Nation: the Defeat of Canadian Nationalism*, first published in 1965, Grant combined an explanation of the particular failures of Diefenbaker's conservative administration with an analysis of the way in which the forces of liberalism and modern technology had subverted the possibility of genuine national community in Canada, so that Canada suffered the more general American fate.

In the period since then Grant has drawn upon Nietzsche and Heidegger to develop a systematic critique of modernity, one that makes it urgent to identify what resources from the past are left to us which will enable us to preserve traditions of justice and civility in dark times. It is to this task that *English-Speaking Justice* is devoted. First published in 1978 by Mount Allison University at Sackville, New Brunswick, it is the written version of the Josiah Wood Lectures delivered at that university in 1974. The editors of the *Revisions* series are grateful for permission to reprint it. The only changes from the original version consist of one correction of a minor typographical error and of fuller references in a few footnotes.

Grant's judgments may perhaps sometimes strike members of the academic community in the United States as harsh and even peremptory. It is important to remember that he is speaking politically and practically and out of a deep loyalty to a tradition of thought and practice which he believes to be deeply endangered.

Stanley Hauerwas
Alasdair MacIntyre

Josiah Wood Lectureship

The following comprises the main portion of the deed of gift from the Honourable Josiah Wood, D.C.L., dated May 28, 1925:

As we grow older there is a danger of looking back on our early days and considering them much better than the present; but even the optimistic will admit that in recent years spiritual and moral progress has not kept pace with material advancement.

Since the infirmities of my advancing years have obliged me to live retired at my home in Sackville, and I have been largely confined to the house, with leisure to read the paper, I have been surprised at the wrong-doing and crimes that have been almost daily recorded in them. I have been impressed with the fact that the stern integrity of our fathers has been gradually weakened, and in many cases has entirely disappeared. Occupations and pleasures which, in their days, would have been regarded as wrong are without hesitation indulged in. In business, profit is the first consideration, and little thought is given to the moral character of the transactions. Indeed, wilful fraud and deliberate crime have been frequently discovered and exposed.

When I was a member of the Canadian Senate I did not draw all the money to which I was legally entitled.

I did not then intend that it should be taken from the public treasury. During my retirement, however, I have felt a desire to do something with this money which would have a tendency to lessen evil, and to benefit society generally. In this way it seemed possible to make this money practically useful. Upon mature reflection it has appeared to me that to establish a foundation for a lecture course in connection with Mount Allison University at Sackville will meet my views. The principal is to be invested and to be kept invested in securities which are at the time legal investments for trust funds in the Province of New Brunswick. The income is to be appropriated, partly as an honorarium for one or more lectures each year, and partly in the printing and distribution of the lectures. The lectures shall be delivered by men of high standing and exceptional ability. The lecturer shall be free to deal with his subject as he thinks best, keeping in mind the fundamental idea for which this foundation is established, namely, to impress on our students and citizens generally the absolute necessity of honesty and honour, of integrity and truthfulness, of an altruistic public spirit, of loyalty to King and Country and of reverence for God; in short, of all those virtues which have long been recognized as the very basis of the highest type of citizenship. I desire that a copy of the lectures be given to each student and Professor in the University and a copy be sent free to every University library in Canada. Other copies may be sold, in so far as there is a demand for them.

My desire is to assist in carrying out the purpose which the late Charles F. Allison had in mind in founding an Educational Institution in Sackville. These lectures are, therefore, always to be delivered in connection with the Foundation there bearing his name. The President of the University with the Treasurer of the Board of Regents and one other appointed each year by the Regents shall be trustees who will be responsible for arranging the lectures year by year and carrying out the terms of this bequest. This trust shall be know as the Josiah Wood Lectureship.

Part I

During this century western civilisation has speeded its world-wide influence through the universal acceptance of its technology. The very platitudinous nature of this statement may hide the novelty which is spoken in it. The word 'technology' is new, and its unique bringing together of 'techne' and 'logos' shows that what is common around the world is this novel interpenetration of the arts and sciences. As in all marriages, this new union of making and knowing has changed both parties, so that when we speak 'technology' we are speaking a new activity which western Europeans brought into the world, and which has given them their universalising and homogenising influence. Kant's dictum that 'the mind makes the object' were the words of blessing spoken at that wedding of knowing and production, and should be remembered when we contemplate what is common throughout the world.

The first task of thought in our era is to think what that technology is: to think it in its determining power over our politics and sexuality, our music and education. Moreover we are called to think that technological civilisation in relation to the eternal fire which flames forth in the Gospels and blazes even in the presence of that determining power.

We English-speakers have a particular call to contemplate this civilisation. We have been the chief practical influence in taking technology around the world. Russians and Chinese have often communicated with each other in the language of a small island off the west coast of Europe. Bismarck said that the chief fact of nineteenth century politics was that the Americans spoke English. To assert this practical influence does not imply the absurd suggestion that technological civilisation is mainly a product of the English-speaking world. Names such as Heisenberg and Einstein remind us that the crowning intellectual achievement of modernity was not accomplished by English-speakers. Descartes and Rousseau, Kant and Nietzsche, remind us that those who have thought most comprehensively about modernity have often not been English-speaking. Nevertheless, in theory and practice we English-speakers have universalised technological civilisation; we have recently established its most highly explicit presence in North America. In the very fullness of this presence we are called to think what we are.

As a small part of this multiform task, I intend in these Wood lectures to start from one fact of our situation: the close relation that there has been between the development of technology and political liberalism. By thinking about that relation, I hope to throw light on the nature of both, our liberalism and technology.

Over the last centuries, the most influential people in the English-speaking world have generally taken as their dominant form of self-definition a sustaining faith in a necessary interdependence between the developments of technological science and political liberalism. Most of our scientists have been political (and indeed moral and religious) liberals; the leading philosophic and journalistic expounders of liberalism have nearly always tied the possibility of realising a truly liberal society to the potentialities of modern mastering science. Indeed that close interdependence appears most obviously in the way that some convinced modern liberals put forth their creed as if it were a product of modern science itself; that is, speaking about it in the very language of objectivity which is appropriate to scientific discoveries, but not to an account of the political good. The expression of that close relationship has greatly varied. On the one hand there have been those who held the identification because they believed political liberalism was the best means of guaranteeing the progress of science. (Freedom's great achievement was that it allowed modern technology to appear.) On the other hand, there have been those who emphasised that modern science was a means of actualising the good which was liberal society. (Technology's great achievement was that it allowed freedom to flourish.) Whatever these differences of emphasis, however that close identification rested finally in a widely shared belief that the same account of reason which resulted in the discoveries of science, also expressed itself humanly in the development of political regimes ever more congruent with the principles of English-speaking liberalism. This assumed relation of modern science and modern liberalism is still our dominant form of public self-definition, whatever vagaries it has suffered in the twentieth century. Indeed, what do we English-speaking people possess of the political good, if we do not possess what is given in our particular liberalism?

It might be argued that I am incorrect to summon forth one side of that relation by the word 'liberalism'. It is indeed true that North American journalists often obscure practical issues by opposing 'liberalism' to 'conservatism'. A clearer way of speaking is to call the practical opposite of 'conservatism' 'progressivism'. Liberalism in its generic form is surely something that all decent men accept as good—'conservatives' included. In so far as the word 'liberalism' is used to describe the belief that political liberty is a central human good, it is difficult for me to consider as sane those who would deny that they are liberals. There can be sane argument concerning how far political liberty can be achieved in particular times and places, but not concerning whether it is a central human good. It may seem therefore that the use of the word 'liberal' about our explicit political faith during the last centuries does nothing to specify that faith clearly, other than to state the platitude that it was part of the broad tradition of sane discourse in the western world. Would it not be better to use for the purposes of general description the phrase 'English-speaking progressivism'? Despite this argument, I will use the phrase 'English-speaking liberalism', because it makes clear the two following points. First, the institutions and ideas of the English-speaking world at their best have been much more than a justification of progress in the mastery of human and non-human nature. They have affirmed that any regime to be called good, and any progress to be called good, must include political liberty and consent. It is not simply a racialist pride in our own past that allows us to make that boast. This must be reaffirmed these days, when our tradition seems often to have degenerated into an ideology the purpose of which is to justify the uninhibited progress of cybernetics, and when therefore it is very easy for decent men to attack English-speaking liberalism as a shallow ideology. Secondly, the use of the word 'liberalism' rather than 'progressivism' emphasises the necessary point that our English-speaking variety is not liberalism itself, but a particular species of it. This is often forgotten amongst us with the result that our account of liberalism is taken to be the only authentic account, rather than a particular expression of it. This arrogance has often made us depressingly provincial, especially in our philosophising.[1]

Two general propositions seem true about our contemporary liberalism. On the one hand, it is the only political language that can sound a convincing moral note in our public realms. On the other hand, there are signs that modern liberalism and technology, although they have been interdependent, may not necessarily be mutually sustaining, and that their identity may not be given in the nature of reason itself. These two propositions are fundamental to this writing.

The first appears to me indubitable. If argument is to appear respectable and convincing publicly, it must be spoken within the broad assumptions of modern liberalism. Arguments from outside this tradition are put out of court as irrational and probably reactionary. This response is so part of the air we breathe that we often forget its existence. For example, reactions against liberalism emerge on our continent based on local patriotisms and parochialities. These reactions are rarely able to sustain any national control of public policy, partially because the moral language in which they express themselves can easily be shown to be 'irrational' in terms of liberal premises, by the dominant classes of our society and their instruments of legitimation. Or again, the language of traditional religion can sustain itself in the public realm only insofar as it responds to issues on the same side as the dominating liberalism. If it does, it is allowed to express itself about social issues. But if there is a conflict between the religious voices and the liberalism, then the religious voices are condemned as reactionary and told to confine themselves to the proper place of religion, which is the private realm. It was not surprising that an influential liberal philosopher defined religion as what we do with our solitude, and in so doing turned around the classical account of religion. Or again, people who wish to justify certain moral positions are forced to pay lip service to modern liberalism if their arguments are to be convincing. The paying of lip service is always evidence of the dominance of a particular way of thought. There was a time when lip service had to be paid to Christianity. In our present world, lip service must be paid to liberalism.

For example, the bell of liberalism sounded in the fall of Nixon. The waves of public indignation which made possible his fall were too sustained to have been produced simply because the wind machines were owned by his enemies. The fact that so many had an obvious interest in bringing about his fall must not allow one to forget that they finally depended for their success on the disinterested voices of those who truly believed in the universal principles of liberal government. Indeed, the surprise in other parts of the world that the Americans were getting rid of an effective president, simply because of a few domestic crimes, showed unawareness of the strength of political liberalism in the heartland of that empire. Those who were surprised showed that they only understood the United States as an object—that is, from outside.

The reason why modern liberalism is the only language that can seem respectable in the public realm is because the dominant people in our society still take for granted that they find in it the best expression of moral truth. This must be stated unequivocally because some of us often find ourselves on the opposite side of particular issues from that espoused by the liberal majority, and do not accept the deepest premises, which undergird liberalism, concerning what human beings are. It is disturbing to find that a belief that does not appear to one rationally convincing is nevertheless the dominating belief in the world one inhabits.

If one wants to communicate, it is constantly necessary to use language which cannot express one's own grasp of reality. The escape from this can be paranoia, which expressed itself in the U.S. as the belief that the dominance of modern liberalism was produced simply by a conspiracy of 'intellectuals', 'media people', 'the eastern establishment' etc. Paranoia in any form is always the enemy of sanity and charity. This particular paranoia is especially dangerous because it closes the eyes to the essential fact that modern liberalism has been dominant because the dominant classes in our society have taken for granted that it expressed what is good. For a century the majority of people have at the centre of their education received the belief that the modern liberal account of justice is the best account. To accept the implications of the fact is a 'sine qua non' of any sane vision of English-speaking societies.

To turn to the second proposition: it is not difficult to point to facts which suggest that technological development does not sustain political liberalism. Abroad, the tides of American corporate technology have not washed up liberal regimes on the shores of their empire. Indeed, to put it mildly, the ferocious determination of the Americans to keep Indo-China within the orbit of their empire made clear that the rights to life, liberty and the pursuit of happiness might be politically important for members of the domestic heartland, but were not intended to be applicable to the tense outreaches of that empire. In the light of these facts, the argument is still presented by liberals that unfree regimes arise in colonial areas when they are first being modernised, but that in the long run they will develop into liberal domocracies. By this argument the identity of technological advance and liberalism is preserved in thought. The strength of the argument is necessarily weakened, however, as fewer and fewer colonial regimes remain constitutional democracies. The question is then whether the argument is an appeal to progressivist hope, or to facts; or whether progressivist faith is indeed fact.[2]

However, it is in the heartlands of the English-speaking empire that the more fundamental facts appear which put in question the mutual interdependence of technological and liberal reason. The chief of these facts is that the development of technology is now increasingly directed towards the mastery of human beings. In the words of Heidegger, the sciences are now organised around cybernetics — the technology of the helmsman. To state part of what is given in that thought: technology organises a system which requires a massive apparatus of artisans concerned with the control of human beings. Such work as behaviour modification, genetic engineering, population control by abortion are extreme examples. The machinery reaches out to control more and more lives through this apparatus, and its alliance with the private and public corporations necessary to technological efficiency. The practical question is whether a society in which technology must be oriented to cybernetics can maintain the institutions of free politics and the protection by law of the rights of the individual. Behind that lies the theoretical question about modern liberalism itself. What were the modern assumptions which at one and the same time exalted human freedom and encouraged that cybernetic mastery which now threatens freedom?

Moreover, what can be the place of representative government in the immense society ruled by private and public corporations with their complex bureaucracies?[3] The great founders of our liberalism believed that the best regime required that the choices of all its members should have influence in the governing of the society. It was also hoped that free and equal individuality would be expressed in our work as a field for our choices. The free society would require the overcoming of the division of labour, so that our individuality could be expressed in an egalitarian variety of work. How are either of these possible when the dominant decisions come forth from private and public corporations? In this situation, the institutions of representative government seem increasingly to wither in their effectiveness. Lip service is paid to them; but institutions such as elections and parliaments seem to have less and less constitutive authority. The work of most human beings is intensely specialised, and proceeds from routines which have little to do with individual spontaneity. The widespread concentration of most North Americans on private life, and their acceptance that the public realm is something external to them, takes us far away from the original liberal picture of autonomous and equal human beings participating in the government and production of their society.

Indeed, the current concentration on private life, and the retreat from the public realm as something which is other, raises questions beyond the practical failures of our liberalism. It raises fundamental questions about what is being spoken about human beings in that liberalism. Its theoretical founders asserted that justice was neither a natural nor supernatural virtue, but arose from the calculations necessary to our acceptance of the social contract. In choosing the benefits of membership in organised society, we choose to obey the contractual rules of justice. But is not the present retreat into the private realm not only a recognition of the impotence of the individual, but also a desire to leave the aridity of a realm where all relations are contractual, and to seek the comfort of the private where the supracontractual is possible? For example, the contemporary insistence on sexual life as the chief palliative of our existence is clearly more than a proper acceptance of sexuality after nineteenth century repressions. It is also a hunger and thirst for ecstatic relations which transcend the contractual. After all, mutual orgasmic intercourse cannot finally be brought under the rules of contract, because it takes one beyond the realm of bargains. Therefore human beings rely on its immediacy partially as a retreat from the arid world of public contractualism. In this sense, the retirement of many from the public realm raises deeper questions about modern liberalism than its practical failure to achieve its ideals. It raises questions about the heart of liberalism: whether the omnipresence of contract in the public realm produces a world so arid that most human beings are unable to inhabit it, except for dashes into it followed by dashes out. But such a tenuous relation to the public realm is far from the intentions of the early founders of modern liberalism. This leads to asking: was the affirmation by those founders that justice is based on contract ever sufficient to support a politics of consent and justice? This questions modern liberalism at its theoretical heart.

To sum up: we are faced by two basic facts about our moral tradition. First, our liberalism is the only form of political thought which can summon forth widespread public action for the purposes of human good. Secondly, this liberalism seems presently to speak with a confused voice in the face of the technology it has encouraged and this confusion puts in question the theoretical roots of that liberalism. These lectures will, therefore, try to enucleate what is being spoken about human and non-human beings in that liberal tradition. Only in the light of such an enucleation can one turn to the more difficult question of what is the relation between technological reason and modern liberal reason.

Part II

What is being spoken about human beings in our contemporary liberalism now that technology is not simply a dreamed hope but a realising actuality? I will seek this by discussing a recent writing: *A Theory of Justice*, by Professor John Rawls of Harvard. The centre of the English-speaking world has moved since 1914 to the great republic. It is therefore appropriate to listen to contemporary liberalism in an American garb. Harvard has been an intellectual centre of that empire. Since President Eliot, the ends of that university have more and more seemed to be the stamping of liberal ideology on the articulate classes of that empire. A book of six hundred pages about justice is a good place to start. Justice is after all the central political question and a carefully composed theory of it, clearly within contemporary liberal assumptions, allows us to hear much of what is being spoken about human beings in that liberalism.[4]

Rawls affirms that justice can only be truly understood when it is known as rooted in contract. He summons forth as his chief teachers the great contractarian theorists of modern liberalism, Locke,

Rousseau, Kant; he sees his task as expressing their fundamental contractarian truth in terms which will be acceptable to contemporary analytical philsophising. Indeed among those who have written about political liberalism in the English-speaking world there have been two main conceptual schemes: those who have been purely utilitarian and those who have subordinated utilitarianism within a firm contractarian frame. Rawls places his liberalism within such a frame and his book is a sustained criticism of pure utilitarianism as the basis for a free society. It is surely not hard to understand that contractarian theory has always protected the rights of individuals in a way that utilitarian theory does not allow, and that this is a pressing issue at a time such as ours when the rights of individuals are assailed by progressive corporate power, acting under the banner of technological necessities. In terms of utilitarianism's own first principle, why should individuals have inalienable rights, if those rights stand in the way of the greatest happiness of the greatest number? When applied to the actual world of politics, contractarian theory has always supported a legal and political system which grasped the nitty-gritty of justice in its details, while the broad principle of utilitarianism could be used to sweep them away. It is for this reason that contractarian theorists such as Locke and Rousseau have had direct influence on actual politicians to an extent never achieved by utilitarians such as Hume and Bentham. The politicians had to come to terms with the details of justice in terms of individuals. Therefore when Rawls insists on the superiority of Locke to Hume, we seem to be entering a world which is much less flaccid about what can be done to individuals than the world called forth by successors of Hume. Can we do anything to individuals in the name of minimising the misery of the greatest number? In starting from the great contractarians, Rawls gives us hope that we will meet the complexities and difficulties of political justice in a way that is not possible under the principles of mass hedonism.

Contractarian theory may seem an abstraction of philosophers, taking us away from the common sense needs of human beings so obviously faced by the utilitarians in their principle of the greatest happiness of the greatest number. Nevertheless it is more fundamental than utilitarianism because it answers the question: Why should human beings consent to even that minimal social cooperation without which organised society cannot exist? It answers this question in terms of the interests of the free individual. 'Liber' and 'free' are after all synonymous at the literal level. Its answer is that the good society is composed of free individuals who agree to live together only on the condition that the rules of cooperation, necessary to that living together, serve the overall purposes of each member of that society. That agreement or contract, and the calculating implicit in it, is the only model of political relations adequate to autonomous adults. The state must be such that each person can freely agree to the limitations it imposes, and this will only be possible when its free, rational members know that its existence is, in the main, to their advantage. Rawls is in the central tradition of modern liberalism in that his ideal political beings are adult calculators, who freely decide that social cooperation is worthwhile because it is to their individual advantage. It is in this sense that Rawls believes that the true principles of justice depend on a social contract. He believes that if one is to push to the point of philosophic clarity the idea of justice implicit in social cooperation, the conception of social contract becomes necessary, because without the social contract it is not possible to show that the acceptance of justice is to the advantage of the freely calculating individual. The vision of society as a collection of free, calculating individuals puts his book at the heart of modern liberalism. The book is the attempt to make clear the nature of that social contract (a) in the light of the new conditions of advanced technological society and (b) in terms acceptable to modern analytical philosophers.

To explicate Rawls' account of the social contract and to see whether it provides a foundation for the principles of justice he builds upon it, it is necessary to compare Rawls' account with those of his avowed masters, Locke and Kant.[5] Locke's account of the social contract is that it is made by sensible calculating human beings, in the light of their recognition of the way things are in the state of nature. In exemplary consciousness of what he is doing, Locke follows Hobbes in substituting the state of nature for the createdness of nature as the primal truth. From this truth his understanding of politics is derived. In short, Locke's belief in contractual constitutionalism as the best regime is founded upon a new primal teaching about nature which is radically distinguished from that which had been traditional to western Europe. The Aristotelian account of nature (which had been strangely put together with the doctrine of creation in the dominant western tradition) was known by Locke to be untrue, above all because of what was given in a clear philosophic reflection about the discoveries and methods of the new sciences. (It is worth remembering that as a young man Hobbes had served as a clerk in the household of Francis Bacon.) For Locke, the Aristotelian teaching could no longer be the framework for the understanding of either the human or the non-human things. In the old view of nature, human beings were understood as directed to a highest good under which all goods could be known in a hierarchy of subordination and superordination. Our lesser goods were seen as pale participations in that highest good. To Locke, the untruth of the traditional teaching means that there is no such highest good given to human beings in their recognition of the way things are. Nevertheless the understanding of the way things are — the state of nature — remains for him the only basis from which a true account of the best political regime can be understood. Put negatively then, for Locke the great question about justice must be: how can the foundations of justice be laid when rational human beings are not given the conception of a highest good? His answer to that question is that justice is contractual, not natural. The state of nature does not provide us with the conception of a highest good; but it does provide us with knowledge of the greatest evil, and the desire to escape that evil. The calculating individual knows that the worst evil is death, and that although we cannot finally escape it, we must escape as long as we can. We must preserve ourselves — if possible comfortably. Reflection on the state of nature makes us recognise this given end (albeit negative) and from it a new political teaching can be laid down. In the social contract, we agree to government and its limitations upon us because it is to our advantage, in the sense that it protects us from the greatest evil. That contract is the source of our rights because we have consented to be social only upon certain conditions, and our rights are the expressions of those limiting conditions. All members of society are equal in the possession of these rights, because whatever other differences there may be between human beings, these differences are minor compared to the equality in our fundamental position: to be rational is to be directed by the dominating desire for comfortable preservation. Justice is those convenient arrangements agreed to by sensible men who recognise the state of nature, and what it implies concerning the greatest evil. Because of his bland and indirect rhetoric, Locke was to be the chief theoretical influence on generations of English-speaking bourgeois, persuading them to give their allegiance to the new form of liberalism. In so far as they understood his teaching as more than immediate political prescriptions, they came to recognise that in accepting that liberalism they were giving up the doctrine of creation as the primal teaching.

To be aware of what is being spoken by Rawls about human beings, it is necessary to state where his account of the social contract differs from that of Locke. Rawls' central teaching is that the principles of justice are not self-evident to our 'common sense'; the positing of an 'original position' enables us to formulate them. The original position is an imagined situation in which an individual is asked to choose principles of justice for his society under a 'veil of ignorance'. This veil conceals from him his particular circumstances, and therefore eliminates from his choosing those motives of self-interest which otherwise would corrupt the fairness of his judgement. In the original position we all would choose fairly because we would be abstracted from knowing the detailed facts about our condition in the real world. Because we would not know who we were in detail (we might be people in the most miserable conditions) we would therefore have an interest in choosing the universal principles of our society which would be good for all its members, not simply to the advantage of some. As we choose under a veil of ignorance, we would choose principles which would be good for all, because we might be one of those to whom partial principles did not apply. Chosen from this abstracted position, the principles of justice are the basis for the constitution of any just society in any time or place. The original position is Rawls' basic theoretical teaching because from it we can derive universal principles of justice acceptable to all rational human beings. All human beings can agree to say 'yes' to a society so based, because it is the one most likely to serve their advantage.

It is important to recognise that in Rawls' account of justice as fairness human beings remain essentially calculators of their own self-interest in the original position. When Rawls speaks of human beings as rational, he means that they are able to calculate their self-interest. The calculations of our self-interest are concerned with what Rawls calls 'the primary goods'. These are those goods such as wealth, liberty, status, etc. which all sensible human beings will agree are good, however much they disagree as to what is the highest good or whether there is a highest good. Calculation concerning these goods is the central activity of the original position, because in it individuals know that they have self-interest, and know the general content of those self-interests. What they do not know is the particularities of those self-interests. They do not know their place in society e.g. wealth, skills, inclinations, ambitions, private philosophies of life, etc. Indeed the original position is made timeless and ahistorical in that it does not include knowledge of the level of technological development the particular society has reached. In two essential ways Rawls' teaching is close to that of Locke's social contract. (1) For both Rawls and Locke the primary political act from which justice is derived is an act of individualist calculation of self-interest. (2) What men primarily calculate about are those good things which lead to comfortable self-preservation.

Nevertheless Rawls' teaching differs in substance from that of Locke. 'The original position' is an abstraction from life, according to Rawls; 'the state of nature' is the way things are, according to Locke. Nobody has ever actually lived in the original position; all reflective people are aware that they could easily find themselves in Locke's state of nature, if the conventions of civil society were wiped away. What holds us in society according to Locke is our consciousness of what we have to lose (life itself) if we do not put up with the convenient rules of the game. The fear of violent death is the reason for setting up those rules and it remains the final reason for staying with them. Rawls' original position is not concerned with the way things are, it is an imagined abstraction from that. Justice is as much a matter of convenient rules of the game as it is in Locke's teaching. But the rules of the game are derived from a quite different situation from that described by Locke. They are reached from a stance set up to achieve fairness. Clearly there is a great gulf fixed between a contract for rules of the game founded on a calculation of individual self-interest which is always aware that its chief end must be self-preservation, and a contract concerning the rules of the game founded on an imagined stance abstracted from the way things are.[6]

One clear cause of this gulf between earlier contractarian teaching and that of Rawls is that Rawls defines the activity of philosophising in a quite dif-

ferent way from Locke and Hobbes. It is not my
business here to describe the history of English-
speaking philosophy in the last centuries, or its subtle
copenetration with changes in the continental account of philosophy. In journalistic terms, it suffices
to state that since 1900 the 'subject' has been increasingly practised in English-speaking universities
within a rubric that can be crudely labelled as 'the
analytical'. Rawls practises philosophy within the
broad outlines of that rubric; so what he thinks he
is doing is clearly differentiated from what Locke
thought he was doing.[7] In the sphere of morals and
politics, analytical philosophers have often expressed
their teaching within the negative principle known
as 'the naturalistic fallacy': that propositions concerning how human beings ought to act cannot be
derived solely from factual propositions about nature. Clearly the contractarian teaching of Hobbes
and Locke is an example of 'the naturalistic fallacy',
because what they both say about justice is founded
upon what they claim to know about the way things
are. The regime founded upon the social contract
is the best regime because of the way things are in
the state of nature. Locke unfortunately practised
philosophy before the discovery of 'the naturalistic
fallacy', the divisions between 'nature' and 'freedom',
between 'is' and 'ought'. Rawls is the inheritor of
these later explications. According to him the principles of justice cannot be derived from such metaphysical propositions as the state of nature. To put
his difference from Locke in terms of the history of
ethical theory, his doctrine of the original position

may then be taken as the attempt to preserve the advantages of contractarian over utilitarian foundations for liberal justice, while avoiding 'the naturalistic fallacy' (call it if you will the metaphysical foundations) upon which Locke's contractarian teaching is based.

With the division between nature and freedom, 'is' and 'ought', we enter the world of thought dominated by Kant. It is indeed appropriate that in the preface of Rawls' book we read that his theory "is highly Kantian in nature" (viii), and that in his index we find more references to Kant than to any other thinker. Kant has been the German philosopher who over long and changing generations has most sustained his influence over English-speaking academics. That influence continued even in the years since 1870 as the English and the Germans moved into increasingly explicit economic and political conflict, and their intellectual worlds became further separate. In the public world, Kant's great political teacher, Rousseau, exerted a greater influence, first through the French revolutionists, and more recently through Marxism. But it was through the thought of Kant that the tradition of continental liberalism most firmly touched our universities. Generations of professors studied and taught Kant's writings, so that his influence penetrated the form of our education. For example, when we think about the origins of the distinction between judgements of fact and of value, we are apt to impute the formulation of this assumption to the work of Max Weber. Yet not only did Weber's formulation arise from his study of Kant, but also in our world the long influence of Kant on academic philosophers had prepared the ground for the dominance of this distinction in the social sciences. What is being attacked as 'the naturalistic fallacy' is avoided by the distinction between judgements of fact and of value.

Indeed Rawls' notion of justice as fairness seems on first view to take us into the political world of rational choice which was so wonderfully explicated by Kant. The free power of human reasoning is seen not only as overcoming the deficiencies of nature by developing the arts and sciences, (technology), but also as showing us, in its impartial universalising power, why these arbitrary and deficient allocations of nature ought not to be allowed to continue. We not only transcend nature in our technological ability to correct its deficiencies, but also in our moral willing which is the statement that they ought to be corrected. The human species depends for its progress not on God or nature but on its own freedom, and the direction of that progress is determined by the fact that we can rationally give ourselves our own moral laws. Within this view of freedom as transcending nature, the principle of equality is extended to realms unthought of in the earlier contractualism of Hobbes and Locke. It becomes no longer simply a matter of equality in legal rights, but an equality also of goods and powers to be distributed fairly by the rational will of the community. At the simplest level of interpretation, the greatness of Kant's account of justice lies in his assertion that it is irrational for human beings to make favourable exceptions of themselves. It is irrational to ask for goods from our communities that we do not will for other people. Rawls' account of justice as fairness is obviously close to that Kantian assertion. In the immediate political scene, the equality he advocates is an equality defined in the tradition of Rousseau, not of Locke. It is an equality not only of legal rights but of substantive goods, towards which all communities ought to strive. Such an equality is considered a sane political goal, not only because the progress of technology allows us to put right the blindness and deficiencies of nature, but also because reason teaches us that these deficiencies ought not to be.

Yet despite Rawls' continuous appeals to Kant, it is a dimmed and partial Kant which emerges. Kant is quite clear why the contractually based state founded on the rights of man is the best state. The first sentence of *The Laying of the Foundations of the Metaphysics of Morals* expresses the ontological basis of that affirmation. "Es ist überall nichts in der Welt, ja überhaupt auch ausser derselben zu denken möglich was ohne Einschränkung fur gut könnte gehalten werden, als allein ein **guter Wille**." It is not pedantry which makes me write this sentence in German. The ring of its affirmation is lost in all English translations I have read or attempted. "It is impossible to conceive anything at all in the world, or even out of it, which can be taken as good without qualification, except a good will." Yes, but not quite.[8] According to Kant we can know this to be so, because as he says in *The Critique of Practical Reason*, morality is the one fact of reason. Facts are given and our rationality gives us the very form of justice for all our actions. Indeed, as justice is present to our wills in the mood of command, reason commands us to the faith that justice is what we are finally fitted for. Our other activities may be what we are fitted for under certain circumstances, but they may not be under other circumstances. Justice is always good and is the final court of appeal for the judging of the goodness of any act. In the command to be just, given us in our very reasons, we are also given the idea that being fitted belongs essentially to us. All the uncertainties about whether we are fitted for anything which arises for us from our sense of nature's arbitrariness, our knowledge of its mechanism and the relativities of our desires, are overcome in the command, beyond all bargaining, to be just. The categorical imperative presents to us good without restriction. Moreover that justice which is our good depends upon our willing of it. We are the makers of our own laws; we are the cause of the growth of justice among our species. We are not only the species whose good is justice, but also the species who are the cause of the coming to be of our own good. According to Kant, in our ability to will justly we are both timelessly rational, outside the world where everything is relatively good and where reasoning is simply calculation; we are also utterly in the world of time where we make history, where what happens matters absolutely and depends upon our autonomous willing. What it means to say that the good will is the only good without restriction is both the traditional doctrine of the timeless factuality of the moral law; but also the new idea that as makers of our own laws we are called upon to realise justice progressively in history.[9]

Kant's account of the political in his shorter writings is firmly related to the affirmation that the good will is the only good without restriction. Kant took the contractarian teaching of Hobbes and Locke which was based on the passions of nature and founded it rather on the freedom of human beings to legislate a timeless rational morality which quite transcended nature. It may be said that he sacralised the contractarian teaching. From the side of will in the phrase 'the good will', the social contract represents the consent necessary in any regime proper to human beings whose essence is their autonomous freedom. Because the highest purpose of human life is to will autonomously, the best political regime must be such as could be willed rationally by all its members. In this sense, consent becomes the very substance of the best regime. It must be a state based on 'the rights of man', that is, giving the widest possible scope to external freedom, because any limitations on external freedom stand in the way of the exercise of our autonomy. These rights must be universal throughout society, because all human beings are equal in the sense that they are all open to the highest human end of willing the moral good. Inequalities between human beings are only concerned with lesser goods, such as intellectual or artistic powers. Concerning what matters absolutely we are all equal in the fact that the rational willing of our duty is open to all.

From the side of good in the phrase 'the good will', Kant's contractarian teaching leads to a sharp division between morals and politics, and therefore to a strict limitation on the powers of the state given in the social contract itself. Properly understood, morality is autonomous action, the making of our own moral laws. Indeed any action is not moral unless it is freely legislated by an individual. Therefore the state is transgressing its proper limits when it attempts to impose on us our moral duties. Our autonomous choices of timeless good cannot be so imposed. Indeed, Kant more than any other political philosopher, lays before us that side of liberalism which says that the state should not interfere with the actions of its citizens, except when those actions infringe the external freedom of other citizens. The state is concerned with the preservation of the external freedom of all, and must leave moral freedom to the individual. It is concerned with the relativities of nature understood by Kant within the non-teleological and non-substantialised view of nature given us in modern science. When in his *Perpetual Peace* he states that the hard problem of organising a good regime can be solved even for a race of devils, as long as they are intelligent, he is asserting that the state must be limited to those natural relativities, and that the ability to calculate is an adequate account of reason when one is concerned with those relativities. Nowhere is Kant's affirmation that the world of nature is strickly relative more lucidly put before us than in his definition of marriage as a life-time contract for the mutual use of the genitals. But the limitations of the state to contracts concerning these relativities is necessary in order to guard the individual's willing of the timeless good, in which he quite transcends those relativities. It is on moral grounds that the morally neutral state is the best state. The state is limited in the social contract because the good will is the only good without restriction.[10]

For all Rawl's appeals to Kant, the central onto-logical affirmations of Kant are absent from Rawls. Clearly in Rawls' account of philosophy there can be no fact of reason. Justice, therefore, cannot be justified as coming forth from the universal moral-ity given us in reason itself. Rawls cannot make the affirmation that the good will is the only good with-out restriction, or that the good will is that which wills the universal moral law. His account of philos-ophy does not allow him such statements about the supreme good.

What Rawls takes from Kant is partial in a way common among contemporary English-speaking teachers of philosophy. The central import of the critical system is interpreted in a way that leaves Kant essentially a precursor of modern analytical philos-ophy. His tribute to Hume as having awakened him from his dogmatic slumbers is emphasised; his stronger, more positive and more often repeated tributes to Rousseau seem to have been forgotten. It is only necessary to quote one of these tributes to make clear that Kant does not take as limited an account of the scope of philosophy as is usual among English-speaking academics: "Newton was the first to discern order and regularity in combination with great simplicity, where before him men had encountered disorder and unrelated diversity. Since Newton the comets follow geometric orbits. Rousseau was the first to discover beneath the varying forms human nature assumes, the deeply concealed essence of man and the hidden law in accordance with which Providence is justified by his observations."[11]

When Kant is taken as essentially a precursor of modern analytical philosophy, certain sides of his thought are being correctly grasped. Obviously he is a great philosopher of science and the greatest critic of traditional western metaphysics. There is no more wonderful account than his of the darkness in which we find ourselves when we attempt to apply the conception of final cause to the understanding of nature. Our fate is to find ourselves agnostic (in the literal sense) about the purpose of the way things are. He enucleates how that agnosticism has been presented with a new certainty to educated people through the discoveries of modern science. He is as aware as Hobbes or Locke of the consequences of the Galilean physics for our practical lives. Our knowledge of justice cannot be derived from our knowledge of nature (as some once believed) because our knowledge of nature is not teleological. Indeed Kant has as often been taken as a precursor of modern existentialism, as of modern analytical philosophy. We are thrown into a world of otherness. Yet, and it is an enormous 'yet', across the darkness of that agnosticism there is thrown, according to Kant, the beacon light of our knowledge of what is required of us concerning justice. That requirement is presented to all human beings from the earliest days of their reasoning, in the categorical commands of our reason itself. According to Kant, we are not in darkness concerning the one thing absolutely needful for us all. Because there is that beacon (the one fact of reason), Kant's purpose is not simply to criticize metaphysics as such, but out of his criticism of the traditional metaphysics to lay the foundations of the new one. As he makes consummately clear in the preface to the 2nd edition of *The Critique of Pure Reason*, metaphysics must become Rousseau's 'Socratic wisdom'. It is the laying of the metaphysical foundations necessary to protect that beacon light of justice. These protecting foundations are necessary on the one hand against the intellectual extremities of dogmatists who would deny our moral autonomy in denying our darkness; and on the other hand against the sceptics who would deny that there is this beacon light of justice. This 'Socratic wisdom' requires that we affirm statements which are 'beyond physics' — statements about God and about freedom. Clearly the proposition that the good will is the only good without restriction is an ontological proposition. To interpret Kant as if he were simply a precursor of modern analytical philosophy is to lay him upon a bed of Procrustes and cut his thought down to a required ametaphysical shape. Rawls passes beyond this in taking Kant as an ethical theorist whose love of egalitarian justice he admires. But by cutting Kant's ethics off from its ontological foundations, he nevertheless proceeds to the work of Procrustes upon that analytical bed.

Rawls' difference from Kant is seen in his account of 'the free and rational person'. According to Rawls, rationality is analytical instrumentality; freedom means that we cannot avoid choices. This is different from Kant's account of our free moral self-legislation as participation in the very form of reason itself. This difference becomes obvious when it is cashed in political effect around the question of equality. Why is it good that all human beings should live in a society to which they can give consent and in which they are guaranteed an equality of political liberties? Why is it good that human beings should have political rights of a quite different order from members of the other species? Why should equality in legal rights stand above and not be influenced by the obvious inequalities in contribution to progress whether in production, in the arts or in the sciences? To Kant, the answer is quite clear. The only good without restriction is the good will, and that is open to all human beings irrespective of their other differences. Our differences in talent, in education and social contribution count as nothing against fundamental equality, because we are equal in what is essential. In our moral willing we take part in the very form of reason itself. But why does Rawls' account of the 'person' make equality our due? Why are beings who can calculate and cannot avoid choices worthy of equal inalienable rights? After all, some humans can calculate better than others. Why then should they not have fuller legal rights than the poor calculators? Why do either of these human abilities justify the primacy of equality, or the different level of our rights compared with those of other species?

Nor can it be said that Rawls' use of the word 'person' illuminates his position. Indeed his use of the word seems at odds with his analytical account of philosophy. To call human beings 'persons' is clearly not a scientific description. What is it then? If the word is a true description but not scientific, is it not then one of these supra-scientific metaphysical terms which analytical philosophy would have us eschew? One may be glad that Rawls has inherited the noble belief in political equality, and the belief that 'the free and rational person' is 'valuable' in a way quite different from members of other species. But in an era such as ours, we cannot help hoping that he will tell us why it is so. His writing is typical of much modern liberal thought in that the word 'person' is brought in mysteriously (one might better say sentimentally) to cover up the inability to state clearly what it is about human beings which makes them worthy of high political respect. Where Kant is clear concerning this, Rawls is not.

In short, Rawls affirms a contractarian as against a utilitarian account of justice, but wishes to free that contractarian teaching from the metaphysical assumptions upon which it was founded in the thought of its greatest exponents. To state how successful he is in this attempt, it is necessary to return to Rawls' account of how the question of justice arises, and how his teaching concerning 'the original position' claims to answer it.

According to Rawls, the question of justice arises because all sensible people know that they have interests, and also know that these interests are sometimes going to be in conflict with those of other people. They also know that it is in their interest to live in organised society, not only to protect themselves in the pursuit of their interests against others who may interfere with such pursuits, but also positively to further their particular interests through such means as the division of labour.[12] In the light of this plurality of interests and the plurality of opinion as to what is good, how can we come to agreement about foundational rules for the social system? These foundations must reconcile the need to live in society with the need to pursue our own interests. Such basic rules are what Rawls means by the principles of justice. They are the basis of any decent constitution. Through the constitution they set the limits to positive laws, and therefore the limits within which all public relationships should take place. This account of the political situation in which the question of justice arises in terms of essentially calculating individuals may be described accurately as American bourgeois common sense. So to describe it is not meant simply derisively. It would be foolish to deride the American bourgeois self-image because it has become dominant in most of the western world, and views do not become widely dominant without at least some partial sense in them.

How are we to come to knowledge of such basic rules? Let us imagine, says Rawls, an original position in which human beings are under a veil of ignorance, so that they know that they have interests, and know that these interests are likely to be in conflict with those of other people, but do not know their own particular ones. In such a position, human beings who calculate sensibly would choose a society in which "each person is to have an equal right to the most extensive basic liberty compatible with a similar liberty for others." Rawls' first principle of justice is identical with J.S. Mill's sole principle. Sensible human beings would choose a society founded on such a principle, because under a veil of ignorance they would calculate that such a fundamental rule would allow them to pursue their own interests at least partially. Without such a rule they would chance finding themselves in a situation where they might even be unable to pursue their interests at all. For example, they might be enslaved. From the original position we reach therefore a universal principle of justice. It is universal in that it would be chosen by any sensibly calculating individual if he were in the position of calculating about interests in the abstract; that is, calculating as if he were everybody, and not simply himself or herself. This abstracted calculation is able to provide the universal principle of justice because it is a calculation about calculating which would be made by all good calculators. To repeat, human beings for Rawls are, in their public role, calculators of their interests. The act of thought in the original position might be called disinterested calculation because it is made outside any knowledge of particular interests; it is not disinterested, however, in that the calculation of interest in general is its very centre. Substantively it provides a first principle of justice because it comes to terms with the basic difficulty of any political thought. It shows how consent can be reconciled with the necessity for organised society. Consent is only possible when we know that the society is organised for the pursuit of individual interests in general.

It is important to emphasise that this account of the derivation of the first principle of justice appears to Rawls to have the enormous advantage of not requiring any knowledge of the way things are beyond common sense. It does not depend on our being able to attain any knowledge of what human beings are fitted for. Our legal rights, so derived from the original position, in no way depend on any public affirmations concerning what is good. Indeed it would appear that according to Rawls enlightened human beings are quite clear that it is not possible to have knowledge of the highest good. But if many citizens (perhaps even the majority) misguidedly think such knowledge possible, this opinion need not affect the morally neutral state, because its principles of justice can be clearly determined quite outside any opinions concerning that possibility. Indeed the doctrine of the original position claims that at one and the same time it preserves the state as morally neutral, yet also guarantees that such a state protects the rights of free and equal citizens. Moral pluralism about 'life-plans' is guaranteed by the law so long as those plans do not harm other people or interfere with their basic liberties. We are thus freed from the bad old days when the powers of the state were used to enforce the monistic opinions of some concerning goodness, on the unwilling lives of others. We are able to achieve this tolerance without sacrificing our certainty about the superior justice of the liberal regime. Moreover in terms of modern theory the chief advantage of the original position is that it enables us to free ourselves from all the difficulties and disagreements of the traditional political philosophy, which arose from its dependence on metaphysical assumptions. We free ourselves from that burden of speculation while remaining quite certain about the principles of political justice. Philosophy or religion become comparable to the question of sexual habit. They are simply a matter of private pursuit, unless their conclusions interfere with the liberty of others. We can think what we like metaphysically or religiously (if we have a taste for that kind of thing) as long as we recognise that these thoughts are our private business, and must have no influence in the world of the state. Philosophy and religion can be allowed to be perfectly free because their conclusions are perfectly private. On the other side of the same coin, the principles of justice so derived will remain utterly impervious to anything we know through scientific discovery. Let us say we reach the conclusion, because of the discoveries of modern science, that human beings are accidental occurrences which have arisen in a world which is completely explainable in terms of necessity and chance. This gives us no reason to doubt that all human beings should have the free and equal rights of the liberal regime. As the principles of that regime are derived solely from abstracted calculation about obvious human interests, they will stand as self-evidently true, however the world be explained, or whatever it be.

Rawls derives much more than the regime of political rights from the 'original position'. Justice requires a regime which pursues equality in all aspects of life, social and economic as well as political. He shows this in terms of what he calls 'primary goods', and our calculation about them in the original position. Primary goods are those goods which any sensible person will know he will need, whatever may be his particular 'life-plan'. To repeat, according to Rawls we cannot know what is the highest good for human beings, or whether there is such. Nevertheless all sensible persons know that certain goods are necessary to any way to life. At an obvious level, these are such things as food, shelter and safety. Rawls, however, adds a long list of liberties and powers beyond these immediacies, stretching from civil liberties all the way to the provision of self-respect. Under the veil of ignorance in the original position, the calculating individual is not ignorant of the fact that he needs as much as possible of these primary goods. He also knows that there are unlikely to be enough of them to go around. What he does not know is the details of his particular possession of those goods. Neither does he know the stage of technological development in his particular society. In this partial ignorance, therefore, the calculating individual decides for a system which strives toward equality in these primary goods. This is a rational calculation because if he were to choose any other regime he would be likely to find himself in a position where he got less rather than more of the pie. Indeed, in certain stages of technological development, if he did not so choose he would be likely to find himself without even a sufficiency. From this rational calculation under the veil of ignorance we reach his second principle of justice. "Social and economic inequalities are to be arranged so that they are both: (a) to the greatest benefit to the least advantaged, — and (b) attached to offices and positions open to all under conditions of fair equality of opportunity."[13]

In making substantive equality necessary to the content of justice in his second principle, Rawls passes beyond the bourgeois political common sense of his first principle to what may be called American progressivist common sense. In practical terms, what he is saying is that the works of F.D. Roosevelt must be carried to their completion, probably by the Democratic party. Welfare egalitarianism can be united with the individualist pluralism of the constitution in an advanced technological society. The difficulties between liberty and equality raised by de Tocqueville must be overcome; justice requires the union of equality and liberty. Although this progressivism has its own American style, it finds its justification in European philosophy. Nature does not supply fairly. The arbitrary deficiencies of nature

and society are to be overcome in history in the name
of equality. The very definition of history as progress is the coming to be of equality. This philosophic liberalism reached its apogee in Marx. Technology and equality go so closely together as almost
to be considered one. It must be said that Rawls
takes only partially this European progressivism,
because he is always attempting to unite it with
bourgeois common sense. This can be seen in the
limits he puts on substantive equality compared with
Marxism in its originating form. At the centre of
Marxism is the belief that the realisation of equality will require such a prodigious event as the overcoming of the division of labour. This kind of question is just not present for Rawls. His acceptance
of progress as equality is restrained from that hope
by his bourgeois common sense. To put it crudely,
the overcoming of the division of labour is not likely
to be within the imaginative limits of the Harvard
professor. Substantive equality yes, but only at the
level of consumption and welfare.

Indeed what makes Rawls' book worthy of study
is that it is so typical of current liberalism in both
the intellectual and practical English-speaking
worlds. His book combines a theory of justice with
an account of the substance of justice. His theory
of justice attempts to come to terms with the intellectual difficulties which analytical philosophy has
brought against any theory of justice which transcends the analytical. His account of the substance
of justice puts together the claims of bourgeois individualism and progressive equality, typical of of-

ficial American liberalism. This strange mixture has
only lately begun to be faced by its contradictions,
both from the 'left' and the 'right'. However, his
book is a confident exemplar of what has been the
dominant moral strain in our politics.

In terms of what is happening in advanced societies, it is indeed not difficult to ridicule Rawls'
hopes concerning this union of individualism and
egalitarianism. The contradictions in this union have
been made explicit both by 'the left' and 'the right'.
Rawls' account of justice seems simply to abstract
from the fact that liberty and equality now have to
be realised in a society largely shaped politically by
the cooperation between massive private corporations and the public corporation which coordinates
their welfare. Indeed his thought seems to abstract
from the very existence of these dominating powers.
Can his calculating individualism bring forth a doctrine of the common good strong enough to control
the ambitions of these mammoths? Can the calculating individual be a citizen in such a world, or does
this account of human beings only lead to individuals
concerned with consumption — above all entertain-
ment and the orgasm as consumption?

Even more surprising than Rawls' lack of interest
in such powers within his own country is his abstraction from their influence in the world as a whole.
That is, his theory of justice is written in abstraction from the facts of war and imperialism. He only
deals with war around the question of the right of
the individual to refuse the claims of the state. The
abstraction from the facts of war and imperialism

is particularly emptying when one remembers that the modern liberal English-speaking regimes have both been great imperial powers. Moreover, his book was written during the period when his country was embarked on a savage imperial adventure carried out under the regimes of Kennedy and Johnson, who advocated domestically the same welfare equality and individualism which he is advocating. Indeed his abstraction is even more surprising when one remembers that the Vietnam war was justified in terms of liberal ideology, was largely planned by men from the liberal universities, the most influential of whom were from Rawls' own university. Paradoxically, however, Rawls' abstraction from war and imperialism makes his work even more typical of our liberalism. Most American liberals have discussed the questions of world order under the rubric of internationalism and the relation between equal sovereign states, when in fact they lived at the centre of a great empire. After all, that archetype of modern liberalism, F. D. Roosevelt, used forceful language against war and imperialism at the very time when he was consolidating an empire. Be that as it may, Rawls' theory of justice is enormously weakened by his failure to relate it to the facts of imperialism or of domestic corporate power.

Such criticisms of Rawls concerning his apprehension of the technological society must not, however, divert us from the fundamental question about his theory. This question is the following: can the content of justice he advocates be derived from his contractual theory? He advocates many liberties and equalities as the necessary content of a just regime. Sensible people can disagree with Rawls about the details of these liberties and equalities; but surely any decent human being will agree that liberty and equality are at the heart of political justice. Any English-speaker who cares about our tradition must be glad that our regimes have, at their best, attempted to realise such justice. But Rawls' book claims to be more than a catechism of such goods; it claims to be a theory of justice. That is, it claims to be giving us knowledge of what justice is, and how we know that a regime of liberty and equality is its core. He meets the demands of that claim by stating that we will know what justice is and why liberty and equality are necessary to it when we think the calculation of everybody's self-interest in general, abstracted from any self-interest in particular. The fundamental question about Rawls' book is whether such justice can be derived from calculation of self-interest in general.

Rawls characterises his account of justice as 'justice as fairness'. Sometimes in the reading of this long and complex book it may seem that we are being asked to play the old shell game. When we look for the bean of justice under the shell of self-interest, it has moved under the shell of altruism, and vice versa. Nevertheless when we are really able to pay attention to the mover's hands, we find that the bean is always under one shell — the shell of self-interest. Justice as fairness is under it. Justice is derived from calculation about self-interest in general. The fundamental question about Rawls' book is then whether justice as fairness can be so derived. Is it possible to believe that the complex apparatus necessary to preserving and extending liberty and equality in the midst of the technological society can be known as necessary to the best regime simply by thinking through the calculation of self-interest in general?

It must be insisted (yet once again) that this calculation is carried out within a particular account of what we can know about self-interest. Indeed, Plato's account of justice might be sensibly described as known by a calculation concerning self-interest. When Socrates tells us that it is better to suffer injustice than to inflict it, he is saying that it is always in our interest to be just. But in his account our interests are known through our knowledge of the nature of things. Justice is what we are fitted for. We come to know that through the practice of philosophy, which gives us knowledge of the nature of things, of what we are fitted for and what the consequences are for our actions in being so fitted. In philosophy we are given sufficient knowledge of the whole of the nature of things to know what our interests are, and to know them in a scheme of subordination and superordination. In this account, justice is not a certain set of external political arrangements which are a useful means of the realisation of our self-interests; it is the very inward harmony of human beings in terms of which they are alone able to calculate their self-interest properly. The outward regime mirrors what is inward among the dominant people of that regime, and vice versa. Within that account, justice could then be described as the calculation of self-interest, as long as it is understood that at the centre of that self-interest is justice itself. For justice is the inward harmony which makes a self truly a self (or in more accurate language which today sounds archaic: Justice in its inward appearance is the harmony which makes a soul truly a soul).

Obviously Rawls means something very different by the calculation of self-interest. His analytical account of philosophy does not allow him to think that our knowledge of self-interest can be derived from what knowledge we have of the way things are as a whole. Such knowledge is not possible according to his account of philosophy. Nor (as has been argued previously) can analytical philosophy allow him even that knowledge of self interest which Locke claims can be derived from our knowledge of the nature of things as a whole. According to Locke, we can place self-interest in an order of subordination and superordination, because our knowledge of the way things are as a whole (the state of nature) tells us that everybody's chief interest is the avoidance of violent death. Justice is derived from that knowledge of our highest self-interest.[14] For Rawls the calculated self-interest in general is not derived from any such knowledge. It is avowedly not derived from any contemporary philosophic or scientific knowledge. Our self-interests are "the primary goods", and these are simply accepted as obviously our interest, whatever may be the nature of things as a whole. Indeed, much of Rawls' book is taken up with show-

ing the superiority of his contractarianism to utilitarianism. Nevertheless his account of 'primary
goods' is hard to distinguish from the utilitarian account of pleasure. As far as the calculation of the
political contract is concerned, self-interest in general
is the maximising of the cosy pleasures. It is taken
as self-evident that this is everybody's self-interest,
irrespective of what anybody may claim to know
about the way things are as a whole. I do not imply
that there is anything bad about cosy pleasures.
Much of our life is concerned with them. The point
is, however, that Rawls derives justice from a
calculation which is in terms of them alone. What
kind of regime will result?

What must be asked then about Rawls' theory is
not only whether justice as liberty and equality can
arise from a social contract reached from a calculation of self-interest in general; but also whether it
can be derived from a calculation in which the interests are self-evidently independent of any account
of the way things are as a whole. After all, the first
question has been on the agenda of political philosophy since our contractarian theory was first enucleated by Hobbes and Locke: is justice simply pursued because we calculate that it is the most convenient means to our self-interest? Rawls raises nothing
new about that question. What he adds, however,
is the attempt to justify this contractarianism within
analytical assumptions: Is justice pursued because
of convenience, even when the calculation is in terms
of an account of self-interest reached in abstraction
from any knowledge of the way things are as a

whole? Is such justification of justice able to support the pursuit of liberty and equality at a time when the conveniences of technology do not seem to favour them?

It may be argued that I have made too much of one academic book. One swallow does not make a summer; one academic book does not make an autumn of our justice. However, theories are at work in the decisions of the world, and we had better understand them.

Part III

Why is it that liberalism remains the dominating political morality of the English-speaking world, and yet is so little sustained by any foundational affirmations? At the level of immediate historical cause, this is not difficult to understand. The long ascendency of English-speaking peoples, in the case of England since Waterloo, and the United States since 1914, was achieved under the rule of various species of bourgeois. Members of classes are liable to consider their shared conceptions of political goodness to be self-evident when their rule is not seriously questioned at home, and when they are successfully extending their empires around the world. Those shared conceptions of constitutional liberalism seemed to be at one with technological progress, particularly as this progress was being achieved above all by English-speakers. This unity between progress in liberty and in technology, under English-speaking guidance, was often further guaranteed by being enfolded in such doctrines as the ascent of man.

In the case of England, the victory of the Whigs in 1688, and the almost unopposed consolidation of that victory after 1715, provided the political and ideological setting for the development of the first industrial society with its maritime empire. English constitutional liberalism was immensely flexible under Whig guidance. As new bourgeois classes appeared in the quick changes of a technological society, they were allowed near power, and persuaded to loyalty to the Whig constitution. The constancy among the articulate classes concerning what constituted the best regime was such that there was little need to wonder as to what was being said about human and non-human nature in the foundations of that liberalism. It was so assumed and so successful that it did not need to be thought.

In that bourgeois dominance the notes of comfort, utility and mastery could alone ring fully in the public realm. Among those who wrote political philosophy since Hobbes and Locke, there has been little more than the working out in detail of variations on utilitarianism and contractualism, their possible conflicts and their possible internal unclarities. What do Bentham or J. S. Mill or Russell add to Locke at the level of fundamental political theory? Indeed it is better to put the question: what has been lost in them of his comprehensiveness, subtlety and depth? The confidence of that Whig dominance is illustrated by the way that Burke has been interpreted since his day. He has been taken as our chief 'conservative' in contradistinction of our 'liberals'. In fact he was in practice a Rockingham Whig, and did not depart from Locke in fundamental matters, except to surround his liberalism with a touch of romanticism. That touch of the historical sense makes him in fact more modern than the pure milk of bourgeois liberalism. Such figures as Swift and Johnson and Coleridge, who attempted (in descending order of power) to think of politics outside the contractarian or utilitarian contexts, were simply taken as oddities dominated by nostalgia for a dying Anglicanism, and having no significance for the practical world.

This great confidence in bourgeois liberalism explains why the new continental philosophies of politics, from later stages of the age of progress, never seem to have exerted much influence in English intellectual life. Rousseau's account of contractarianism, based on freedom, which dominated Europe through the work of Kant and Hegel and Marx, only touched English thought in an academic way. What influential English thinker has ever come to terms with Rousseau's fundamental criticism of Hobbes and Locke? Indeed, till recently, Marxism has had little influence in England, even among the abused proletariat of the first industrial society. Since this European liberalism of freedom little penetrated English thought, it is not surprising that English thinkers hardly recognised at all the attack on that liberalism of freedom which arose in Germany. Nietzsche was not taken by the English as the great critic of Rousseau's politics, but as an obscurantist pseudo-poet. They did not need to look at his lucid analysis of what we were being told about human and non-human beings in the advancing technological society. Both for good and ill, the English thinkers were sheltered from the extremities of European political thought because of their successes under bourgeois constitutional liberalism. This was for good because the pursuit of comfortable self-preservation, though not the highest end, is certainly more decent and moderate than the extremities of communism or national socialism. There are worse things than a nation of shopkeepers. This sheltered confidence had the ill effect of leaving English intellectuals singularly unprepared to understand the extremities of the twentieth century, particularly because it had weakened the theoretical tradition in its cosy embrace.

Indeed English political philosophy has been little more than a praise of the fundamental lineaments of their own society, spiced by calls for particular reforms within those lineaments. Thinkers such as Mill or Russell were too much at home in their world to be political philosophers in the classical meaning of that term, which always implied that qua philosophers, they transcended the opinions common to their society. Even the philosophic radicals had drawing rooms. As late as our generation, after the results of two world wars had sapped the confidence of many Englishmen, and when the possibilities of technological tyranny had become obvious, the most popular academic theorising about politics went no farther than the decent prescription that we ought to pursue 'piecemeal social engineering' so as to 'minimise misery'. The only purpose of political philosophy was the valid negative task of freeing us from the delusions of general statements which might encourage a more than piecemeal engineering. Our tradition of justice was so blandly self-evident as to be in no need of further justification.

It must be insisted, however, that this long consensus about political good, and the resulting poverty of thought, did much to innoculate the English from those theoretical viruses which have plagued continental Europeans. The very weakness of philosophical life protected them from its modern extremities. The fact that the English received modern political thought in an early form from Hobbes and Locke, and continued to be generally content with that form, meant that they were free from the much more explicit modernity which arose first in France and later in Germany. Their very confidence in their liberalism saved them from taking seriously the traditions which proceeded either from Rousseau or from Nietzsche. They were for example saved from such a manifestation of those political philosophies as ideology. Clearly one of the uniquely modern phenomena has been ideologies, either of the 'left' or of the 'right'. Ideology is here defined as surrogate religion masquerading as philosophy. All forms of it have been destructive of social moderation. Its modern appearance has been chiefly caused by confusion concerning the related but distinct roles which religion and philosophy play in good societies. This confusion originated above all in the false formulation of these roles made during the French and German enlightenments. The fact that the dominant English political philosophy came from a period before those enlightenments has helped till recently in insulating the English from this virus. As illustration, the greater prestige given to scholars and artists in the German world has often resulted in an ideological politics in that country. Hitler was after all an ideologue who conceived himself as the artist in politics. The very disinterest in philosophy among the English has saved them in the past from that lack of moderation which is inherent in modern political philosophy and technology.[15]

To rise above the scholars, Churchill's writings may be taken as an example of this confidence in liberalism which did not need thought, even at a late date in that British destiny. After 1945 he wrote *A History of the English-speaking Peoples*. Here we might expect to find English liberalism lying before us as 'monumental history'. We might even expect to find a Thucydidean telling of why the deeds of those whom he had loved and to whom he had belonged had been both great and good. We might expect a telling freed from that attenuated ignorance of the heat of practice, so common in academic history. Churchill, like Bertrand Russell, came from one of the great landed families who in their rule of England and its imperial expansion had been responsible, more than any other class, for the incarnation of modern principles of liberty into the English constitution. His class had believed profoundly in the inter-dependence of commerce, domestic liberty and scientific progress. Indeed in Churchill's life of his founding ancestors, both the man and the woman, he had shown them to be substantially responsible for the origins of that Whig rule. He was a modern liberal in the sense that in domestic politics he had been an enthusiastic member of that Liberal government which first brought nationalism, social welfare and democracy together. He was a liberal in that he always maintained that superior contempt for the traditional religion, except as a useful political tool in times of emergency.[16] Churchill has often been described as a conservative, but he was only that because he appeared at a time of conflict, when his nation's constitutionalism was threatened by new alternatives—Marxist communism and national socialism. His intransigent opposition to these alternatives was expressed not only in writing but in war. Indeed he showed himself more than an English nationalist in that he believed that the American experiment was the authentic continuation of English liberalism, and was willing to sacrifice much of his country's greatness to guarantee that the torch of world leadership should be passed in our era to the capitalist republic.

One might therefore expect Churchill to state in such a late writing what it was about English-speaking liberalism which had made it worthy of loyalty such as his. One could expect an account of substantive loyalties to community goods, which is indeed not philosophy, but the only soil out of which political philosophy can arise. Such accounts carry in themselves an incipient recognition of what is said in philosophy. Particularly at that late date, one might have expected from Churchill such 'monumental history', when the ambiguity of his career must have lain before him. His career had been given to the perpetuation of English power, and yet had led to the decline of that power. However, a presentation of these loyalties in their substance and meaning is quite absent from his book. English-speaking institutions are glorified in the description of deeds, but we are not given the substance of those deeds which made them both great and loveable, other than they just happen to have been our own. Indeed the pure distance in Churchill's book between his account of action, and what good was being lived and thought in those actions, is seen in the fact that Locke is mentioned only once in the book, and then because of his work on the reformation of the coinage. The most influential thinker of the good of capitalist liberalism is not understood in relation to the deeds of that liberalism, but simply as one of those academics with which influential families decorate their lives. It seems indeed that Churchill's book is finally an appeal to pure racial will. However, such a reading would be unfair, because his failure to present good does not come from crude arbitrariness of will. He was no existentialist, but a gentleman whose loyalties transcended will. Rather it is the givenness and certainty of his loyalties which does not allow him to present those goods. Even as late as 1945, his confidence in English political greatness, and in the obvious truth of the superiority of constitutional liberalism, so enfolds him that there is no need to articulate what is good and great in the deeds he is describing.

The leading makers of the American constitution conceived themselves as influenced by political philosophy, which they took in its modern form. The

love of English political philosophy among the
French of the enlightenment came back into English-
speaking explicitness among the lawyers and intellectuals of the new world, rather than among the more
rooted English rulers. The legal and political forms
of the U.S. are more purely founded on constitutional contractualism than those of the country
where that modernism was first thought comprehensively. The pioneering expansion into an unexploited
continent gave American liberalism a greater egalitarian tint than in England. However, the coin-
cidence of that expansion with the development of
increasingly powerful forms of industrial capitalism
always resulted in these egalitarian influences being
safely confined within the practical and ideological
bounds of a given bourgeois liberalism. The egalitarianism of Paine and the egalitarianism of populism
were always subsidiary. Indeed, political contractualism and its resultant private pluralism fitted the
long term public needs of the later immigrants of
non-English traditions. The very pressures of pluralism have encouraged that interpretation of their constitution which would see it as a sheerly contractual
document. Issues in the political realm could be
decided in terms of the contracted constitutional
rights of individuals, while the denser loyalties of
existence were left supposedly untouched within
pluralism. The ideology of pluralism suited both the
institutions of industrial capitalism and the immigrant groups. It helped both the unrestrained
monistic power of the corporations, and at the same
time the entrance of members of many races (at least

those of European origin) into the freedom of the
common heritage, seemingly without losing their
private traditions. Increasingly, the substance of the
common good was expressed rationally only as contractual reason, to the exclusion of those loyalties
which gave content to that good in more traditional
societies. American nationalism, with effective sense
of a righteous destiny, has had to be explicitly affirmed so as to provide for the conception of the
common good a substance which transcended the
simply contractual. Contractualism was less inhibited even than in capitalist England, where certain disappearing classes maintained remnental
reverences from before the age of progress. In the
United States such remnants as Anglican poetry and
piety were largely squashed with the revolution, and
reverences brought by later immigrants were easily
engulfed and legitimised into the public contractual
framework. The crossing of the Atlantic to a society
which had no history of its own from before the age
of progress brought a flowering of the contractual
principle in its purest form.

In the first half of this century the expansion of
the United States around the world, as the great
capitalist empire, was so fast and successful that the
constitutional principles of bourgeois hegemony became even more self-evident.[17] Even more than in
the case of England, the domestic and foreign successes of their system put contractualism safely beyond any serious thought. However much Americans have been impregnated by modern negations
in other spheres of existence, there is little serious

alternative to the fundamentals of their legal and political framework. Many are still able to exalt themselves as the country of freedom, and in that exaltation it is the essentially contractual which is being glorified.

While the theoretical foundations of our justice came increasingly to be understood as simply contractual, nevertheless decent legal justice was sustained in our regimes. This can only be comprehended in terms of the intimate and yet ambiguous co-penetration between contractual liberalism and Protestantism in the minds of generations of our people. I am not capable of enucleating the nature of that relation, and it can only be hinted at here. Indeed one can use of that co-penetration the words of one who battled with it in his own being: there is "the sense, in the whole element, of things too numberous, too deep, too obscure, too strange or even simply too beautiful, for any ease of intellectual relation."[18] Perhaps more than any other European country, England's practical flesh and bones have been fed till recently by its remarkable religious traditions. They may not have been the home of much philosophy, but they were a deeply religious people. The more uncouth and less integrated Protestantism of North America has sustained certain forms of justice, at least for those of European origin. Several elementary comments about liberalism and Protestantism are necessary to the understanding of our surviving justice.

To start at the surface: it is clear why the English free church tradition feared established Christianity, or any close connection between church and state. The Calvinists had only gained political control for a very short period. They therefore saw in the secularization of the state a means to their freedom against established religion. Beyond the political, moreover, the fearful solitariness in the Calvinists' account of the meeting between God and his creatures encouraged that individualism which was at home with a politics essentially defined in terms of individual right. It is not necessary to enter the debate between Marxist and Weberians to recognise the truth understood by both: namely that Calvinist individualism and the development of capitalism went hand in hand, and that the contractualist political regime was a useful expression for both. Indeed one can say that the extraordinary compact between God and man in Calvinism strangely prepares people for contractual human relations. As secular liberalism became increasingly progressivist, the millenarianism in extreme forms of Protestantism often seemed to be saying the same thing as the secular idea of progress. The religion which has in its heart "He has put down the mighty from their seats and has exalted them of low degree" must have some connection with equality. Less obviously, there was an intimate relation between the development of modern positive science and the positivist account of revelation in Calvinism.[19] It is often forgotten by those outside theology that English Protestantism was overwhelmingly Calvinist or Anglican, not Lutheran. Such fates are consummate. Modern European history brings forth the comparison: Germany with

its philosophy and music, its political immaturities
and extremities; England with its poverty in music
and contemplation; its political moderation and
judgement. Whatever forces were operating, one of
them was their differing Protestantisms. Indeed in
England the long consensus about political good,
which was sustained by this ambiguous union between Protestantism and secularity, had much to do
with protecting that civilisation from the worst extremities of the twentieth century. Whatever else may
be said about England, there has been more moderation in its domestic politics so far than in any of the
other dominating western societies. The English
were indeed willing to be more extreme towards non-
Europeans than they were at home; but there were
some restraints even in their imperial adventures. In
his fight for Indian independence, Gandhi had to deal
with Lord Halifax, not with Himmler or Beria.

In the United States, the Protestantism was of
a more unflinching, more immoderate and less
thoughtful sort than in England. The Puritan seekers
after a new world were escaping the public demands
of an Anglicanism which at its heart was not Calvinist. This rougher Protestantism was more suited
to the violent situation of conquering a new continent, first emptied of its French and Spanish opposition and some easily conquered Indians. Indeed the
Puritan interpretation of the Bible produced more
a driving will to righteousness than a hunger and
thirst for it. As it became secularised in America,
that will became the will of self-righteousness, and
produced its own incarnation in Emerson. Never-

theless, even in the immoderation — indeed the ferocity — which has been so manifest in American history, that Protestantism gave a firmer and more unyielding account of justice to its country's constitutionalism than would have been forthcoming from any simply contractual account. The continuing power of American Protestantism in popular life today comes from the fact that it has been a less thoughtful species of religion than the originating Protestantism of Europe, and therefore less vulnerable to modernity. That Protestantism is today above all pietist. This has given it the strength to continue even through all the modernising of rural and small town America. But this pietism has little intellectual bite compared to the Calvinism it replaced, so that its direct practical effect on the control of technology (the central political question) is generally minimal.

All this can be easily said by modern historians. It is more important to recognise the dependence of secular liberalism for its moral bite upon the strength of Protestantism in English-speaking societies. Most of our history is written by secularists who see the significant happening as the development of secular liberalism. They are therefore likely to interpret the Protestants as passing if useful allies in the realisation of our modern regimes. This allows them to patronise Protestant superstitions in a friendly manner, as historically helpful in the development of secularism. To put the ethical relation clearly: if avoidance of violent death is our highest end (albeit negative), why should anyone make sacrifices for the common good which entail that possibility? Why should anyone choose to be a soldier or policeman, if Lockian contractualism is the truth about justice? Yet such professions are necessary if any approximation to justice and consent are to be maintained. Within a contractualist belief, why should anyone care about the reign of justice more than their life? The believing Protestants provided that necessary moral cement which could not be present for those who were consistently directed by contractualism or utilitarianism or a combination of both. This fundamental political vacuum at the heart of contractual liberalism was hidden for generations by the widespread acceptance of Protestantism. At one and the same time believing Protestants were likely to back their constitutional regimes; yet they backed them without believing that the avoidance of violent death was the highest good, or that justice was to be chosen simply as the most convenient contract.

The word 'dialectic' used about 'history' has had such cruel consequences for so many people that one is loath to use it even loosely. Nevertheless the relation between Protestants and the growing explicitness of secular liberals can be expressed in the political dialectic between them. The more Protestants came to be influenced by the theoretical foundations of the liberalism which they had first accepted for practical reasons, the less were they able to sustain their prime theological belief which had allowed them to support justice in a more than contractual way; therefore they were less able to provide the moral cement which had given vigour to the liberal regimes. The more secular liberals were able to make explicit that their belief in freedom was not simply a matter of political consent, but implied that human beings were the makers of their own laws, the less could they receive from their Protestant supporters that moral force which made their regimes nobler than an individualism which calculated its contracts.

The long history of the gradual secularising of Protestant faith would require a detailed discussion of its relation to the discoveries of modern science and the formulations of modern philosophy. Protestant faith was not only undermined by the objective discoveries of the sciences, but equally by the affirmations concerning humanity in the dominant philosophies. On the scientific side, for example, it was Darwinism which gave Protestant faith its intellectual 'coup de grace' among so many of our bourgeois. On the philosophic side, as 'enlightened' human beings came to express their self-understanding as autonomy—that is, to believe themselves the makers of their own laws—any formulation of Christianity became unthinkable.

This co-penetration of Protestantism and liberalism must not be understood in terms of a simply passive overriding in which Protestantism gradually lost itself. It was a veritable co-penetration in which Protestantism shaped as well as being shaped. In writing of the positive influence of Protestantism on our liberalism, one is forced to touch, however hesitantly, upon the most difficult matter which faces anybody who wishes to understand technology. This is the attempt to articulate that primal western affirmation which stands shaping our whole civilisation, before modern science and technology, before liberalism and capitalism, before our philosophies and theologies. It is present in all of us, and yet hidden to all of us; it originates somewhere and sometime which nobody seems quite to know. Nobody has been able to bring it into the full light of understanding. In all its unfathomedness, the closest I can come to it is the affirmation of human beings as 'will', the content of which word has something to do with how westerners took the Bible as a certain kind of exclusivity. The Calvinist form of Protestantism was a strong breaking forth of that primal and unfathomed affirmation, because 'will' and exclusivity were so central to its theology. Calvinist theological voluntarism made it utterly a modern western theology as distinguished from the theologies of the Platonic world. Hooker saw this with hard practical clarity when he wrote against the Calvinists at the time of their beginnings: "They err who think that of the will of God to do this or that, there is no reason beside his will."[20] In that sense Calvinists were not simply the passive victims of secularisation, but were formulators of it even in their definitions of God and humanity as 'will'. Calvinist secularism is as useful a substantive as secularised Calvinism. Because of their rootedness in what is thought in the word 'will', these Calvinist secularists were particularly open to that definition of will as autonomy. This openness is central to the nemesis of their faith. But in that very nemesis, Calvinism remained a continuing influence in formulating our new 'self-definitions'. An intellectual example from Europe is the fact that thinkers such as Rousseau and Sartre, who were such formulators of human beings as freedom, were both impregnated with Calvinism in their origins. A more important and immediate example is the sheer conflict of competing wills which has characterised the history of American contractualism. "Winning isn't everything; it's all there is."

To turn back from the depths of technology's origins, it may be said simply that the nobility of English-speaking Protestants often lay in what was given them in the word 'freedom', and the consequences of this for the political realm. Nevertheless what was there given them made them prone to take the meaning of the will to be autonomy. But clearly once that Rubicon is crossed, no form of Christianity can consistently stand. As the Protestants accepted the liberalism of autonomous will, they became unable to provide their societies with the public sustenance of uncalculated justice which the contractual account of justice could not provide from itself.

This ambiguous relation between Protestants and secularisation was expressed academically in the influence of Kant among generations of professors — particularly those making the first or second steps away from the pulpit, and finding in the teaching of philosophy an acceptable substitute for preaching. Intellectuals wanted to seem emancipated from Protestantism, even as they were strongly held by it. They liked to see themselves as the friends of freedom and the new technologies, while at the same time they needed to believe that the new society would incorporate the 'absolute moral values' of Protestantism. They could not accept the account of liberalism given in its strictly worldly forms. Kant seemed to tell them how all these needs could be met.

They could be moderns and maintain the 'values' of their past. He seemed to show them how they could believe in freedom as autonomy and in an 'absolute morality' as well. He offered them a Protestantism purified of superstitions and open to progress. A comparison can be drawn between the hopes of these gentle ministers-cum-professors and the more tragic history of the relations between philosophic Jews and German society. The most remarkable of the 'neo-Kantians' was Hermann Cohen, and as late as this century he seems to have been close to identifying the coming of the Messiah with the full realisation of the German liberal state.

In the United States, contractualism was later to be buttressed by other forms of Biblical religion which came with the later immigrants. Both Judaism and Roman Catholicism gave a firmer bite to the political justice lived out under the American constitution than that implied by contractualism. Nevertheless, because the primal formation of that constitutionalism was in the meeting of Protestantism and secular accounts of legality, it cannot be my purpose here to describe how the later immigrant forms of Biblical religion gave force to justice in those institutions, nor to describe how those religions were transformed by existing within English-speaking institutions.[21]

To sum up: the principles of our political and legal institutions did not need to be justified in thought,

because they were justified in life. They were lived
out by practical people for whom they provided the
obvious parameters of any decent society. Anyone
who wished to act outside these parameters had
rightly to feel or assume shame. They were identified
with the coming to be of progressive technological
society; they justified and were justified by that coming to be. Through that long period when our bourgeois societies were not only stable at home but
increasingly dominant throughout the world, the
liberalism could simply be lived in without contemplation. If those who considered themselves political
philosophers questioned whether decent rules of
justice could be expected to come forth from the
foundational affirmation that political relations are
simply calculated contracts, they were cushioned
from clarity by a long tradition of justice otherwise
sustained, and new progressivist hopes. Such intellectuals lived in societies which were enfolded in a suf-
ficiently widespread public religion to produce be-
lievers who accepted the liberal state, and yet did
not believe that justice was good simply because it
was the product of calculated contract. The story
has been told many times of how most intellectuals
in our societies scorned the fundamental beliefs of
the public religion, and yet counted on the contin-
uance of its moral affirmations to serve as the convenient public basis of justice. Clever people generally believed that the foundational principles of
justice were chosen conveniences, because of what
they had learnt from modern science; nevertheless
they could not turn away from a noble content to

that justice, because they were enfolded more than they knew in long memories and hopes. They were so enfolded even as they ridiculed the beliefs that kept those memories alive among the less articulate. Intellectual oblivion of eternity could not quickly kill that presence of eternity given in the day to day life of justice. The strength of those very memories held many intellectuals from doubting whether justice is good, and from trying to think why it is good in the light of what we have been told about the whole in modern science. This combination of the public successes of liberalism with these memories and hopes inhibited the thought which asks if justice is more than contractually founded, and whether it can be sustained in the world if it be considered simply a chosen convenience. The very decency and confidence of English-speaking politics was related to the absence of philosophy.

Part IV

English-speaking contractualism lies before us in the majority decision of the U.S. Supreme Court in "Roe vs. Wade". In that decision their highest court ruled that no state has the right to pass legislation which would prevent a citizen from receiving an abortion during the first six months of pregnancy. In that decision one can hear what is being spoken about justice in such modern liberalism more clearly than in academic books which can be so construed as to skim questions when the theory cuts. Theories of justice are inescapably defined in the necessities of legal decision.

Mr. Justice Blackmun begins his majority decision from the principle that the allocation of rights from within the constitution cannot be decided in terms of any knowledge of what is good. Under the constitution, rights are prior to any account of good. Appropriately he quotes Mr. Justice Holmes to this effect, who, more than any judge enucleated the principle that the constitution was based on the acceptance of moral pluralism in society, and that the pluralism was finally justified because we must be properly agnostic about any claim to knowledge of moral good. It was his influence in this fundamental step towards a purely contractual interpretation of their constitution that has above all enshrined him in American liberal hagiography.[22] In the decision, Blackmun interprets rights under the constitution as concerned with the ordering of conflicting claims between 'persons' and legislatures. The members of the legislature may have been persuaded by conceptions of goodness in passing the law in question. However, this is not germane to a judge's responsibility, which is to adjudicate between the rights of the mother and those of the legislature. He adjudicates that the particular law infringes the prior right of the mother to control her own body in the first six months of pregnancy. The individual who would seem to have the greatest interest in the litigation, because his or her life or death is at stake, — namely the particular foetus and indeed all future U.S. foetuses — is said by the judge not to be a party to the litigation. He states that foetuses up to six months are not persons, and as non-persons can have no status in the litigation.

The decision then speaks modern liberalism in its pure contractual form: right prior to good; a foundational contract protecting individual rights; the neutrality of the state concerning moral 'values'; social pluralism supported by and supporting this neutrality. Indeed the decision has been greeted as an example of the nobility of American contractarian institutions and political ideology, because the right of an individual 'person' is defended in the decision against the power of a majority in a legislature.

Nevertheless, however 'liberal' this decision may seem at the surface, it raises a cup of poison to the lips of liberalism. The poison is presented in the unthought ontology. In negating the right to existence for foetuses of less than six months, the judge has to say what such foetuses are not. They are not persons. But whatever else may be said of mothers and foetuses, it cannot be denied that they are of the same species. Pregnant women do not give birth to cats. Also it is a fact that the foetus is not merely a part of the mother because it is genetically unique 'ab initio'.[23] In adjudicating for the right of the mother to choose whether another member of her species lives or dies, the judge is required to make an ontological distinction between members of the same species. The mother is a person; the foetus is not. In deciding what is due in justice to beings of the same species, he bases such differing dueness on ontology. By calling the distinction ontological I mean simply that the knowledge which the judge has about mothers and foetuses is not scientific. To call certain beings 'persons' is not a scientific statement. But once ontological affirmation is made the basis for denying the most elementary right of traditional justice to members of our species, ontological questioning cannot be silenced at this point. Because such a distinction between members of the same species has been made, the decision unavoidably opens up the whole question of what our species is. What is it about any members of our species which makes the liberal rights of justice their due? The judge unwittingly looses the terrible question: has the long tradition of liberal right any support in what human beings in fact are? Is this a question that in the modern era can be truthfully answered in the positive? Or does it hand the cup of poison to our liberalism?

This universal question is laid before us in the more particular questions arising from the decision. If foetuses are not persons, why should not the state decide that a week old, a two year old, a seventy or eighty year old is not a person "in the whole sense"? On what basis do we draw the line? Why are the retarded, the criminal or the mentally ill persons? What is it which divides adults from foetuses when the latter have only to cross the bridge of time to catch up with the former? Is the decision saying that what makes an individual a person, and therefore the possessor of rights, is the ability to calculate and assent to contracts? Why are beings so valuable as to require rights, just because they are capable of this calculation? What has happened to the stern demands of equal justice when it sacrifices the right to existence of the inarticulate to the convenience of the articulate? But thought cannot rest in these particular questionings about justice. Through them we are given the fundamental questions. What is it, if anything, about human beings that makes the rights of equal justice their due? What is it about human beings that makes it good that they should have such rights? What is it about any of us that makes our just due fuller than that of stones or flies or chickens or bears? Yet because the decision will not allow the question to remain silent, and yet sounds an ambiguous note as to how it would be answered in terms of our contemporary liberalism, the decision "Commends th' ingredients of our poison'd chalice/ To our own lips."

The need to justify modern liberal justice has been kept in the wings of our English-speaking drama by our power and the strengths of our tradition. In such events as the decision on abortion it begins to walk upon the stage. To put the matter simply: if 'species' is an historical concept and we are a species whose origin and existence can be explained in terms of mechanical necessity and chance, living on a planet which also can be explained in such terms, what requires us to live together according to the principles of equal justice?

For the last centuries a civilisational contradiction has moved our western lives. Our greatest intellectual endeavour — the new co-penetration of 'logos' and 'techne' — affirmed at its heart that in understanding anything we know it as ruled by necessity and chance. This affirmation entailed the elimination of the ancient notion of good from the understanding of anything. At the same time, our day-to-day organisation was in the main directed by a conception of justice formulated in relation to the ancient science, in which the notion of good was essential to the understanding of what is. This civilisational contradiction arose from the attempt of the articulate to hold together what was given them in modern science with a content of justice which had been developed out of an older account of what is.

It must be emphasised that what is at stake in this contradiction is not only the foundations of justice, but more importantly its content. Many academics in many disciplines have described the difference between the ancient and modern conceptions of justice as if it were essentially concerned with differing accounts of the human situation. The view of traditional philosophy and religion is that justice is the overriding order which we do not measure and define, but in terms of which we are measured and defined. The view of modern thought is that justice is a way which we choose in freedom, both individually and publicly, once we have taken our fate into our own hands, and know that we are responsible for what happens. This description of the difference has indeed some use for looking at the history of our race, — useful both to those who welcome and those who deplore the change of view. Nevertheless, concentration on differing 'world views' dims the awareness of what has been at stake concerning justice in recent western history. This dimming takes place in the hardly conscious assumption that while there has been change as to what can be known in philosophy, and change in the prevalence of religious belief among the educated, the basic content of justice in our societies will somehow remain the same. The theoretical differences in 'world views' are turned over to the domain of 'objective' scholarship, and this scholarship is carried out in protected private provinces anaesthetised from any touch with what is happening to the content of justice in the heat of the world. To feel the cutting edge of what is at stake in differing foundations of justice it is necessary to touch those foundations as they are manifested in the very context of justice.

The civilisational contradiction which beset Europe did not arise from the question whether there is justice, but what justice is. Obviously any possible society must have some system of organisation to which the name 'justice' can be given. The contradiction arose because human beings held onto certain aspects of justice which they had found in the ancient account of good, even after they no longer considered that that account of good helped them to understand the way things are. The content of justice was largely given them from its foundations in the Bible (and the classical philosophy which the early Christians thought necessary for understanding the Bible), while they understood the world increasingly in terms of modern technological science.

The desire to have both what was given in the new knowledge, and what was given us about justice in the religious and philosophical traditions, produced many conscious and unconscious attempts at practical and theoretical reconciliations. It is these attempts which make it not inaccurate to call the early centuries of modern liberal Europe the era of secularised Christianity. It is an often repeated platitude that thinkers such as Locke and Rousseau, Kant and Marx were secularised Christians. (Of the last name it is perhaps better to apply the not so different label — secularised Jew.) The reason why an academic such as Professor Rawls has been singled out for attention in this writing is as an example of how late that civilisational contradiction has survived in the sheltered intellectual life of the English-speaking peoples.

Indeed the appropriateness of calling modern contractualism 'secularised Christianity' may be seen in the difference between modern contractualism and the conventionalism of the ancient world. Although the dominant tradition of the ancient world was that justice belonged to the order of things, there was a continuing minority report that justice was simply a man-made convention. But what so startlingly distinguishes this ancient conventionalism from our contractualism is that those who advocated it most clearly also taught that the highest life required retirement from politics. According to Lucretius, the wise man knows that the best life is one of isolation from the dynamism of public life. The dominant contractualist teachers of the modern world have advocated an intense concern with political action. We are called to the supremacy of the practical life in which we must struggle to establish the just contract of equality. When one asks what had been the chief new public intellectual influence between ancient and modern philosophy, the answer must be western Christianity, with its insistence on the primacy of charity and its implications for equality. Modern contractualism's determined political activism relates it to its seedbed in western Christianity. Here again one comes upon that undefined primal affirmation which has been spoken of as concerned with 'will', and which is prior both to technological science and to revolution.

This public contradiction was not first brought into the light of day in the English-speaking world. It was exposed in the writings of Nietzsche. The Germans had received modern ways and thought later than the French or the English and therefore in a form more explicitly divided from the traditional thought. In their philosophy these modern assumptions are most uncompromisingly brought into the light of day. Nietzsche's writings may be singled out as a Rubicon, because more than a hundred years ago he laid down with incomparable lucidity that which is now publicly open: what is given about the whole in technological science cannot be thought together with what is given us concerning justice and truth, reverence and beauty, from our tradition. He does not turn his ridicule primarily against what has been handed to us in Christian revelation and ancient philosophy. What was given there has simply been killed as given, and all that we need to understand is why it was once thought alive. His greatest ridicule is reserved for those who want to maintain a content to 'justice' and 'truth' and 'goodness' out of the corpse that they helped to make a corpse. These are the intellectual democrats who adopt modern thought while picking and choosing among the ethical 'norms' from a dead past. Justice as equality and fairness is that bit of Christian instinct which survives the death of God. As he puts it: "The masses blink and say: 'We are all equal. — Man is but man, before God — we are all equal.' Before God! But now this God has died."

Particularly since Hume, the English moralists had

pointed out that moral rules were useful conventions, but had also assumed that the core of English justice was convenient. Hume's 'monkish virtues'—the parts of the tradition which did not suit the new bourgeoisie—could be shown to be inconvenient; but the heart of the tradition could be maintained and extended in the interests of property and liberty. It could be freed from its justification in terms of eternity, and its rigour could be refurbished by some under the pseudo-eternity of a timeless social contract. But Nietzsche makes clear that if the 'justice' of liberty and equality is only conventional, we may find in the course of an ever changing history that such content is not convenient. He always puts the word 'justice' in quotation marks to show that he does not imply its traditional content, and that its content will vary through the flux of history. The English moralists had not discovered that realm of beings we moderns call 'history', and therefore they did not understand the dominance of historicism over all other statements. Their social contract was indeed a last effort to avoid that dominance, while they increasingly accepted the ways of thought that led ineluctably to historicism. The justice of liberty and equality came forth from rationalists who did not think 'historically'. For whom is such justice convenient when we know that the old rationalism can no longer be thought as 'true'?

However, it is Kant who is singled out by Nietzsche as the clearest expression of this secularised Christianity. Kant's thought is the consummate expression of wanting it both ways. Having understood what is told us about nature in our science, and having understood that we will and make our own history, he turned away from the consequence of those recognitions by enfolding them in the higher affirmation that morality is the one fact of reason, and we are commanded to obedience. According to Nietszche, he limited autonomy by obedience. Because this comfortable anaesthetising from the full consequences of the modern was carried out so brilliantly in the critical system, Nietzsche calls Kant 'the great delayer'. Kant persuaded generations of intellectuals to the happy conclusion that they could keep both the assumptions of technological secularism and the absolutes of the old morality. He allowed them the comfort of continuing to live in the civilisational contradiction of accepting both the will to make one's own life and the old content of justice. He delayed them from knowing that there are no moral facts, but only the moral interpretation of facts, and that these interpretations can be explained as arising from the historical vicissitudes of the instincts. Moral interpretations are what we call our 'values', and these are what our wills impose upon the facts. Because of the brilliance of Kant's delaying tactics, men were held from seeing that justice as equality was a secularised survival of an archaic Christianity, and the absolute commands were simply the man-made 'values' of an era we have transcended.

Nietzsche was the first to make clear the argument that there is no reason to continue to live in that civilisational contradiction. Societies will always need legal systems — call them systems of 'justice' if you like the word. Once we have recognised what we can now will to create through our technology, why should we limit such creation by basing our systems of 'justice' on presuppositions which have been shown to be archaic by the very coming to be of technology? As we move into a society where we will be able to shape not only non-human nature but humanity itself, why should we limit that shaping by doctrines of equal rights which come out of a world view that 'history' has swept away. Does not the production of quality of life require a legal system which gives new range to the rights of the creative and the dynamic? Why should that range be limited by the rights of the weak, the uncreative and the immature? Why should the liberation of women to quality of life be limited by restraints on abortion, particularly when we know that the foetuses are only the product of necessity and chance? Once we have recognised 'history' as the imposing of our wills on an accidental world, does not 'justice' take on a new content?[24]

Against this attack on our 'values', our liberalism so belongs to the flesh and bones of our institutions that it cannot be threatened by something as remote as ontological questioning. The explicit statements of the American constitution guard their system of justice; the British constitution guards the same shape of rights in a less explicit but in a more deeply rooted way. These living forces of allegiance protect the common sense of practical men against the follies of ideologues. Anyway, did not the English-speaking peoples win the wars against the Germans, and win them in the name of liberalism, against the very 'philosophy' that is said to assail that liberalism?

It is also argued that the very greatness of American pluralism, founded upon the contract, is that out of it have come forth continuous religious revivals which produce that moral sustenance necessary to the justice of their society. Is it not a reason for confidence that in the election of 1976 the two candidates competed in allegiance to the traditions of religion, and that there is a renewed interest in religion among the young in the contractual society? Where is the atheism of the right in the United States? Does not the greatness of the American constitution lie in the fact that the general outlines of social cooperation are laid down and maintained by a secular contract, while within those general rules the resources of religious faith can flourish, as long as such faiths do not transgress that general outline? The greatness of the system is that the tolerance of pluralism is combined with the strength of religion. God has not died, as European intellectuals believed; it is just that our differing apprehensions of deity require that the rules of the game are not defined in terms of any of them. The rules of the game are defined in terms of the calculation of worldly self-interest; beyond that, citizens may seek the eternal as they see fit.

Indeed, any sane individual must be glad that we face the unique event of technology within a long legal and political tradition founded on the conception of justice as requiring liberty and equality. When we compare what is happening to multitudes in Asia who live the event of technology from out of ancient and great traditions, but without a comparable sense of individual right, we may count ourselves fortunate to live within our tradition. Asian people often have great advantages over us in the continuing strength of rite; our advantage is in the continuing strength of right. Also our liberalism came from the meeting of Christian tradition with an early form of modern thought, so that our very unthinking confidence in that liberalism has often saved us from modern political plagues which have been devastating in other western societies. At the practical level it is imprudent indeed to speak against the principles, if not the details, of those legal institutions which guard our justice.[25]

Nevertheless, it must be stated that our justice now moves to a lowered content of equal liberty. The chief cause of this is that our justice is being played out within a destiny more comprehensive than itself. A quick name for this is 'technology'. I mean by that word the endeavour which summons forth everything (both human and non-human) to give its reasons, and through the summoning forth of those reasons turns the world into potential raw material, at the disposal of our 'creative' wills.[26] The definition is circular in the sense that what is 'creatively' willed is further expansion of that union of knowing and making given in the linguistic union of 'techne', and 'logos'. Similar but cruder: it has been said that communism and contractual capitalism are predicates of the subject technology. They are ways in which our more comprehensive destiny is lived out. But clearly that technological destiny has its own dynamic conveniences, which easily sweep away our tradition of justice, if the latter gets in the way. The 'creative' in their corporations have been told for many generations that justice is only a convenience. In carrying out the dynamic convenience of technology, why should they not seek a 'justice' which is congruent with those conveniences, and gradually sacrifice the principles of liberty and equality when they conflict with the greater conveniences? What is it about other human beings that should stand in the way of such convenience? The tendency of the majority to get together to insist on a contract guaranteeing justice to them against the 'creative' strong continues indeed to have some limiting power. Its power is, however, itself limited by the fact that the majority of that majority see in the very technological endeavour the hope for their realisation of 'the primary goods', and therefore will often not stand up for the traditional justice when it is inconvenient to that technological endeavour. The majority of the acquiescent think they need the organisers to provide 'the primary goods' more than they need justice.

In such a situation, equality in 'primary goods' for a majority in the heartlands of the empire is likely; but it will be an equality which excludes liberal justice for those who are inconvenient to the 'creative'. It will exclude liberal justice from those who are too weak to enforce contracts — the imprisoned, the mentally unstable, the unborn, the aged, the defeated and sometimes even the morally unconforming. The price for large scale equality under the direction of the 'creative' will be injustice for the very weak. It will be a kind of massive 'equality' in 'primary goods', outside a concern for justice. As Huey Long put it: "When fascism comes to America, it will come in the name of democracy". We move to such a friendly and smooth faced organisation that it will not be recognised for what it is. This lack of recognition is seen clearly when the President of France says he is working for 'an advanced liberal society', just as he is pushing forward laws for the mass destruction of the unborn. What he must mean by liberal is the society organised for the human conveniences which fit the conveniences of technology.

As justice is conceived as the external convenience of contract, it obviously has less and less to do with the good ordering of the inward life. Among the majority in North America, inward life then comes to be ordered around the pursuit of 'primary goods', and/or is taken in terms of a loose popular Freudianism, mediated to the masses by the vast array of social technicians.[27] But it is dangerous to mock socially the fact of contradiction. The modern account of 'the self' is at one with the Nietzschian account. This unity was explicitly avowed by Freud. With its affirmation of the instrumentality of reason, how can it result in a conception of 'justice' similar to that of our tradition? In such a situation, the majorities in the heartlands of the empires may be able to insist on certain external equalities. But as justice is conceived as founded upon contract, and as having nothing to do with the harmony of the inward life, will it be able to sustain the inconveniences of public liberty?

In the western tradition it was believed that the acting out of justice in human relationships was the essential way in which human beings are opened to eternity. Inward and outward justice were considered to be mutually interdependent, in the sense that the inward openness to eternity depended on just practice, and just practice depended on that inward openness to eternity. When public justice is conceived as conventional and contractual, the division between inward and outward is so widened as to prevent any such mutual interdependence. Both openness to eternity and practical justice are weakened in that separation. A. N. Whitehead's shallow dictum that religion is what we do with our solitude aptly expresses that modern separation. It is a destructive half-truth because it makes our solitude narcissistic, and blunts our cutting edge in public justice.

Above all, we do not correctly envisage what is happening when we take our situation simply as new practical difficulties for liberalism, arising from the need to control new technologies, themselves external to that liberalism. Such an understanding of our situation prevents us from becoming aware that our contractual liberalism is not independent of the assumptions of technology in any way that allows it to be the means of transcending those technologies. Our situation is rather that the assumptions underlying contractual liberalism and underlying technology both come from the same matrix of modern thought, from which can arise no reason why the justice of liberty is due to all human beings, irrespective of convenience. In so far as the contemporary systems of liberal practice hold onto the content of free and equal justice, it is because they still rely on older sources which are more and more made unthinkable in the very realisation of technology. When contractual liberals hold within their thought remnants of secularised Christianity or Judaism, these remnants, if made conscious, must be known as unthinkable in terms of what is given in the modern. How, in modern thought, can we find positive answers to the questions: (i) what is it about human beings that makes liberty and equality their due? (ii) why is justice what we are fitted for, when it is not convenient? Why is it our good? The inability of contractual liberals (or indeed Marxists) to answer these questions is the terrifying darkness which has fallen upon modern justice.

Therefore, to those of us who for varying reasons cannot but trust the lineaments of liberal justice, and who somehow have been told that some such justice is due to all human beings and that its living out is, above all, what we are fitted for, — to those of such trust comes the call from that darkness to understand how justice can be thought together with what has been discovered of truth in the coming to be of technology. The great theoretical achievements of the modern era have been quantum physics, the biology of evolutionism, and the modern logic. (All other modern theoretical claims, particularly those

in the human sciences, remain as no more than pro-
visional, or even can be known as simply expressions of that oblivion of eternity which has characterised the coming to be of technology.) These are
the undoubtable core of truth which has come out
of technology, and they cry out to be thought in harmony with the conception of justice as what we are
fitted for.

The danger of this darkness is easily belittled by
our impoverished use of the word 'thought'. This
word is generally used as if it meant an activity
necessary to scientists when they come up against
a difficulty in their research, or some vague unease
beyond calculation when we worry about our existence. Thought is steadfast attention to the whole.
The darkness is fearful, because what is at stake is
whether anything is good. In the pretechnological
era, the central western account of justice clarified
the claim that justice is what we are fitted for. It
clarified why justice is to render each human being
their due, and why what was due to all human beings was "beyond all bargains and without an alternative". That account of justice was written down
most carefully and most beautifully in "The Republic" of Plato. For those of us who are Christians, the
substance of our belief is that the perfect living out
of that justice is unfolded in the Gospels. Why the
darkness which enshrouds justice is so dense — even
for those who think that what is given in "The
Republic" concerning good stands forth as true — is
because that truth cannot be thought in unity with
what is given in modern science concerning necessity

and chance. The darkness is not simply the obscurity
of living by that account of justice in the practical
tumult of the technological society. Nor is it the im-
possibility of that account coming to terms with
much of the folly of modernity, e.g. the belief that
there is a division between 'facts' and 'values'; nor
the difficulty of thinking its truth in the presence of
historicism. Rather it is that this account has not
been thought in unity with the greatest theoretical
enterprises of the modern world. This is a great
darkness, because it appears certain that rational beings cannot get out of the darkness by accepting
either truth and rejecting the other. It is folly simply
to return to the ancient account of justice as if the
discoveries of the modern science of nature had not
been made. It is folly to take the ancient account
of justice as simply of antiquarian interest, because
without any knowledge of justice as what we are fitted for, we will move into the future with a 'justice'
which is terrifying in its potentialities for mad in-
humanity of action. The purpose of this writing has
been to show the truth of the second of these propositions. In the darkness one should not return as
if the discoveries of modern science had not taken
place; nor should one give up the question of what
it means to say that justice is what we are fitted for;
and yet who has been able to think the two together?
For those of us who are lucky enough to know that
we have been told that justice is what we are fitted
for, this is not a practical darkness, but simply a
theoretical one. For those who do not believe that
they have been so told it is both a practical and

theoretical darkness which leads to an ever greater oblivion of eternity.

In the task of lightening the darkness which surrounds justice in our era, we of the English-speaking world have one advantage and one great disadvantage. The advantage is practical: the old and settled legal institutions which still bring forth loyalty from many of the best practical people. The disadvantage is that we have been so long disinterested or even contemptuous of that very thought about the whole which is now required. No other great western tradition has shown such lack of interest in thought, and in the institutions necessary to its possibility. We now pay the price for our long tradition of taking the goods of practical confidence and competence as self-sufficiently the highest goods. In what is left of those secular institutions which should serve the purpose of sustaining such thought — that is, our current institutions of higher learning — there is little encouragement to what might transcend the technically competent, and what is called 'philosophy' is generally little more than analytical competence. Analytical logistics plus historicist scholarship plus even rigourous science do not when added up equal philosophy. When added together they are not capable of producing that thought which is required if justice is to be taken out of the darkness which surrounds it in the technological era. This lack of tradition of thought is one reason why it is improbable that the transcendence of justice over technology will be lived among English-speaking people.

Notes

1. This second point, which would appear to be obvious, has been greatly obscured by recent propagandists for English-speaking liberalism, who in their desire to defend that tradition have denied that other traditions of liberalism have any right to be called 'liberal' at all. At its silliest this kind of writing is to be found in Professor K. Popper's "The Open Society and Its Enemies", particularly in its polemics against Plato and Hegel. It is obviously the proper work of political philosophy to argue, as Montesquieu does so brilliantly in "The Spirit of the Laws", that the modern English polity is a higher regime than the Athenian polis, and that modern philosophers understand the good of liberty in a fuller way than the ancients. Whether Plato understood the good of liberty as well as Locke is a question for serious and difficult argument. But to argue, as Popper does, that Plato and Hegel denied that political liberty was a central human good, and were indeed progenitors of modern totalitarianism, must have required such a casual reading of these two writers that his book can only be considered trivial propaganda. How is it possible to read through "The Apology" or "The Philosophy of Right" and believe that the writers of either did not believe that political liberty

was a central human good? Rather similar arguments have been advanced by English-speaking liberals against the tradition of European liberalism which originates with Rousseau. See for example Bertrand Russell's account of Rousseau in his "History of Western Philosophy" or J. L. Talmon's "The Origins of Totalitarian Democracy". The danger of such writings is that they have encouraged in our universities a provincial approach towards the history of political thought, just at a time when our situation required the opposite. For the continuing health of the liberal tradition, what we least needed was a defensive exclusion of the classical and European traditions from the canon of liberalism. At a time when massive technological advance has presented the race with unusual difficulties concerning political liberty, what was needed from our academics was an attempt to think through all that was valuable from the great western traditions which could help us in dealing with these difficulties. Instead, what we got from men such as Russell and Popper was a procrustean affirmation of the self-sufficiency of English liberalism. To put the matter crudely: in a time of great intellectual confusion, our crimes at home and abroad should not prevent us from trying to see what good is present in English-speaking liberalism, any more than the crimes of the Soviet Union should prevent us from trying to see what good is present in the tradition that proceeds from Rousseau, or indeed any more than ancient slavery and imperialism should prevent us looking clearly at classical political philosophy.

2. It is of course true that the dilemma arising within liberalism, because of its imperial as well as its domestic role, existed as much in the European empires of the nineteenth century as in the American. Indeed, Plato's sustained attacks on Athenian imperialism, and its close rela-

tion to democracy, deals with a comparable situation, except for the presence of technology in our day. In England, modern liberalism was above all the creed of the new bourgeois, in that the insistence on political liberties was related to the liberation of dynamic commercial technology, and thus with the expansion of that dynamism around the world. The claim to legal and political freedoms at home was not a claim that could be universally applied abroad to alien races who had to be made the subjects of that commercial technology. This was an even more pressing difficulty for the French, because after the revolution their ideology more explicitly universalised the rights of man. Western principles of right in claiming universality became at one and the same time the basis for anti-imperialism both at home and abroad, yet also a justification for western expansion as the bringing of enlightenment into 'backward' parts of the world. Liberalism as a justification for imperialism can be seen very clearly in the work of Macauley. His account of English history is a panegyric to modern liberalism, with the world-historical good of England's greatness. In India he was the chief instrument in westernising education, and above all for substituting English for Sanskrit in that education. He once said that "All the lore of India is not equal to Aesop's fables". In the intense competition for the world's crassest remark, this one has a high claim. On the other hand, as imperialism developed, the western critique of it came forth largely in the name of liberalism. The antiprogressivist critics of imperialism, such as Cunningham Graham, spoke after all in voices which were not easily understood in modern Europe. Indeed the dilemma became increasingly obvious; in so far as modern liberals put their trust in the development of commerce and technology, they were inevitably identifying themselves with the spread of imperialism; in so far as liberalism became explicitly a universal doctrine of human rights, the liberals had to become critics of their imperialism. A similar dilemma was present from the beginnings of American imperialism, and erupted into immediate political significance over the Vietnam war. The part of F. D. Roosevelt at one and the same time was domestically the liberal part, and abroad established the highest tide of American imperialism. Yet the dominant force in the American protest against that war came from people who protested in the name of liberalism. However ashamed we English-speaking people should be of that war, it should not be forgotten that the strongest anti-imperialist protest in western history occurred in the U.S.A. It may be that the majority of protesters accepted the high consumption due to their imperialism, nevertheless that protest says something about the authenticity of American liberalism.

3. The word 'hierarchy' is still often used as the political opposite to 'equality'. This is bad usage because the subordinations and superordinations of our bureaucracies are not intended to be 'sacred orders' given in the nature of things. There seems to be no current positive word which expresses clearly the opposite of equality. Is this because our liberal language has become increasingly egalitarian, and the lip service we pay to this principle makes it impossible to find accurate words to express what is happening in our institutions?

PART II

4. That Rawls writes within the assumptions of modern liberalism is evident in every page of his writing. Not only does he appeal to Locke, Rousseau and Kant

as his masters, but he covers extensively contemporary English-speaking writing on his subject, not only that of fellow teachers of philosophy, but also that of social scientists interested in theories of justice. All this literature lies within the assumptions of liberalism. To put the matter negatively: Rawls does not give any account of those theoretical positions about morals and politics which in the western world have stood as alternatives to our liberalism. These alternatives can be divided simply into two groups. The first of these is the political philosophy of Plato and Aristotle and the modification of that teaching worked out by their Christian and Jewish followers. This group is temporarily antecedent to our liberalism. The second group is temporarily consequent. It may be quickly typified by calling it the thought dependent upon Marx and that dependent upon Nietzsche. All that need be said about Rawls' approach to classical political philosophy is that in a book on justice there are four times as many references to a certain professor Arrow as there are to Plato. It would appear that for Rawls the classical teaching about moral and political good is simply a dead alternative of only antiquarian interest. Rawls' appeal to Aristotelian psychology is used by him as if that psychology did not live as part of the whole body of Aristotle's teaching. This appeal is therefore not to be taken as an exception to Rawls' disregard of the ancients. As for the great contemporary alternatives to our liberalism, Marx and Marxism are disregarded and Nietzsche is only casually mentioned. For example, the difficulties which historicism presents for moral and political philosophy — difficulties which have engrossed generations of continental European thinkers since Nietzsche — are not discussed. The advantage of this procrustean stance is that it allows Rawls to hold English-speaking liberalism before us for our undivided attention. We swim in a particular bay whose contours we can come to know intimately, and we are never asked to swim out into the ocean the immensities of which can easily overwhelm us. Reading Rawls' book is comparable to reading a contemporary book of Roman Catholic thought in which the issues are presented as the differences of interpretation between Maritain and Teilhard, Rahner and Lonergan. In the same way in Rawls' book we are not diverted from the details at issue within our contemporary liberalism, so that it lies before us to tell us what it is.

5. It might be thought that the names of Hobbes and Rousseau should be added. Rawls finesses the thought of Hobbes in a footnote, saying that there are unspecified 'difficulties' in that thinker. He takes Locke as his master, not Hobbes. Also, why Kant rather than Rousseau? Rousseau was after all the thinker who reformulated contractarian doctrine in the light of his profound criticism of Hobbes' and Locke's account of the origins of human beings. Be that as it may, there are more references to Kant in Rawls' book than to any other thinker. It is well to remember in this connection Kant's continual statements of his debt to Rousseau. English-speaking academics have been apt to regard Kant as a critical epistemologist, to emphasise his debt to Hume and to disregard the fact that his continual tributes to Rousseau are wider than his tribute to Hume. For one of these tributes, see p. 30 of this text. As the subject of this writing is the interdependence between technological reason and reason as political liberalism, it is well to remember that Kant's dedicaton of "The Critique of Pure Reason" to Francis Bacon is combined with his tribute to Rousseau. One partial way of looking at his three "Critiques" is surely as

the attempt to lay before us modern liberalism and technological science as unified in his account of reason. In
this sense Rawls is surely right to turn to Kant as his chief
master.

6. For a brilliant and extended account of the difference between the state of nature and the original position see A. Bloom's article, "John Rawls vs. The Tradition of Political Philosophy" American Political Science
Review, June, 1975.

7. It is indeed little more than journalism to state that
in the English-speaking world since 1900 there has been
a dominating account of what it is to do philosophy and
that the best label to pin upon these complex phenomena
is 'analytical'. To become wary of simplifications in this
matter, it is only necessary to think of the differences in
interest, in method and in doctrine between such disparate
practitioners as Russell and Wittgenstein, Quine and
Austin; or to think of the subtle intermingling of continental logistics and native English empiricism. Nevertheless it is accurate to say that when youngsters come
to study philosophy at our universities they generally meet
a curriculum and teachers who require of them certain
assumptions as to what that study is. It may be helpful
here to remember Walter Rathenau's aphorism: "There
are no specialists, there are only vested interests."

8. The underlining is Kant's. "The Groundwork of the
Metaphysics of Morals" translated H. J. Paton, Harper's
Torchbooks, 1964 p. 61. Also the translation of 'Grun-
dlegung' as 'Groundwork' or elsewhere as 'Fundamental
Principles' loses the sense of the enormity of the claim
made in the title. Why does Kant have to lay new foundations for the metaphysics of morals? — because all the
previous foundations will not do. They will not do be-

cause freedom has not been understood as autonomy, nor the human species understood as the cause of its own development.

9. It is not my business here to describe the holding in unity of these two sides—timeless good and historical will—as it is laid before us through an account of the modern sciences and arts, in the edifice of Kant's three Critiques. However, in an era when oblivion of eternity has almost become the self-definition of many of us, it is necessary to insist on the side of timeless and universal good in Kant's system. Indeed this side is shown with startling clarity by Kant, when despite all the causes which might lead him to propound the philosophy of history, as an essential part of any true philosophical teaching, he turns back from possibility of such an enterprise because it would involve our moral choices depending on knowledge other than the timeless fact of reason itself. See The Critique of Judgement paras. 83 and 84.

10. There is no clearer example of how the vagaries of intellectual history turn inside out the teachings of a great philosopher than the way that Kant's assertion that the morally neutral state is the best state is now generally taken by his liberal successors. For Kant the morally neutral state is advocated on the basis of an egalitarian moral absolutism; today it is often advocated on the basis of moral relativism. The morally neutral state based on sceptical grounds is the strange progeny of the morally neutral state based on absolutist grounds. Perhaps the fate of Kant's doctrine on this matter may be taken to illustrate the fate of inadequate teachings.

11. P. 630 'Fragmente aus dem Nachlasse' in vol. 8, *Immanuel Kant's Sämmtliche Werke*, edited by Gustav Hartenstein, Leipzig, 1968.

12. In describing Rawls account in terms of 'interests'

rather than 'goods', I am not denying that these interests are often unified into the pursuit of what he calls 'life-plans'. I use the word 'interests' to exclude any implication that the word 'good' is used by him in the traditional sense of 'what we are fitted for', or any implication that he believes that we can have knowledge of the highest good for human beings in general. The word 'good' allows Rawls to make use of Aristotle's teaching, through which he attempts to deepen his essentially utilitarian account of happiness by seeming to undergird it with Aristotle's very different account. Commentary on Rawls' version of Aristotle would require the gifts of Dean Swift.

13. I have omitted the words 'consistent with the just saving principle' from Rawls' formulation of his second principle, because they are confusing without a long account of his vague descriptions of his compromises between capitalism and socialism, and of the consequent relation he maintains between economics and politics. Such an account is not essential to my present purposes.

14. The strangest part of Rawls' book is his appeal to Kant as his chief master. The very core of Kant's thought is his sharp division between self-interest and fairness. The moral law of fairness appears to us as categorical command, and therefore simply cuts across the claims of self-interest. It is because of the very great difference between Rawls and Kant on this key issue, and because of Rawls' claim that his theory "is highly Kantian in nature", that I have used the unfriendly metaphor of the shell game about his book.

Part III

15. As in the previous paragraph I have ridiculed Sir Karl Popper's political thought, it is necessary to say that

what is good in his writing is just his trust in the strength
of English liberalism to combat the plague of ideology.
Foolishly he has combined this trust with an inability to
distinguish ideology from philosophy. This is above all
evident in his crass writing about Plato.

16. This contempt for Christianity lies at the heart of
the division between modern liberalism and the earlier
liberties of English history. See for example Churchill's
letter to the Times 'On praying for rain'. Both in substance
and style this letter might have come from Russell.

17. It is worth repeating that one of the strangest combinations of events in American life was the way that the
brutality of their crimes in Vietnam was followed by the
very careful protection of domestic rights in the affair of
Watergate. To many Americans the victory of their congress and courts over their President seems to have been
above all a means of justifying their own self-righteousness, to the end of forgetting what had happened in Vietnam. To understand how that purging worked as an
anodyne would require an understanding of the relation
between modern liberalism and imperialism.

18. Henry James' preface to "The Aspern Papers".
That relation has been illumined by the massive historical
scholarship about it in the last generation; but such a relation clearly cannot be fathomed by scholarship. Even
Weber or Troeltsch, as they move beyond scholarship
towards philosophy, are still unable to catch that self-
definition of our wills which arose from the co-penetration. For my comments see *Technology and Empire:
Perspectives on North America*, Toronto, 1969.

19. In the fine writing on this matter recently, e.g.,
the books of Trevor-Roper, Webster, Yates, etc., it is still
necessary to single out the early articles of M.B. Foster

as most theoretically illuminating. See Mind 1934-35-36.
    20. The Laws of Ecclesiastical Polity, Book I, chap. 2.
    21. It is often pointed out that Jewish people remain
the most fervent and articulate advocates of our contractualism. Therefore a word must be appended about the
relation between Judaism and modern English-speaking
regimes. It is obvious why the Jewish community has
always welcomed and supported modern liberalism. In
western and eastern Europe, Jews had lived for centuries
under regimes in which some form of Christianity was
the official religion, and under which their survival required both fortitude and patience. As the regimes became
secularised, they presented Jews with the possibility of
living openly in the civil society. Beyond this obvious fact,
it is necessary to understand the deeper question of why
Jews have exerted such a formative influence on American
society, far beyond their percentage of the population.
Perhaps it is that in Judaism worship of God is closely
bound together with the existence of a particular historical nation, and that this sense of being a people has given
Jews sources of strength when they move out into the im-
personal and individualistic public realm consequent on
contractualism. Its members have been able to live force-
fully in the unblinking public light, because they could
retire into the shade of a community not only based on
the universality of religion, but on the particularity of na-
tionhood, and these two bound together in a quite unique
way. In a society in which contractual relations define
more and more human encounters, the Jews have maintained a public force from that given union of worship
and nationality, which could only exist sporadically
among Christians because of the very nature of Christ's
message.

Part IV

22. Blackmun's appeal to Holmes illustrates the uncertainties in current American usage of the words 'liberal'
and 'conservative'. His decision about abortion has been
put in the 'liberal' column, when it is in fact based on
a strict construction of contractualism which is generally
put in the 'conservative ' column. It is well to remember
that Blackmun is a Nixon appointee, and tends in his interpretation of the constitution towards 'strict constructionism', and away from that interpretation according to
the changing consensus of a progressing people, which
characterised the Warren Court. Nixon consistently advocated over many years that the progressive historicism
which dominated the Warren Court should be rectified
by the appointment of justices who followed the theory
of strict constructionism. This involved that their constitution be conceived as a foundational contract which
established certain rights unaffected by the passage of
time. But the difference concerning judicial interpretation
does not alter the fact that both sides to it appeal to a
contractual view of the state, related to the acceptance
of the consequences of moral pluralism in society. A foundational contract which is viewed as timeless may seem
less oblivious of eternity than an historically developing
contract; but in both views justice is considered contractual. Indeed, what is meant in the U.S. by 'conservative'
is generally a species of modern 'liberal'.. 'Conservatives'
want to hold onto certain consequences of the earlier
tradition of our liberalism which more modern 'liberals'
are willing to scrap in the interest of the new and the progressive. It is this usage which can be so confusing to people from other countries who may identify 'conservatism'
with those who have some memories from before the age

of progress. But the indigenous memories in the U.S. are never from before the age of progress. Thus American 'conservatives' can advocate the most modern technological proposals in the name of 'conservatism'. At the judicial level, this strange usage led certain progressivists to call Mr. Justice Frankfurter a 'conservative' when he became the clearest advocate of strict constructionism on their court.

23. In discussing this case I am not concerned to elucidate the complex question of justice in abortion, whether in individual conduct or positive law. If I were so concerned, I would have to expound these facts of embryology.

24. To put the matter politically: the early public atheism of Europe generally came from 'the left'. Its adherents attacked the traditional religion while taking for granted almost unconsciously that 'the right' would continue to live within its religious allegiances. 'The left' could attack religion partially because it relied on 'the right' having some restraint because of its religion. Philosophers cannot be subsumed under their political effects, but with Nietzsche the atheism of 'the right' enters the western scene. One definition of national socialism is a strange union of the atheisms of 'the right' and of 'the left'.

25. It is well to remember that the greatest contemporary philosopher, Heidegger, published in 1953 "An Introduction to Metaphysics" in which he wrote of National Socialism: "the inner truth and greatness of this movement (namely the encounter between global technology and modern man)". One theoretical part of that encounter was the development of a new jurisprudence, which explicitly distinguished itself from our jurisprudence of rights, because the latter belonged to an era of

plutocratic democracy which needed to be transcended in that encounter. Such arguments must make one extremely careful of the ontological questioning of our jurisprudence, even in its barest contractual form.

26. See M. Heidegger *Der Satz Vom Grund*, Pfullingen, 1957.

27. We are fortunate these days when the social technicians are controlled by something as human as popular Freudianism. Whatever its defects, popular Freudianism is surely superior to the 'new brutalism' of behaviour modification carried out by behaviourist techniques.